The RealAge®

Makeover

The RealAge®

Makeover

take years off
your looks and
add them to
your life

Michael F. Roizen, M.D.

A completely revised and
updated edition of *RealAge*®

Collins
An Imprint of HarperCollins*Publishers*

A hardcover edition of this book was published in 2004 by
HarperResource.

HarperCollins books may be purchased for educational, business, or
sales promotional use. For information please write: Special Markets
Department, HarperCollins Publishers Inc., 10 East 53rd Street,
New York, NY 10022.

First Collins edition published in 2005.

Designed by Ellen Cipriano

Library of Congress Cataloging-in-Publication Data

Roizen, Michael F.
    The realAge® makeover : take years off your looks and add them to
your life / Michael F. Roizen.—1st ed.
        p.   cm.
    Complete revision and updated edition of: RealAge® : Are you as
young as you can be?
    Includes bibliographical references and index.
    ISBN 0-06-019682-3(hc.)
    1. Rejuvenation. 2. Aging—Prevention. 3. Self-care, Health.
4. RealAge. 5. Aging—Computer programs. 6. Longevity—
Computer programs. I. Title: Real age makeover. II. Roizen,
Michael F. RealAge. III. Title.

RA776.75.R653   2004
613'.0434—dc22

                                                        2004040502

ISBN-10: 0-06-081702-x (pbk.)
ISBN-13: 978-0-06-081702-2 (pbk.)

06 07 08 09 WBC/RRD 10 9 8 7

This book is dedicated to my family, for their enthusiasm for RealAge and their patience with the project. They not only help me stay young but are the reason I want to be young. I also dedicate the book to Marty Rom and Charlie Silver, my partners in introducing so many people to RealAge; and to all who enjoy RealAge, including the fifty or so Makeovers who inspired this work and are living younger. May you always have the RealAge you desire.

All case studies portrayed in this book are based on real people. Details not significant to the use in this book have been changed to protect the identities of the individuals involved. In some cases, two or more similar stories have been combined into one story. Only references to my father, my daughter, and myself should be considered clearly identifiable. Any other likenesses are purely coincidental.

In certain instances, I have listed products, such as medications, by their brand names, because that is how they are commonly known. On occasion, I have also included the names of companies and products if I thought such information would be relevant for the reader. To my knowledge, I have no connections to any of the companies or brand-name products listed in this book, with the exception of RealAge, Inc., the company I helped establish for the express purpose of developing the RealAge computer program. RealAge and Age Reduction are trademarks and service marks of RealAge, Inc., which currently directs the RealAge website (*www.RealAge.com*).

This book is intended to be informational and should not be considered a substitute for advice from a medical professional, whom the reader should consult before beginning any diet or exercise regimen, and before taking any dietary supplements or other medications. The author and publisher expressly disclaim responsibility for any adverse effects arising from the use or application of the information contained in this book.

Contents

Acknowledgments

First and foremost, I would like to thank the patients, the many physicians, and thousands of people who sent questions, notes, cards, and e-mails, and transformed themselves with Makeovers. They inspired me to write this book, encouraged further development of the RealAge ideas, and motivated the passion that created this book. I hope the book will help them live younger longer. That would be the best reward any physician could have.

I am grateful to the many, many other people who contributed to this book. Some deserve a very specific thank you: Candice Fuhrman, for making it happen; Elsa Hurley, who rewrote and edited more than sixteen editions of each chapter; Pauline Snider, my editor for over twenty-five years, for keeping the English crisp and the grammar and style appropriate and consistent; Elizabeth Stephenson, my partner in the first RealAge book, who encouraged this work; Tracy Hafen, who taught me a tremendous amount about exercise and wrote descriptions of the exercises in Chapter 9; Sukie Miller, whose passion for the project proved to be the consistent encouragement I needed; Anita Shreve, for saying the RealAge book was possible and that the chapters were just what she wanted to read; the many gerontologists and internists who read sections of the book for accuracy; Mehmet Oz, Jack Rowe, Jeremiah Stamler, Linda Fried, and the many investigators of the Iowa Women's Health Study, the Nurses' Health Study, and the Physicians' Health Study, for invaluable research and advice that improve the science in this book; others on the RealAge scientific team who helped analyze the research, especially Keith Roach, a consistent partner in this work since 1994; those on the RealAge team who helped validate and verify the content, including Shelly Bowen; Michelle Lewis, for her endless patience and good humor in producing the manuscript; Charise Petrovitch, for improving the charts and slides; Anne-Marie Prince, for doing so much so well, and for doing it so calmly in the midst of a constant storm; Sally Kwa, Arline McDonald, Tate Erlinger, Linda Van Horne, Jeremiah Stamler, Mark Rudberg, Mike Parzen, and especially Axel Goetz and Harriet Imrey, for their roles as scientific partners in evaluating the data and scientific content of RealAge; Leo Vivona, Dr. Robert Genco, and Dr. John Vasselli for educating me about gum care and air pollution; Sidney Unobskey and Martin Rom, who inspired the process and named it; Charlie Silver, who funded the research and assembled the innovative RealAge team that continually evaluates and updates RealAge and its website; and especially Megan Newman, who believed in this book. I owe a special gratitude to Kathy Huck who repeatedly told me how to improve each chapter; she made each chapter better, and not just a little, and not just once. She conveyed her excitement to me and to the book. I would not passionately believe that RealAge could change the health of the world without her excitement and encouragement about the project.

Finally, I would like to thank you my wife, Nancy, for her constant love and support, and my children, Jeffrey and Jennifer, for their encouragement and patience. The book is dedicated to them, to my partners who founded RealAge, and especially to the millions of people who use the RealAge ideas to improve their health. Thank you for keeping the passion burning. May you be inspired to have the RealAge you desire.

Preface

Dear RealAge.com,

I hope you'll encourage Dr. Roizen to write an update to the book *RealAge: Are You as Young as You Can Be?* It would be of great service to the medical profession. He has helped me motivate my patients, as well as helping me make myself healthier and younger.

—A physician, via e-mail

Dear RealAge Team,

I'm a general surgeon and true believer in the RealAge program. I've given a dozen copies of *RealAge: Are You as Young as You Can Be?* to friends. I've convinced several dozen patients to buy and read the book, and they've praised it to the skies.

I hope that an updated version of this important book will be available soon—I know that there have been lots of great studies, and lots of important new health information, since *RealAge* was first published.

If Dr. Roizen and his staff were to do nothing else but establish this important resource as a standard format released every two or three years, he would have made an enormous contribution to the health of our country. Many thanks for this seminal publication.

—A physician, via e-mail

I care passionately about people's health and well-being. As a doctor, I find it enormously satisfying to help people overcome illness, disease, and disability. And, of course, nothing is more meaningful than actually saving a life. At the same time, life as a doctor can have its darker side. As a specialist in both cardiovascular anesthesiology and internal medicine, I spend much of my working life with patients who are among the sickest of the sick, such as people who need emergency bypass surgery to fix potentially fatal aneurysms. The physical and emotional distress I witness is made even more painful by the knowledge that so much of my patients' suffering could have been prevented.

Back in 1994, when the RealAge concept first began, I was starting to feel frustrated at witnessing so much preventable illness. After spending so much time in the operating room with these people, it pained me not to be able to do more for them. At the same time, on some level I was mad as heck. So many of these people were sick because they had mistreated their bodies over time by eating unhealthy foods, smoking, and leading sedentary lives. Furthermore, every single one of them knew better.

Why were so many people—smart, educated, thoughtful people—not doing the things it takes to live a long, healthy life? It would have been easy to blame the patients. *But it wasn't their fault.* My colleagues and I were failing to communicate as well as we should what was important and what wasn't. I was desperate for a way to get out the message.

Granted, at the time, almost none of us had any idea exactly to what extent patients themselves could prevent illness in the first place. But as the RealAge program began to develop, and data from studies slowly began to reveal the extraordinary power of specific lifestyle choices in keeping us young and vibrant, all that changed—and I became enormously excited.

At the time, I was chairman of the Department of Anesthesia and Critical Care at the University of Chicago, and I had just started running a program in my second specialty, internal medicine, that focused on comprehensive preventive health. I'd always worked long hours—80 to 90 hours a week on average, and sometimes as many as 100. However, I was so excited about the RealAge program that I threw myself into research and began working 120 hours a week.

My wife, Nancy, has always been my greatest cheerleader, but even she got a little concerned. One day she asked me, "Mike, what are you doing? You're killing yourself with work."

"I know, but I think it's worth it," I told her. "I truly believe that RealAge could change the health of the world! I just have to find an effective way to get the information out of my office and into mainstream culture."

I was truly driven to share all that I'd learned about how easy it is for people to keep themselves young and vibrant. I care deeply about the health not only of my own patients but of all people, and I was sure that the RealAge program could make a radical difference in the health of the whole nation.

Then it occurred to me that a book that explained the RealAge program could be just what this country needed. As we all know, many Americans suffer the tragic debilitation that comes with strokes, cancers, and other serious illness. A book that would show them how to implement the RealAge program in their own lives could help them turn their health around. They could give themselves a makeover in the truest sense of the word. They could look younger and healthier not because of makeup or plastic surgery, but because they actually *are* younger and healthier from the inside out.

However, faced with the thought of actually writing such a book, I had some concerns. It is rare for physicians—or at least it was then—to try to help people with a popular book that explains science. I worried that I wouldn't be able to write a book well, and questioned whether I could really convince readers that the program would work. Many doctors consider it unprofessional and self-promoting to try to motivate people other than one's own patients. I feared losing the respect of my colleagues.

However, the reaction to the book after its publication in 1999 quelled all of those fears. To my surprise and delight, the book became a *New York Times* bestseller. I was a guest on several national television shows including *Oprah*, where I was lucky in two very special, unexpected ways (anyone is lucky to get on Oprah's show; she brings out the best in her guests). First, her producers put together a magnificently wonderful show. Second, as fate would have it, a huge snowstorm hit the East the day the program aired, so people were home in front of their televisions and the rating were huge. Then the show was aired a second time, the same week that *RealAge* was featured on *20/20,* and so many people bought the book that it temporarily knocked *Harry Potter* off the number one spot on *Amazon.com.* The media exposure jump-started the RealAge Revolution: hundreds of thousands of people were transforming themselves by using the power of RealAge to take control of their rate of aging.

As for my fears about losing the respect of my professional colleagues, that hasn't happened. Several months after release of the book, I gave a lecture on RealAge to a large group of family physicians and internists. At the book signing after the lecture, I was gratified to see physicians standing in line for over an hour and a half. Most physicians won't wait for more than three milliseconds for anything. The fact that they waited so patiently reassured me that my fears had been unfounded.

However, it wasn't the experience of going on television, keeping the esteem of my colleagues, or even the commercial success of the book that has given me real joy. Rather, it's been witnessing how thousands of people across the nation have been using the RealAge program to make themselves younger, healthier, and happier. It's been a remarkable transformation, this RealAge Makeover: people are making choices that cause them to look, feel, and actually *be* many years younger. It's a true makeover from the inside out, the way it should be. No expensive beauty treatments or invasive plastic surgery are needed. You look and feel your best naturally.

More than ten million people have taken the RealAge test in one form or another, and nearly two million subscribe to the free RealAge "Tip of the Day." Thousands and thousands have e-mailed me about simple changes in their lives that have made them healthier, younger, and more vibrant. The RealAge website received more than one hundred fifty "thank-you" e-mails each and every day, seven days a week, for more than a year after the first *RealAge* book was released.

In the years since then, while taking pleasure in following these success stories, I have also followed the exciting new information emerging from numerous health studies. These studies have investigated many issues such as nutrition, exercise, and lifestyle choices, and how they affect our health. In some cases, the data proved beyond a doubt what we already suspected to be true. In other rarer cases, it gave us new understanding that actually contradicted what we had previously believed. Whatever the case, enough new information emerged to convince me that a revised version of the book was needed, so that my readers could make choices based on the most up-to-date information.

Other health professionals agreed. I received numerous e-mails like the two at the start of this book encouraging me and the entire RealAge scientific team to write a revised version of the book incorporating the new health information we now have. I also owe a great deal to a huge number of physicians and other health professionals—nurses, dieticians, nutritionists, exercise physiologists—and especially just plain folk who told me through e-mails and the website how much they appreciated the motivation and the understanding RealAge gives them. It is their personal stories that have inspired me, and their transformations that make me believe in the power of RealAge more than ever.

Over half of this revised book is new, as are many of the patient stories that illustrate key RealAge principles and, I hope, inspire you to give yourself a Real-Age Makeover.

I want to motivate *you* by making medical knowledge understandable, and to show how simple changes in the way you live can make you one, two, ten or more years younger. Also, I want you to know that your future health is not in the hands of fate: it's in your own hands. There are simple and concrete things you can do today to prevent that heart attack, disease, or stroke down the road.

Knowledge really is power when it comes to your own health. Many people have become motivated by the knowledge that the choices they make in their lives can help them live better, healthier, and younger. You can live better, healthier, and younger, too, by joining the RealAge Revolution. You can give yourself the gift of a RealAge Makeover and start looking, feeling, and actually *being* years younger. It's the best gift of all.

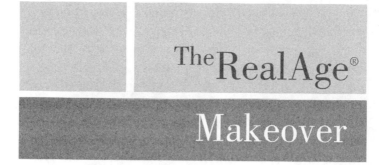

The RealAge® Makeover

Look Younger, Live Longer

Give Yourself the Energy and Looks You Had Ten or Twenty Years Ago

Thousands of Americans are younger today than they were five years ago. How is that possible? They have joined the Real-Age Revolution. They have given themselves a makeover from the inside out. By following the specific age-reversing recommendations in my book *RealAge: Are You as Young as You Can Be?*, people who were previously much older physiologically than their calendar age have now taken ten, fifteen, up to forty years off their biologic age. (Men can be twenty-five years younger and women, twenty-nine years younger than their calendar age.) This is what we call giving yourself a RealAge Makeover: you can significantly transform your health, looks, and life.

And it can be so easy. For example, just developing the habit of calling friends in times of stress can actually make a real difference in your health and longevity. As word about the RealAge concept spread, and Americans started to see firsthand how small but simple—and often fun!—changes in their daily lives could transform their health, so many people have gotten the RealAge bandwagon that it's become a kind of revolution—a revolution back to great health. And nobody has been more thrilled to see it happen than I.

Since publication of the first book, we've learned more about the process of aging. While our team has been hard at work interpreting data from the latest clinical trails to keep the RealAge program on the cutting edge, readers of *RealAge* have been hard at work getting younger. For example:

- Katherine M., a forty-eight-year-old nurse with a busy schedule and a RealAge of fifty-five, knew she wasn't getting healthy nutrition. So she started taking calcium, vitamin D, magnesium, and folate supplements. In addition, she added lycopene to her diet by having spaghetti with marinara sauce once a week. As a result, even though she now has a calendar age of fifty-one, her RealAge is forty-five. She has an added bounce in her step and feels the ten years younger she has become. (She made her RealAge ten years younger as she went from a RealAge of 55 to one of 45.)

■ Kenny T., a high-powered attorney of fifty-eight with a RealAge of sixty-six, started a stress-reduction program that included yoga and meditation. In addition, he began walking and paying more attention to safety issues such as wearing a seat belt while driving and a helmet when bicycling. These combined factors made his RealAge six years younger.

■ I am most proud of Betty G., who works in my old department. Betty had a three-pack-a-day smoking habit that made her RealAge eight years older than her calender age of thirty-nine. She felt more than fifteen years older, and looked it, too. No one thought she could quit. She'd frequently be seen outside on a smoke break with cigarettes in both hands. Betty eventually got fed up with feeling so old and tired, and decided to give herself a makeover. She started a walking program; then she quit smoking. It wasn't easy, but she did it with the method described in Chapter 6. After five years completely smoke-free, she is well on her way to shedding seven of the eight years she had originally aged due to smoking. She now looks twenty years younger than she did. In fact, her RealAge is fourteen years younger than it was just three years ago (she did more than just quit smoking). She has literally made herself over. Friends who have not seen her in three years have asked how she was able to afford plastic surgery. She is proud to tell them she hasn't had any surgery; instead, she has changed her appearance from the inside out.

I find it incredibly exciting to see people making such changes—some easy, some difficult, but all crucial toward living younger, longer, healthier lives. This book updates what's been learned in the past several years and gives you all the information you need to transform yourself with a RealAge Makeover.

There's a lot in the realm of health and medicine we don't know, but we *do* know more than 80 percent of how to postpone, delay, or avoid the onset of age-related disease and the disability it causes. That's extremely exciting news! (It's different, however, from postponing aging itself. Postponing aging would mean living at the top of your curve to one hundred twenty or one hundred fifty years after your birth—something very different from what we can do now.) We now know how to delay until age ninety or ninety-five those age-related diseases that keep us from living at the top of the quality-of-life curve. And that's what the goal of the RealAge program is all about.

What Is RealAge?

It's most common, of course, when someone rudely asks you your age, to think in terms of calendar age. You are very aware (and may even grumble) when you pass the big milestones—for example, when you turn thirty, forty, fifty, sixty, seventy, eighty, or ninety. But this way of thinking—couching age only in terms of calendar age—does not do justice to the complex (and, happily, often reversible) process of aging. You have an age that more truly reflects how much your body has aged: your RealAge. It can be many years older or younger than your calendar age, depending on your choices—how well you care for your health and well-being. If your RealAge is five years younger than your calendar age, for example, it means that your rate of aging is such that you are in the same shape physiologically as the average person who is five years younger than you. Likewise, if your RealAge is five years older than your calendar age, you have aged to the same biologic condition as someone who is five years older. But you do not have to despair; the great thing about the science of the last twenty years is it shows you how to slow and yes, even reverse your aging. How to do that is the subject of this book. Instead of the one-size-fits-all nature of calendar age, RealAge reflects you as a unique individual, and the choices you've made for yourself.

When we consider this concept—that different people of the same calendar age may actually be older or younger depending on the state of their health—most people instinctively accept this is true. We've all had the experience of meeting someone we assume is one age, only to find out he or she is actually much older or younger. Perhaps you've met a new employee at your company who you thought was in her early thirties, only to discover later that she's actually in her mid-forties. Or perhaps you assumed your postal carrier was in his sixties, nearing retirement, and then were surprised to learn he's only fifty-five. What may be more surprising is that the calendar age you estimated for people is not that far from their RealAge (physiologic age).

Some people are young for their age: they are physiologically and mentally as active and vibrant as someone chronologically younger, because they've slowed the pace of aging by making healthy lifestyle choices that can help prevent age-related diseases. Others are old for their age: they have abused their bodies with unhealthy lifestyle choices, causing them to age much faster than they should have.

Despite how logical and intuitive the concept of RealAge is, it actually flies in the face of much of what was previously believed about aging. For far too long, the medical community had assumed that how a person will age is "written in the genes." But the more we know about genetics, the more we know that this is not true. Studies continue to show that for most of us, lifestyle choices and behaviors have far more impact on longevity and health than our genetic inheritance. Studies of twins in Denmark, Finland, the United States, and Asia all show the same thing: about 25 percent of how we age is in our genes and 75 percent results from our choices. Genes define basic biology, but how you interact with the world around you—whether through food choices, exercise, or social connections—is how you control the way your genes will affect your body.

In fact, behavioral choices account almost entirely for a person's overall health and longevity by age sixty. The older you are, the more your choices determine how long and how well you live. People who are still able to live young even when their calendar age is old weren't necessarily born with good genes nearly so much as they have made good choices. They exercise, eat lots of fruits and vegetables, and keep their minds engaged. It doesn't sound too hard, does it? And that's because it isn't. The RealAge program shows every single one of us just how simple it is to become one of those people who really are younger than their years.

By taking the RealAge test, you'll find out exactly how young or old you are. You'll get specific tips on how you can make your RealAge younger. Essentially everything you do contributes to or prevents aging. Eating a diet rich in healthy fats, exercising, and quitting smoking are lifestyle choices you probably already know are good for you and—you may never have thought about it exactly this way—prevent aging. But did you know that flossing your teeth nightly or using a cell phone can make a big difference in how fast you age? Flossing regularly can make your RealAge as much as 6.4 years younger (see Chapter 5). And did you know that folate, aspirin, and tomato sauce can help your arteries stay young? Getting 800 micrograms (μg) of folate a day reduces arterial aging and the chance you might develop colon or breast cancer, making your RealAge nine months to as much as four years younger (see Chapter 10).

Many, many of the choices that help prevent aging are easy to put into effect, yet have far-reaching effects on your health. For example, RealAge tells you the habits and foods that increase and decrease the rate of growth of specific cancers, and by how much, so you can choose what you want to do. These recommendations are not based on wishful thinking. Each is backed by data confirmed in four or more studies that looked at outcome, survival, or quality of life in human beings, not animals.

RealAge lets you know what your choices are and the relative value of each, so you can make the choices that are best for you. It's much less work than you think. It's often just a matter of being mindful and adopting easy good habits, instead of living without thinking about choices and accidentally adopting aging choices. Thinking consciously about the wide variety of choices in your daily life lets you adopt as habits those that consistently give you a Makeover from the inside out, your RealAge Makeover.

As I described in *RealAge: Are You as Young as You Can Be?*, published in 1999, the RealAge concept came to me when a friend, Simon Z. (a lifelong smoker), developed severe arterial disease. For some reason, stepping out of my role as doctor and into my role as friend made the concept flash in my head: people need to understand that because of the lifestyle choices they were making, their true age was actually different than their calendar age.

I had tried everything to get my friend Simon to quit smoking, with no success. Suddenly, I thought I might have the key.

"Simon," I asked him, "how old are you?"

"Mike, you *know* I'm forty-nine," he grumbled.

"Simon, this isn't a joke," I replied. "How old are you *really*? Did you know that all that smoking has made you older?" I asked him. "Eight years older. Right now, you may be forty-nine, but your body is as old as someone who is fifty-seven, maybe more. For all practical purposes, your age *is* fifty-seven."

"I *can't* be fifty-seven!" he said. "No man in my family has ever lived to fifty-eight."

That did it. Simon quit smoking. He began exercising and eating right. He reduced his RealAge and began celebrating "years-younger" parties rather than his usual "one more year over the hill" birthday parties. Over time, he became younger.

After years of tracking patients who have used the method, I am thrilled to share their success stories. Simon is himself a great success story. His RealAge is an astonishing nine years younger than it was eighteen years ago—an improvement of twenty-seven years. That is, he made himself at least twenty-seven years younger than he would have been.

Simon chose to take a different route from the one he had followed before. The fact that we have choices that affect the speed of our aging is a crucial Real-Age concept which contradicts of the belief that aging is a constant, inevitable, downward pattern of physical decline. We have the scientific data to prove it, too. Consider the following:

Figure 1.1. Quality of Life, Measured by Performance, as We Age

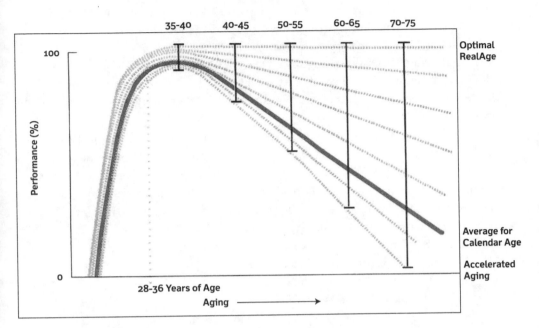

What do the quality-of-life curves mean in Figure 1.1? They mean that we decline in a variety of ways, not just one. The solid line is average performance by an age group—almost all of our functions decline at 5 percent (between 3 and 6 percent) every ten years. What declines on average of 5 percent every ten years after age 30 or 35? Almost everything: your heart function, your lung function, your kidney function, your bone mass, your muscle mass, even your IQ. The dotted lines represent the range within that group: some much better, some much worse. As you can see, the older the chronologic age, the greater the variation within it. Which curve you are on—the same kind of decline you will experience—is largely up to you. Will you live at the top of your curve until you're near the end, or will you decline like the average person, at the rate of 5 percent loss of function in each capacity every ten years, as illustrated by the darkest line? It's up to you.

To illustrate that we can age at different rates, consider the results of tests of IQ and other cognitive functions of Harvard physicians since the early 1950s (see Figure 1.2). Averaged out, the results reflect the previously mentioned 5 percent decline every ten years. However, the amazing thing is how extremely variable the change in IQ has been among the physicians: some have experi-

Figure 1.2. The Change in IQ of Physicians as They Age Varies Greatly

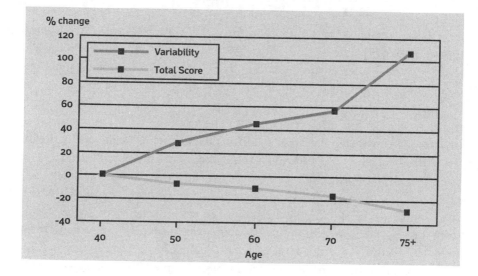

enced a great decrease, while others have experienced almost none. Clearly, average rates are subject to a myriad of individual exceptions. The less steeply declining lower line, which represents the average change in IQ, shows what we would expect: a slow but steady decline. The upper line, however, shows us something very surprising: the rapid incline demonstrates the extremely wide range of variation of the results of those being tested. In other words, while a mathematical average could be found for the results, the results were actually wildly disparate among individuals—some faring much better, some faring much worse. What we now know is you can largely control which curve you are on and how fast or slowly you decline.

A Question of Age: What Does It Mean to Get Old?

If you want to safeguard your health, one of the best ways to do so is by slowing or reversing the process of aging. Almost without exception, a younger body means a healthier body. The diseases that we fear the most, such as cancer and heart disease, are overwhelmingly more likely to strike an older body than a younger one. Not to mention that a younger body tends to feel better, and to have more energy.

Although both the lay public and the medical community are highly aware of the process of aging, exactly how and why it occurs is still a mystery. At best, scientists have been able to offer several theories, all of which have at least some credibility. One theory is that the body is programmed to die: our genes program the cells to divide a certain number of times, and once that maximum number has been reached, the body begins to fail. This is known as the *telomere* theory. (Telomeres are genetic elements that lose DNA—deoxyribonucleic acid—each time a cell divides.) Another theory is that our neurologic and hormonal systems wear out over time, making us more susceptible to a variety of diseases. A third hypothesis is the "wear-and-tear" theory: that living itself makes us old. A fourth theory is that over the years the body eventually accumulates so many toxins and waste products that its systems begin to shut down. The fifth theory is popularly known as the "free radical theory of aging:" The body builds up specific toxins, free radical oxidants, that damage the organs and DNA, causing us to age. A related theory is the glucose toxicity theory, which also involves waste buildup in the body. The seventh theory of aging derives from the law of entropy: within the universe there is continual movement from order to disorder, and in our bodies, that movement is experienced as aging. An eighth theory, the mitochondrial aging theory, is gaining prominence—the mitochondrial energy plants lose their ability to efficiently produce or deliver energy to the rest of the cell. If this last theory proves correct, it will have a radical effect on our future. Imagine staying as young as you are at fifty to age one hundred twenty or one hundred fifty. Just contemplating such a possibility requires a total shift in our way of thinking. Of course, we've already gone through radical shifts in our thinking about longevity. In the 1900s, people hoped to stay vigorous to age forty-five. In the 1960s, they hoped to stay vigorous to sixty or sixty-five. Now most of us want to stay vigorous to ninety or ninety-five.

The new change could be even more dramatic if the mitochondrial aging theory proves correct. This theory relates to the energy sources of our cells and to the second set of DNA in human cells. Most cells have DNA in both their nucleus and other structures called mitochondria, which govern energy transformation. Simply stated, our cells are in a constant state of division and renewal, during which mistakes can occur. And mistakes with the cellular (non-nuclear) DNA may have a big effect on our health and rate of aging. For example, our DNA is continually being replicated, and if we don't have enough folate—and vitamins B_6 and B_{12}—the replication can occur with errors or abnormalities, some which may possibly lead to cancer. The great news is that some genes, drugs, or supplements may be able to keep the mitochondrial DNA much younger.

If so, we might be able to keep ourselves at the top of our quality-of-life curve with the energy and vigor of someone much younger, assuming we keep age-related diseases, such as arterial aging (stroke, memory loss) and immune aging (cancer, infections) at bay as well. Within five to twenty years, it may be possible to be as young at one hundred twenty as most people now are at forty or fifty! So it's even more important to keep your RealAge young now, because how young you are in five to twenty years may determine how young you can be in the next seventy years. Steps as simple as taking acetyl L-carnitine, or lipoic acid, or resveratrol, as well as more folate (see Chapter 10), may keep this part of our DNA healthy. Furthermore, keeping our energy system young may in fact be part of the way of avoiding the essential process of aging. (Even though we feel excitement at these new possibilities, we must remember that they are still just theories.)

What Role Do Your Genes Play in the Aging Process?

Worried about your genes? The fact that you made it into the world at all means that all of your essential genes are working just fine. To develop from an egg to a fetus requires incredible genetic coordination. Simply being born means that everything went pretty much correctly. Also, as most people with severe genetic illness have their illness in childhood, reaching adulthood is an even greater indicator that your genes are working as they should.

In 1990, the Department of Energy and the National Institutes of Health launched an enormously ambitious and groundbreaking 13-year program called the U.S. Human Genome Project. The goals of the project were, among other things, to identify all genes in human DNA and to determine the sequences of the 3 billion chemical base pairs that make up that DNA. Although the project was a great success, and the team of scientists mapped the approximately 30,000 genes much faster than expected, many questions remain. We still don't know exactly what each gene does or how each and every gene affects us. One day we may have all the gene identifiers on a computer chip and, just by putting a drop of blood on the chip, be able to know what age-related diseases present the highest risk for us. But we're not there yet.

For diseases as diverse as diabetes, Alzheimer's, many cancers, and cardiovascular disease, we've long known that genetic components are involved. Some of us are more prone to weight gain, and some are more prone to high cholesterol. Those tendencies can increase the likelihood of certain kinds of disease and aging. Surprisingly, the more scientists have learned about genetics, the more they have also learned just how much environment, and our interactions with it, matter. We all have the genes we were born with, but how we age is largely up to us.

Uncovering our genetic predispositions is difficult. That's probably the greatest promise of the Genome Project. When genes can be analyzed quickly and easily, your predispositions will be identified, and you'll know what to do to make and keep your RealAge as young as it can be. Until there, it's up to you to investigate your genetic inheritance and decide what lifestyle changes to make.

Cardiovascular disease provides an excellent example of the way biologic predispositions and social behaviors interrelate. Some people are *biologically* predisposed to the early onset of arterial aging. They have inherited a tendency to high blood pressure, high cholesterol, or weight gain. Others are *culturally* predisposed to the disease, because factors in their culture or environment make them likely to develop habits such as eating foods high in saturated fat, which can accelerate arterial aging. Finally, we know that there is often, if not usually, a combination of both. The bad habits interact with the biologic predisposition, and cardiovascular aging is accelerated. You feel and look older, and you are older. You may think that this is simply a result of your genes. Most likely, it's a habit or lifestyle choice that is negatively affecting your health, energy level, and even your looks. The great news from the science of the last twenty years is that you can control your genes to a large degree if you want to.

For the most part, when we discuss aging and genetics, we are talking about very subtle differences, not major problems. (See Chapter 5 on cancer genetics and Chapter 12 on evaluating hereditary risks.) While genes are commonly thought to be the overwhelming factor in aging, that is happily not true. Which is not to say they have no effect at all—just that you can lessen that effect through your lifestyle choices. Let's explore how to go about doing just that.

The Three Most Important Factors That Affect Aging

Aging of the Arteries

When it comes to your RealAge Makeover, the single most important part of your body is your arteries. When your arteries are not cared for properly, they get clogged with fatty buildup, diminishing the amount of oxygen and nutrients that can reach your cells. When this happens, your cardiovascular system and entire body age more quickly. Having high blood pressure—a reading over 130/85 mm Hg (millimeters of mercury)—can make your RealAge more than twenty-five years older than having optimal blood pressure (a reading of 115/76 mm Hg). Your arteries deliver blood and its nutrients to your skin, your heart, your brain, your muscles, your gonads, and every cell of your body. Keeping your arteries young is essential for keeping every cell of your body young.

Many people unknowingly suffer from high blood pressure. The good news is that we now know how to decrease arterial aging by 75 to 80 percent. Even if you are genetically predisposed to arterial aging, you can still do much to prevent it, along with the other conditions that often come with it: heart disease, stroke, memory loss, impotence, decay in the quality of orgasm, and even wrinkling of the skin.

Yes, your arteries are essential to your Makeover. Reversing arterial disease gives you more energy and even makes you look younger. And it makes you look younger the right way—due to your arterial health—from the inside out. This book lists a range of actions you can choose to do—everything from taking an aspirin a day to having an alcoholic drink a day—that will make your arteries younger and healthier, and that will make you feel stronger and livelier.

Aging of the Immune System

The immune system is the body's vital self-policing system. It constantly monitors our health and goes into action to thwart any potential problems. When we pick up viruses or bacteria, our immune system works to find and destroy them. When a threat occurs from within the body—such as when a cell becomes malignant—the immune system works to root it out.

Don't let your immune system make you old. When you are young, genetic controls protect your cells—except in relatively rare cases—from becoming cancerous. If one of these cellular controls slips up, your larger immune system identifies precancerous cells in the body and eliminates them. Thus, your body has a double block against cancer, one on the cellular level and one on the organism-wide level. As you age, both the cell-based genetic controls and your immune system become more likely to malfunction, and you become more likely to develop a cancerous tumor. Many types of arthritis are examples of a breakdown of the immune system, which is why arthritis is a disease associated with aging. By keeping your immune system fit, you do your best to avoid such diseases and prevent premature aging. This book tells you which vitamins—and at what doses—help protect your genetic control systems and your immune system. It also describes ways to reduce the stresses in your life that can upset the balance of your immune system, and practices such as strength-building exercises that will help keep your immune system young.

Social and Environmental Factors

It's human nature to think of your health in terms of the big issues, such as whether you can avoid getting cancer. But what you may see as the "little" issues can have a big effect on how young you stay. Much of this involves the way you react to your environment—biologically, psychologically, and socially. Are you happy in your job? Do you get enough undisturbed sleep at night? Do you enjoy stress-reducing time with friends, and lots of laughter? Do you wear a helmet when riding a bike? All of these positive factors involving the environment you live in can increase the likelihood that your life will be longer and less ridden with illness than it might be otherwise.

It's a mistake to think about health only in terms of disease, because when you do you forget about the factors outside your body that can make you healthy. Some choices—for example, becoming a life-long learner by enrolling in classes, reading, playing games on-line, or otherwise stimulating your mind—can help keep you younger longer. Creating a quiet space in your home for daily meditation can do the same. Later chapters discuss the impact of these choices and show you how interacting with your environment in a particular way can keep you young.

Getting Younger: For Life!

Clyde K., a patient of mine, is a perfect example of a RealAge Makeover. He was a very successful executive at one of the large car companies. He first visited me when he was forty-six, because his father had died of a heart attack at that age. Several of Clyde's uncles had also had early onset of severe heart disease, strokes, or peripheral (leg) vascular disease. Clyde weighed 235 pounds, which hung loosely on his six-foot frame. He looked a little paunchy but not obese. His blood pressure was 165/100 mm Hg, the healthy level being 115/76. His blood levels of both C-reactive protein level (a marker of inflammation in the arteries) and "bad" cholesterol (low-density lipoprotein [LDL] cholesterol) were too high. Even though he was not taking any vitamins, his diet was pretty good except for the Mrs. Field's cookies he ate as a snack every morning and afternoon. Clyde was a forty-six-year-old man with a RealAge of fifty-three.

When we discussed his blood pressure and cholesterol, he said he really wanted to control them without pills. Nevertheless, he agreed to start with pills and then wean himself off the pills if he could successfully control his blood pressure with exercise (a course of action I often suggest for patients who have more than one elevated risk factor and a bad genetic heritage). So Clyde started to take medication to control his blood pressure and a small dose of a statin drug to lower LDL cholesterol and raise "good" cholesterol (high-density lipoprotein [HDL] cholesterol). However, the transformation that followed wasn't due to the drugs. It was because he started an exercise regime with plenty of walking. After thirty days, he began lifting weights. After another thirty days, he added treadmill exercises. He also began to enjoy only food that was RealAge-smart. Within six months he had reduced his weight to 180 pounds and had normal blood pressure, normal LDL cholesterol, increased HDL cholesterol, and low markers of inflammation. He was able to stop all medicines. He had transformed himself with a RealAge Makeover: he felt, looked, and *was* younger. By the time two calendar years passed, he had made his RealAge eighteen years younger! He was now forty-eight by the calendar but looked, felt, and truly was thirty-five.

Now feeling so much more energetic, healthy, and vibrant, Clyde's concern turned to the health of his wife of fifteen years, Maureen. As a pharmacy benefits manager at an HMO (health maintenance organization), Maureen K. had to make decisions about drugs based on savings for her company rather than the best interest of the patient. The fact that her choices might potentially harm patients caused her enormous stress. In addition, she hadn't done any regular physical activity for a long time and wasn't making healthy food choices. As a result, she was about fifteen pounds over her desired weight.

Maureen was impressed by her husband's return to youth and was willing to give the RealAge program a try. She found friends to walk with at lunch and started lifting weights three times a week. She started playing tennis again, with Clyde and with her own friends. Within six months, she had lost not only the extra fifteen pounds but another five. As she put it, she had become "a babe again at age forty-six."

With Clyde's support, Maureen made a major decision: to reduce her stress by changing jobs. When I saw her a year after her first visit, she was a new person—a much healthier, happier, and younger one.

Seeing Clyde and Maureen make themselves over in such a significant way by making such wonderful changes in their lives was and is the joy of being a physician—nothing could be greater. But I also got joy from seeing the happiness they themselves felt. They had changed their lives for the better. They felt younger, had a higher quality of life, and would live with less disability and more vitality for much longer.

You can also undergo a RealAge Makeover. Making your RealAge younger doesn't require doing the impossible, but it does involve a commitment to making those changes you decide you are willing to live with. Some are easy, some are more difficult, but all are doable.

A RealAge Makeover Just for You

Another exciting element of the RealAge Makeover is that it's customized just for you and your current lifestyle. You get to decide how you will embark on this new younger and healthier you, by choosing those lifestyle changes with which you feel most comfortable.

In the following chapter I explain how we calculate RealAge, and discuss the science behind the numbers. You will have two options for calculating your own RealAge: the charts provided in this book or, for a more accurate calculation, the computerized survey on the RealAge website, *www.RealAge.com*. Both options provide an individual calculation that distinguishes you from everyone, and also compare you with the health and youth average for your age group. Your RealAge calculation will weigh the risks you face against the health-related behaviors you choose. The end product is a RealAge that is uniquely descriptive of *you*. As you adopt behaviors that change your RealAge (such as eating breakfast every day), you can recalculate your RealAge. With each new calculation, you can chart your progress and watch the years disappear.

How young can you become? When I told a fifty-year-old friend all the things she could do to reduce her rate of aging, she asked, "If I did all of those things, I could have a RealAge of twelve?" Well, for those of us who wouldn't want to relive our teenage years, fortunately, no. In this book, all of the calculations reflect the greatest possible effect of each behavior when no other mediating factors are considered. Both the worksheets in Chapter 2 and the RealAge computer program use a multivariable equation that balances each factor in relation to all the other RealAge factors. This equation evaluates how all of these factors interrelate.

The more Age-Reduction habits you adopt (as described in Chapter 3), the less likely you will be to gain the maximum effect you would from adopting any single practice by itself. However, the more good habits you adopt, the better your across-the-board protection from aging will be, and that advantage will have a cumulative effect over time. Although none of us can be twelve again, it is relatively easy for individuals in their mid-fifties or mid-sixties to make their RealAge five to eight years younger, and only somewhat more difficult to make it fifteen or sixteen years younger. The maximum amount a person can reduce his or her RealAge below his or her calendar age is about twenty-seven years over an entire lifetime. Remember, too, the effect magnifies with age: at fifty, you might have a RealAge of forty-five, but by seventy-five, if you continue on the RealAge program, your RealAge may be only fifty. That means that in twenty-five years, your body may have aged as little as most people age in five.

RealAge is not a guarantee of longevity. In health, there are never guarantees. Nevertheless, RealAge is an accurate reading of your risk. The younger your RealAge, the better the odds that you will have more years left—not to mention higher-quality years—of a younger, healthier, and more energetic life. The calculation of risk is the best approximation we have of the body beneath: the lower the risk, the younger the body. Think of your RealAge as your aging speedometer: it is a reading of how fast you're going. When it comes to aging, slower is better. By making simple decisions, you can ease your foot off the pedal and slow your rate of aging. How fast you age is largely controlled by you.

Getting Younger All the Time

Since I first developed the RealAge concept, I haven't been able to keep quiet. I talk about RealAge to doctors and laypeople all over the country. I have encouraged patients to take the RealAge computer survey and have seen them make the decision to take their aging into their own hands. I have joined people as they have celebrated "years-younger" birthday parties and observed them becoming younger in front of my very eyes.

Since publication of the first edition of *RealAge,* I have joyfully and proudly read over one hundred fifty thank-you e-mails a day. The authors of those emails thanked me for their great, new choices that let them regain years and live more enjoyably. They felt they had achieved a higher quality of life with their younger RealAge. To a doctor, it doesn't get any better than that: people thanking you for helping them live healthier. I feel as though I don't deserve most of the thanks. After all, it was the people themselves who had made the choices and done the work to transform themselves—to give themselves a RealAge Makeover—from the inside out. It was the RealAge scientific team, not I alone, who did the work that provided the information. Still, nothing could make me happier.

Human beings are living longer than ever before. Our life expectancy is increasing, and, barring unforeseen circumstances, most of us can expect to live into ripe old age. Even so, we don't want the last thirty years of our lives to be filled with illness, restricted ability, and dependence on our families or nursing care. We want to be able to play golf, do the tango, or climb mountains right up until the day we die. We want all those extra years to be quality years—years in which we write the novel we've always dreamed of writing, or learn how to paint. We want to have fun with our grandchildren and enjoy our children as adults. With an understanding of the practical steps you can take to make your RealAge younger, all of these things will be possible for you.

What's Your RealAge?

Test Yourself to See How Young You Are

The first step in launching your RealAge Makeover is to determine your current RealAge. There are two ways to do this, depending on how comfortable you are on a computer. If you prefer pen and paper (and a calculator), determine your RealAge by using the charts provided in this book; this will give you a good approximation of your RealAge. If you like to work on-line and have Internet access, go to the RealAge website, *www.RealAge.com*, which will give you a more accurate estimation of your RealAge. By doing nineteen tests and answering 137 simple questions about yourself and your lifestyle, including your health factors, habits, and behaviors, you can determine your RealAge. Once you've done that, you will have the information you need to start your transformation. By selecting among the choices in this book or in your computer printout, you can launch a step-by-step RealAge Makeover best suited to your needs and your present lifestyle.

Two recent e-mails I received illustrate how easy and satisfying it is to calculate your RealAge and to learn how to make it younger:

Dear Dr. Mike,
I first calculated my RealAge last July, and it was four years older than my calendar age. Since using your action plan, I am now three years younger than my birth age with a possible several more to go. I have also managed, with your suggestions, to reduce my weight from 224 pounds to 185 pounds. Every day I look forward to receiving your e-mail "tip of the day."

Thanks, Dean

Dear Dr. Mike,

A friend who saw you on *Oprah* introduced me to your site about two years ago and it's absolutely wonderful. I took the RealAge test and found out I was one year younger but I could get nine additional years younger. I am on my way and am already five years younger. I look forward to my daily RealAge messages and find your selections and content current and informative. Your sources are bona fide, and with the monthly newsletter, it's just enough information without being overwhelming.

I think the best thing about your site is its tone. Everything is stated positively. In other words, "doing this is good," rather than "not doing this is bad." I have signed on to several well-known medical websites, but yours is by far my favorite. And as long as you're in business, and as long as you stay there, I am going to keep making my RealAge younger. Thank you for being so motivating.

Thanks, Kathy

The public response to the RealAge program has been so favorable because it takes health information that might otherwise be confusing or overwhelming and breaks it down into information you can understand and use easily. Still, you might question how we can calculate a number that accurately describes your true physiologic age. How can I say that one sixty-year-old is actually younger than another sixty year-old? Besides, when we talk about the effect of lifestyle on health, we have all witnessed individuals who seem to beat the odds. For example, while so many people who smoke get cancer, there is always one diehard who has smoked a pack a day since he was twelve and is going strong at ninety. So how can we say that quitting a pack-a-day smoking habit will make you seven years younger? Or that taking an aspirin a day can make you 52.8, instead of fifty-five?

The answer lies in two issues: the way science has changed our thinking about aging as a process, and the overwhelming amount of concrete health and lifestyle data the RealAge team has been able to accrue. The RealAge database has become so large (almost 10 million people have taken the RealAge test in one form or another) that we now know a lot more about aging. For example, we have approximately 10,000 people in each ten-year age range after age 25—more than 10,000 in the older age ranges—who have had heart attacks. We found that heart attack victims generally do not make lifestyle changes for the sake of their health until they're over fifty-five. Some don't even make changes after the heart attack, or at least not before they have seen what those changes can mean to their rate of aging and to their RealAge. That is, until they're past age fifty-five, people do not seem to understand that they can easily control their heart health by controlling their arterial aging. It is wonderful to see how much they change after taking the RealAge test. Our huge database, which is probably one of the largest in the world—if not *the* largest—has allowed us to develop important insights that have now been included in the tables in this book.

How We Calculate RealAge

To understand how we calculate RealAge, you will need to know how similar and dissimilar people are to each other as they age. Unless they've inherited a rare genetic disorder or have been in an accident, everyone generally starts aging at a similar rate. Men reach the peak of their performance curve in their late twenties; women, in their mid-thirties. At that point our bodies have fully matured, and we are at our strongest and most mentally acute. Then, somewhere between twenty-eight and thirty-six years of age, most people reach a turning point: they're not just growing anymore; they're aging. One of the most enlightening aspects of giving talks on RealAge is asking people what age they want to be or feel. When I asked people in many parts of the United States, Canada, the Netherlands, Brazil, Argentina, Uruguay, England, and Greece, men want to feel the way they did in their late twenties (specifically, twenty-eight), and women want to feel as they did in their mid-thirties (specifically, thirty-six).

If you track any one function of the human being—whether flexibility of the joints or memory—in the population as a whole you'll see that performance declines with age. In general, after the age of thirty-five, each biologic function decreases 3 to 6 percent per decade. Although these measurements have long been used by scientists to calculate the rate of aging, they can be misleading because they only represent an average, and averages don't take into account how much that rate of decline can vary among individuals. For older populations, especially, the variation is so great that it is often meaningless to calculate an average at all, because averages are only statistically meaningful if the majority of the people studied are reasonably near the midpoint. With aging, this clustering does not happen. In fact, there's such a wide scattering that to present an average is almost meaningless. It is actually misleading: it implies that there is a true average when there is not. In the older populations, there really isn't a meaningful average. Instead, there are people in every age group who fit into every level of function: some show dramatic decline, others show virtually none.

The data from the study we mentioned concerning the IQ of Harvard physicians as they age (Figure 1.2) illustrate this fact. Even though physicians as a group experience a 5 percent decrease in IQ every ten years, the rate of decline varies greatly among individuals. There is a family of curves pertaining to your quality of life, and what we have learned is that *you* can choose which curve you will be on (see Figure 1.1).

The extent to which people vary in their ability to maintain their function extends to all possible results. While some people will lose a function as they age, others will show almost no decline at all. In fact, for certain functions such as mental acuity and IQ, some people can even improve as they progress from calendar age thirty-five to eighty. We can see this in Figure 2.1. If a horizontal line were drawn across the three lines representing the rapid, average, and slow rates of aging (that is, sick, average, and healthy people), you would find that people of very different calendar ages fall at the same place on the curve representing aging.

The question is how can you be one of those people who show almost no decline over time, as young at eighty as you were at thirty-five? The answer starts with a RealAge Makeover. The goal we aspire to through the RealAge program is not just to live longer but to live better, suffering less illness and disability. After a RealAge Makeover, you'll be able to live longer and healthier. You'll look and feel better. And what could be more worthwhile than that?

To more easily understand how the RealAge system works, let's consider a concrete example: the impact of smoking on life expectancy. The average life expectancy of a forty-year-old is seventy-eight years for men and eighty-three years for women, according to the statistics. These numbers include everyone who dies prematurely from health complications caused by smoking. If you remove the data for smokers from the data for the general population, life expectancy becomes substantially greater. Thus, we can infer that smokers have shorter lives and more medical problems than nonsmokers. We can also infer that nonsmokers live longer.

The RealAge team calculates a person's RealAge with respect to smoking by comparing the ten-year survival rate (a calculation of life expectancy) of the smoker with that of the nonsmoker. By calculating the degree of risk and prorating it to the average ten-year survival rate for that person's chronologic age group, we find the number of years smoking can subtract from one's life, and the number of years *not* smoking can add to one's life. We apply this process to a whole range of behaviors and conditions, using a complex routine of statistical techniques to blend them and arrive at a number that reflects your biologic age.

RealAge is a calculation of your relative risk of dying and your relative risk of disability versus those risks for the population as a whole. If your relative risks match those of the average person who is chronologically ten years younger, that is the same as saying your RealAge is ten years younger. You are at the same risk of suffering severe aging or a major health problem as someone that much younger. When it comes to your physiologic age, you are equal.

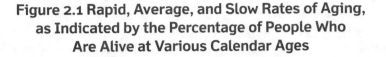

Figure 2.1 Rapid, Average, and Slow Rates of Aging, as Indicated by the Percentage of People Who Are Alive at Various Calendar Ages

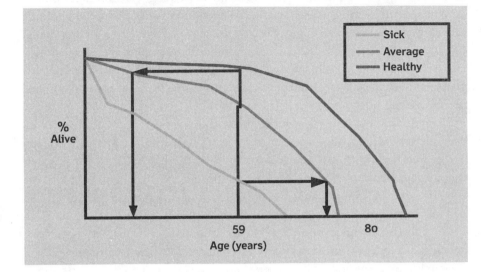

This method of risk-analysis calculation is the clearest measure we have for determining the rate at which you are aging. We draw data from clinical studies that calculate mortality risk for a variety of factors, and integrate the data into survival table analyses. We use these curves to evaluate individual conditions, habits, and other factors that tend to affect physiologic age. Our equations use the most up-to-date and reliable medical information available, which is then modeled by statisticians using the best and most sophisticated formulations for equations dealing with multiple variables.[1]

We start with the most general statistic: the average life expectancy for American men and women. We then break each category into smaller and smaller subcategories. For example, we consider weight-to-height ratios. We calculate

---

[1] The RealAge effects specified in all the other chapters except this one calculate the effects of the factor of interest *individually*—that is, without regard to the existence (and hence the effects) of other factors. Let's take the example of blood pressure. Many factors contribute to your blood pressure reading, such as sodium intake and potassium levels, so that some of the effects attributed to high blood pressure are attributable to other things as well. For example, exercise lowers blood pressure: three of the twelve years' difference in RealAge between a fifty-year-old man who has the ideal blood pressure of 115/76 mm Hg and one who has a high blood pressure of 140/90 mm Hg are attributable to stamina-building exercise. The changes in RealAge described in all of the chapters except this one do not take into account the interaction between factors.

the long-term effects of high blood pressure. We evaluate the benefit people get from taking folate, being physically active, or managing stress. Each breakdown allows us to refine our measurement and to consider how much of an impact each action has on the aging process. Finally, we consider all these categories together, calculating a multivariable equation in which we are able to weigh these multiple and diverse factors together and develop a unique RealAge calculation especially tailored to each person. We integrate the risk calculations for 132 factors and arrive at a number uniquely descriptive of *you*.

Does this process involving multiple variables, statistics, and risk analysis sound complicated? It is. But don't worry. To launch your RealAge Makeover, all you have to do is answer a set of questions that define your RealAge. We'll do everything else.

Where Do We Get the Actual Numbers?

The RealAge team doesn't generate new information. Whereas most medical researchers calculate their statistics in relation to "risk of disease," we have used their data and the data from our own large database of over five million users to calculate and determine the "risk of aging." We interpret the seemingly overwhelming amount of information that has already emerged from numerous published studies, and help you to understand the results. You are getting the best information the medical community has to offer, in a unified and comprehensive form. We can offer you specific recommendations from hundreds of studies, combined into a standardized framework, so you are spared the guesswork. In fact, the majority of the people who e-mail me say, "Thank you very much for providing the RealAge data. It makes it all so simple and clear." Helping to end confusion is the goal of the physicians, epidemiologists, and statisticians who keep the RealAge website current, and who help make the *RealAge* books scientifically correct.

We truly strive to leave no stone unturned. In conjunction with the four other medical experts who form the RealAge scientific advisory team, I have pored over more than 33,000 medical studies, evaluating what they tell us about aging and, more important, about the prevention of aging. Our calculations are based on data from more than 1,200 of those studies, and have been checked against a very large proprietary database. We constantly update our formulas as new research becomes available. As statistics relating to these and other factors change, we recalculate our equations to accommodate the changes. Our on-line RealAge program is also updated whenever new and important research appears. For example, data appeared that vitamins C and E, which retard or reverse arterial aging in most individuals, inhibit the functioning of the cholesterol-reducing "statin" class of drugs, such as simvastatin (Zocor), pravastatin (Pravachol), atorvastatin (Lipitor), and rosuvastatin (Crestor). Thus, if you are taking a statin drug, you should take vitamins C and E in much-reduced dosage; to do otherwise would encourage aging. We modified the RealAge program to reflect this new information, and those changes are included in this book. (See Chapter 10.)

For the most part, the RealAge team uses clinical studies of two types: large-scale risk-factor epidemiology studies, and smaller scale randomized trials. The large-scale epidemiologic studies look at many people, sometimes more than 100,000 individuals, and in one instance as many as 350,000 (the Multiple Risk Factor Intervention Trial on cessation of smoking). The researchers who coordinate these studies track huge populations over a period of time, looking at a certain behavior or testable factor, and evaluate risks associated with that behavior or factor. These studies generate statistics for a large population, and this allows for a more accurate reflection of the variations within the study sample group. The drawback is that they do not provide very detailed information, nor are they controlled studies. That is, the researchers are not able to regulate with any kind of reliability who takes a specific drug or engages in a specific behavior.

A randomized controlled study is quite a different thing. In a controlled study, researchers usually vary just one element. Even though controlled studies can have drawbacks (such as choosing the wrong preparation of progesterone to accompany estrogen, in recent studies on hormone replacement—see Chapter 4), controlled studies are generally much more capable of determining just what the investigator wants to know than are epidemiologic studies. In a randomized controlled study, a study population of any number of people—from a few hundred to 10,000—is randomly divided into groups, and each group is assigned a certain task. For example, one group may be told to take folic acid, and another group may be told to take placebos (harmless sugar pills). In another example, a third of the participants may be given diets devoid of salt, a third may be given diets containing moderate amounts of salt, and a third may be allowed as much salt as they want. Each participant is monitored and tracked for a long period of time, and his or her health conditions are recorded. At the end of the study, the researchers compare the groups and evaluate the effect of the particular behavior on the overall health of each group.

We are rigorous in what we require of data before we include it in the RealAge program. We require that a factor be proven to have an effect on the speed of aging in at least four "peer-reviewed" studies (studies critiqued by other experts on the subject). While this requirement means that some potentially great factors can't yet be part of the RealAge program because they have only been examined in two or three peer-reviewed studies, it helps us feel confident that the information we give you is much more likely to be valid. Science is changing all the time, so three of our earlier recommendations—of more than 132—had to be changed, and we added over 30 factors that hit the four-study validity mark.

One of the most interesting subjects we have been investigating is lycopene—the red stuff in tomatoes. When we first looked at this subject, about five risk-factor epidemiology studies on lycopene had been performed in human beings. Our scientific group has a rule that at least four of the five of us must vote affirmatively for behavior to be said to have a RealAge effect, and be included in the program. Initially, we did not include lycopene consumption because it seemed so outlandish that eating just ten tablespoons of tomato sauce a week would decrease the risk of prostate cancer by 30 to 45 percent. However, the data kept accumulating. When eleven studies associated consumption of lycopene with a decrease in prostate cancer, we included lycopene in the program, but only in relation to prostate cancer. When the prostate cancer studies were followed by seven studies on breast cancer, we voted to include lycopene for breast cancer, too.

At present, three studies on arterial aging show favorable results with lycopene. When a fourth study confirms the effect, we will probably include lycopene consumption as having a RealAge effect on that variable, too. This would confirm lycopene as a much more powerful antiaging agent than it is today. That's right: at present, consuming ten tablespoons of tomato sauce a week makes your RealAge about 1.9 (men) or 0.8 (women) years younger if you're an average fifty-five-year-old. However, if the favorable lycopene effect on arterial aging is confirmed in a fourth study—and the study is a prospective randomized controlled study (data collected during treatment rather than after)—the Real-Age effect of lycopene could jump to more than five years younger. By just eating ten tablespoons of tomato sauce or the equivalent of tomato paste a week (especially if the tomatoes are cooked and eaten with a little olive oil), you could be five years younger! But because the studies are not there yet, at the time of this printing the RealAge effect of lycopene is still 1.9 years for men and 0.8 years for women. (We discuss lycopene in detail in Chapter 5.)

Another interesting factor also seemed unlikely to be meaningful but proved effective. When we considered flossing and customized dental care (see Chapter 5), it took us four meetings to vote these factors into the program because they didn't fit the "medical model." In fact, though, flossing and dental care may be part of the reason that having lower socioeconomic status increases rates of aging. In general, those in lower socioeconomic classes do not take care of their teeth and gums as well as those in higher socioeconomic classes. Data from Great Britain have shown how important good dental care is to cardiac health. Studies there show that individuals who come to emergency departments with chest pain related to the heart also have a high incidence of chronic gum infections. When doctors give these patients an antibiotic specifically for their gum problems at the same time they give aspirin and a beta-blocker (a drug that reduces blood pressure), they decrease the occurrence or recurrence of heart attacks over the next five years by as much as 30 percent!

To be included in the RealAge program, a recommendation must meet the high-quality criterion of confirmation in four peer-reviewed studies. That is why the RealAge program and your RealAge are such powerful, science-based tools.

Time to Start Your Makeover

As we stated previously, calculating your current RealAge is the very first step in your own personal RealAge Makeover. There are two ways you can do so: either by taking the RealAge survey on your computer or by using the chart in this chapter. The computer program is the most accurate method. The charts are accurate too, but will give you a more general approximation of your RealAge. In both versions of the RealAge questionnaire we ask you about 132 detailed questions about a variety of behaviors that are known to relate to aging. Do you eat fish? How often? Are you physically active? Do you regularly get a good night's sleep? Do you own a dog? Do you practice regular stress-reduction methods such as yoga? How long did your mother live? We ask you to answer each question as honestly and completely as you can, without fear of judgment. Your answers to these questions are the raw data we will use to calculate your RealAge.

Your RealAge On-line

If you are comfortable working on-line and have Internet access, you can take the RealAge quiz at *www.RealAge.com*. It's the easiest way to calculate your RealAge, and there is no charge for this service. An added bonus for calculating your RealAge this way is that your account will store your information, so that you can access it as many times as you like. All information you provide is completely confidential and accessible only by you through a password. The computer test takes about forty minutes to complete. As you adopt new Age-Reduction strategies (the plan is in Chapter 3), you can chart your progress and have fun watching yourself become younger.

If at all possible, visit your doctor beforehand to get some vital information that will help you to calculate your RealAge with greater accuracy. Ideally, you'll want to know your blood pressure (systolic and diastolic), heart rate, height, weight, two cholesterol values (total cholesterol, or LDL cholesterol and HDL cholesterol), triglyceride levels, and high-sensitivity C-reactive protein (hs-CRP) level. Also, when you sit down to take the test, you'll want to have a list of the medications you take, and the amounts of any vitamins or other supplements you take. (If you do not know these values, the average values for your gender and age will be used until you provide them.)

Another way to make your RealAge test more effective is to take time before sitting down at the computer to perform some physical tests, such as timing how long you can stand on one leg with your eyes closed (with someone nearby to prevent you from falling). Or you can note how large a drop in your heart rate occurs in the two minutes after you hit your peak exercise heart rate and then stop exercising. These physical tests are not necessary, but can help make your RealAge calculation more accurate. If you do not do one or more of these 19 tests, choose No Change and enter zero in the Tally column for the test you omit.

When you've completed the test, it probably won't take more than two minutes to tabulate your results. After the calculation, the computer will produce a list of Age-Reduction suggestions tailored to your health and behavior profile. These suggestions consist of choices you can make as part of your RealAge Makeover, showing how much each choice would affect your age. Select the suggestions that you would consider adopting. The computer will then recalculate your RealAge, showing what your RealAge will be in three months, one year, and three years if you adopt those behaviors.

The key to success for a RealAge Makeover is to start small and add on. Vary your choices to see which combinations you would be willing to adopt and how each would help you get younger sooner. You can then make informed choices about your health. You can choose which Age-Reduction strategies you want to integrate into your life, and in which order. As you start making healthy changes, you can check back on-line to witness how much younger you have become. Rather than just hoping that all this fresh fruit, leafy greens, and tomato sauce will help you twenty years from now, you can see how much of a difference it is making right now.

Your RealAge on Paper

If you're not a whiz on the computer, don't despair! You can also calculate your RealAge by filling out the chart included in this chapter. You simply respond to the questions asked, choose which answer best describes you, and fill in the corresponding tally column. Because of the complexity of the mathematics involved in calculating RealAge, the chart provides a less accurate reading than the computer program. In fact, RealAge has become possible only because we can now use powerful computers to rapidly make very subtle statistical differentiations, accounting for the interaction of factors and drawing from a huge database of information. However, the chart you fill in by hand provides a relatively accurate reflection of your RealAge. It is modified to account for many interactions and has been tested on more than 3,300 individuals and many, many hypothetical cases, so that it represents the best possible approximation.

When filling out the chart, you will be asked to respond to a list of questions. Possible answers to each question lie to the right of the questions. Choose the box that best describes you. For example, you will be asked if you currently smoke or have ever smoked. The answers range from "less than five cigarettes in life" to "more than twenty pack-years" (a pack-year is one pack per day for one year). Mark the one that describes you best. Then look at the number at the top of the column. It will read, depending on your answer, something like "Years Younger −3" or "Years Older +3." Write the number that corresponds to your answer in the right-hand Tally column, making sure to retain the positive or negative sign. When you have completed the questionnaire, add all the numbers. Remember that a negative number should be subtracted. For example (+2) + (−3) = (−1). When you have added all your answers, you will get a total tally number. Multiply that number by the "multiplier," an age-conversion factor that is provided at the bottom of Chart 2.1, to get your RealAge net change. If that number is a positive number, then your RealAge is that much older than your calendar age. If you get a negative number, then your RealAge is that much younger than your calendar age. For example, if you are now fifty but get a final number of +4, then your RealAge is fifty-four. Likewise, if the final number is −4, then your RealAge is forty-six. The calculation is simple and easy, and taking the quiz and tabulating it should not take more than forty-five minutes.

After you have finished computing your RealAge, review your answers. Any place that you have marked a "plus" number, you have marked a behavior that is causing you to age prematurely. Write down those behaviors. Then read about them in this book to learn how and why those behaviors are causing you to age. Next, you will want to develop a plan for your own RealAge Makeover, as described in the Chapter 3.

What Does Your RealAge Mean to You?

If your RealAge is younger than your calendar age, congratulations! That means that you are already making lifestyle choices that help protect your youth, and are aging more slowly than most of your peers. But that doesn't mean there isn't room for improvement—almost everyone can benefit from a RealAge Makeover, no matter how healthy they are. Keep reading to see what you can do to make your RealAge even younger.

If your RealAge is older, the bad news is that you are aging faster than most of your peers. However, the good news is that you are the type of person who can benefit most from a RealAge Makeover. You've got a chance to witness a true transformation in your life. So instead of getting discouraged, be proactive. Start planning your Makeover today by looking at all your choices and selecting those that you really think you could incorporate into your current lifestyle. Toss in a couple of quick fixes so that you can see right away how easy the Makeover process can be. You have a truly great opportunity in your hands: to slow your rate of aging, bring yourself back in line with your peers, and maybe even get younger. Before you know it, you'll start looking and feeling better. It's a Makeover in the truest sense, from the inside out. All that is required of you is to commit to a few choices.

What are those choices? They vary from simply taking vitamin D, to the difficult one of dropping unwanted pounds. Although a few of these measures may be difficult—overcoming an addiction, for example—the vast majority are simple and much less painful than you ever imagined. Now let's take a look at exactly what options you have.

Chart 2.1   Your Current RealAge: How Old Are You . . . Really?

This chart gives a first approximation for RealAge calculations for both genders between 25 and 100 calendar years of age without acute or chronic diseases. To compute a first approximation of your RealAge and what your health choices and behaviors do to it, begin by filling out the chart as best you can, based on factors below. (If you have no idea for any factor, skip it or estimate it.) Go down the chart, factor by factor. Write the number that best fits in the Tally box at the end of each row. Remember, if your response made you younger, the number in the Tally box should have a negative sign (for example, -1.5).

After you complete this chart, multiply the number at the bottom of the tally sheet by your calendar age multiplier from the box that follows. Then calculate your RealAge by adding or subtracting this number from your calendar age.

HEALTH FACTOR	YEARS YOUNGER -3.0	YEARS YOUNGER -2.5	YEARS YOUNGER -2.0	YEARS YOUNGER -1.5	YEARS YOUNGER -1.0	YEARS YOUNGER -0.5	NO CHANGE	YEARS OLDER +0.5	YEARS OLDER +1.0	YEARS OLDER +1.5	YEARS OLDER +2.0	YEARS OLDER +2.5	YEARS OLDER +3.0	TALLY
TESTS TO DO: Place your hand palm down on a table. Pinch the area between your thumb and your first finger for 5 seconds. See how many seconds it takes for your skin to go back to normal.			Immediately	Calendar age 40 and older, less than 2 seconds	Under calendar age 40, less than 2 seconds	Calendar age 40 and older, 2 to 5 seconds	Under calendar age 40, 2 to 5 seconds; calendar age 40 and older, 5 to 10 seconds	Calendar age 40 and older, 10 to 15 seconds	Under calendar age 40, 5 to 10 seconds; calendar age 40 and older, longer than 15 seconds		Under calendar age 40, 10 to 15 seconds		Under calendar age 40, longer than 15 seconds	
Stand barefoot on a level, uncarpeted surface. With your feet together, close your eyes and raise one foot about six inches off the ground (if you're right-handed, raise right foot). See how many seconds you can stand on one foot with your eyes closed before you have to open your eyes or move your supporting foot. Test three times and take the best score.				Calendar age 40 and older, more than 30 seconds	Under calendar age 40, more than 30 seconds; calendar age 40 and older, 21 to 30 seconds	Calendar age 40 and older, 21 to 30 seconds	Under calendar age 40, 21 to 30 seconds; calendar age 40 and older, 11 to 20 seconds		Under calendar age 40, 16 to 20 seconds	Calendar age 40 and older, 6 to 10 seconds	Under calendar age 40, 11 to 15 seconds	Under calendar age 40, 10 seconds or less; Calendar age 40 and older, 5 seconds or less		
Test your foot flexibility with this test: stand up with bare feet. Place a pen on the floor. Try to pick up the pen with your foot, raising leg until the pen is parallel with floor. Now try it with the other foot.					Can pick up pen more than once	Can pick up pen once	Can pick up pen, but drop it on floor	Can curl toes around pen, but can't pick up	Can't curl toes around pen					

HEALTH FACTOR	YEARS YOUNGER -3.0	YEARS YOUNGER -2.5	YEARS YOUNGER -2.0	YEARS YOUNGER -1.5	YEARS YOUNGER -1.0	YEARS YOUNGER -0.5	NO CHANGE	YEARS OLDER +0.5	YEARS OLDER +1.0	YEARS OLDER +1.5	YEARS OLDER +2.0	YEARS OLDER +2.5	YEARS OLDER +3.0	TALLY
Look at the number 364-2872 for a five-second count. Now look away and cover this spot. In 5 seconds write the number down. Do not look at this number until you have completed the question below.					No mistakes		One mistake		Two mistakes		Three or more mistakes			
Five minutes later write the number on another sheet of paper. Now look at the numbers and pick the box that most closely fits.			No mistakes		One mistake		Two mistakes		Three mistakes		Four or more mistakes			
Find a measured distance, such as around your block or a local track. Using a watch with a second hand, walk as fast and as far as you can in exactly 12 minutes. Calculate the distance you walked.				Calendar age 60 and older: 1.0 mile or more; age 50 to 59: 1.1 miles or more; age 40 to 49: 1.3 miles or more; age 30 to 39: 1.4 miles or more; under age 30: 1.5 miles or more	Calendar age 60 and older: 0.9 to 1.0 mile; age 50 to 59: 1.0 to 1.1 miles; age 40 to 49: 1.1 to 1.2 miles; age 30 to 39: 1.3 to 1.4 miles; under age 30: 1.4 to 1.5 miles		Calendar age 60 and older: 0.8 to 0.9 mile; age 50 to 59: 0.9 to 1.0 mile; age 40 to 49: 1.0 to 1.1 miles; age 30 to 39: 1.2 to 1.3 miles; under age 30: 1.3 to 1.4 miles		Calendar age 60 and older: 0.7 to 0.8 mile; age 50 to 59: 0.8 to 0.9 mile; age 40 to 49: 0.9 to 1.0 mile; age 30 to 39: 1.1 to 1.2 miles; under age 30: 1.2 to 1.3 miles			Calendar age 60 and older: less than 0.7 mile; age 50 to 59: less than 0.8 mile; age 40 to 49: less than 0.9 mile; age 30 to 39: less than 1.1 miles; under age 30: less than 1.2 miles		

HEALTH FACTOR	YEARS YOUNGER -3.0	YEARS YOUNGER -2.5	YEARS YOUNGER -2.0	YEARS YOUNGER -1.5	YEARS YOUNGER -1.0	YEARS YOUNGER -0.5	NO CHANGE	YEARS OLDER +0.5	YEARS OLDER +1.0	YEARS OLDER +1.5	YEARS OLDER +2.0	YEARS OLDER +2.5	YEARS OLDER +3.0	TALLY
Use a heart rate monitor, or see Chapter 9 to learn how to count your maximum heart rate. Do the most strenuous activity you usually do.* Immediately at the end of the most strenuous part of the exercise, stop and take your heart rate. The maximum heart rate** you achieved with this exercise is:					90 percent or greater of age-induced maximum	80 to 90 percent of age-induced maximum			70 to 80 percent of age-induced maximum		Less than 70 percent of age-induced maximum			
Maximum exercise capacity: peak kcals or METs achieved per minute for at least one minute of a 20-minute stamina activity	Men, greater than 11 METs or 14 kcal/min; women, greater than 10 METs or 12 kcal/min		Men, 8.6 to 10.9 METs or 12 to 13.9 kcal/min; women, 8.1 to 9.9 METs or 10.6 to 11.9 kcal/min		Men, 7.3 to 8.5 METs or 10.2 to 11.9 kcal/min; women, 7.0 to 8.0 METs or 9.3 to 10.5 kcal/min		Men, 4.4 to 7.3 METs or 7.8 to 10.1 kcal/min; women, 4.0 to 6.9 METs or 6.2 to 9.2 kcal/min					Men, less than 4.3 METs or less than 7.7 kcal/min; women, less than 3.9 METs or less than 6.1 kcal/min		
Decrease in heart rate in the 2 minutes after a maximum heart rate has been achieved by your most strenuous usual exercise*	More than 66 beats per minute decrease		45 to 66 beats per minute decrease				33 to 44 beats per minute decrease		24 to 32 beats per minute decrease			Less than 24 beats per minute decrease		
Kneel on floor and place hands on either side of chest. You can keep your knees bent on floor, but you must keep back flat throughout the move. Bend elbows into a push-up, touching your chin or chest on floor with each push-up. Do as many as you can until you can't do any more.					Calendar age 60 and older: 30 or more; age 50 to 59: 35 or more; age 40	Calendar age 60 and older: 25 to 29; age 50 to 59: 30 to 34; age 40	Calendar age 60 and older: 15 to 24; age 50 to 59: 20 to 29; age 40	Calendar age 60 and older: 5 to 14; age 50 to 59: 10 to 19; age 40	Calendar age 60 and older: less than 5; age 50 to 59: less than 10; age					

Lie on floor with knees bent and feet flat on floor. With your arms extended, sit up until your hands touch knees. Do as many as you can in one minute.	to 49: 39 or more; age 30 to 39: 44 or more under age 30: 48 or more	to 49: 34 to 38; age 30 to 39: 40 to 43; under age 30: 44 to 47	to 49: 24 to 33; age 30 age 30 to 39: 30 to 39; under age 30: 34 to 43	to 49: 14 to 23; age 30 to 39: 20 to 29; under age 30: 24 to 33	40 to 49: less than 14; age 30 to 39: less than 20; under age 30: less than 24.
	Calendar age 60 and older: 20 or more; age 50 to 59: 25 or more; age 40 to 49: 29 or more; age 30 to 39: 34 or more; under age 30: 38 or more	Calendar age 60 and older: 15 to 19; age 50 to 59: 20 to 24; age 40 to 49: 24 to 28; age 30 to 39: 30 to 33; under age 30: 34 to 37	Calendar age 60 and older: 10 to 14; age 50 to 59: 15 to 19; age 40 to 49: 19 to 23; age 30 to 39: 25 to 29; under age 30: 29 to 33	Calendar age 60 and older: 5 to 9; age 50 to 59: 10 to 14; age 40 to 49: 15 to 18; age 30 to 39: 19 to 24; under age 30: 24 to 28	Calendar age 60 and older: less than 5; age 50 to 59: less than 10; age 40 to 49: less than 15; age 30 to 39: less than 19; under age 30: less than 24.
Perform a single-leg squat to test your knee strength and stability. Try to bend knee until your thigh is parallel with floor. Do not do this to the point of suffering significant pain.	No strain in knee	Slight strain in knee		Heavy strain or dull pain	Sharp pain in knee

HEALTH FACTOR	YEARS YOUNGER -3.0	YEARS YOUNGER -2.5	YEARS YOUNGER -2.0	YEARS YOUNGER -1.5	YEARS YOUNGER -1.0	YEARS YOUNGER -0.5	NO CHANGE	YEARS OLDER +0.5	YEARS OLDER +1.0	YEARS OLDER +1.5	YEARS OLDER +2.0	YEARS OLDER +2.5	YEARS OLDER +3.0	TALLY
To test hip range of motion, lie on floor with one leg straight and bring one leg up toward chest with knee bent. Now open out bent leg slightly from body (if you're lifting right leg, you'll bring it over slightly to right side). Do not do this to the point of suffering significant pain.					No sensation in hip region	A little pressure in the hip region		Dull pain or heavy pressure in the hip region	Sharp pain in the hip region					
Lie flat on back, and raise one leg as far as you can (straight, not bent). Do not do this to the point of suffering significant pain.					More than 90 degrees	90 degrees		75 to 90 degrees	45 to 74 degrees	Less than 45 degrees				
For women only: Think about the muscles that stop your urine in midflow—those are your Kegel muscles, or pelvic-floor muscles. Try squeezing your Kegel muscles for a 10-second hold, then release briefly and squeeze again. Aim for 30 repetitions of this, without feeling pain or fatigue in the area, if you are under 30, 20 if you are 30 and over.				Under calendar age 30: 30 or more; calendar age 30 to 50: 21 or more; over calendar age 50: 12 or more	Under calendar age 30: 25 to 29; calendar age 30 to 50: 18 to 20; over calendar age 50: 12 to 14		Under calendar age 30: 20 to 24; calendar age 30 to 50: 14 to 17; over calendar age 50: 9 to 11		Under calendar age 30: 15 to 19; calendar age 30 to 50: 10 to 13; over calendar age 50: 6 to 8	Under calendar age 30: less than 15; calendar age 30 to 50: less than 10; over calendar age 50: less than 6				

HEALTH FACTOR	YEARS YOUNGER -3.0	YEARS YOUNGER -2.5	YEARS YOUNGER -2.0	YEARS YOUNGER -1.5	YEARS YOUNGER -1.0	YEARS YOUNGER -0.5	NO CHANGE	YEARS OLDER +0.5	YEARS OLDER +1.0	YEARS OLDER +1.5	YEARS OLDER +2.0	YEARS OLDER +2.5	YEARS OLDER +3.0	TALLY
The tape test: On a day you are sunscreen-, makeup-, and moisturizer-free (& shaved more than 2 hours earlier if you are a man) for at least two hours, place a small strip of adhesive tape vertically on the middle of the forehead from scalp to between eyebrows. Move it to these three areas: the outside corners of the eyes, across the apple of each cheek, and above the upper lip. Press gently. Keep it there for a few seconds, then gently remove tape and evaluate the skin's imprint for lines, flakiness, and dehydrated area.			Calendar age 30 to 40: tape is completely smooth; calendar age 40 to 50: tape is completely smooth, or flaky dead skin cells only but no lines; over calendar age 50: tape is completely, smooth, flaky dead skin cells only but no lines, or small lines on one area		Under calendar age 30: tape is completely smooth	Under calendar age 40: flaky dead skin cells only but no lines; calendar age 40 to 50: small lines on one area; over calendar age 50: small lines on two areas		Under calendar age 40: small lines on one area: calendar age 40 to 50: small lines on two areas; over calendar age 50: small lines on four areas	Under calendar age 40: small lines on two areas; calendar age 40 to 50: small lines on three areas.		Under calendar age 40: small lines on three or four areas: calendar age 40 to 50: small lines on four areas.			
Take three deep breaths and hold the fourth breath for as long as you can. Don't force it, just hold your breath naturally.					Under calendar age 40: 2 minutes or more; age 40 to 60: 1 minute, 45 seconds or more; over age	Under calendar age 40: 1 minute, 45 seconds to 1 minute 59 seconds; age 40 to 60: 1	Under calendar age 40: 1 minute, 30 seconds to 1 minute, 44 seconds; age 40 to 60: 1	Under calendar age 40: 1 minute, 15 seconds to 1 minute, 29 seconds; age 40 to 60: 1	Under calendar age 40: less than 1 minute, 15 seconds; age 40 to 60: less than 1 minute; over age					

HEALTH FACTOR	YEARS YOUNGER -3.0	YEARS YOUNGER -2.5	YEARS YOUNGER -2.0	YEARS YOUNGER -1.5	YEARS YOUNGER -1.0	YEARS YOUNGER -0.5	NO CHANGE	YEARS OLDER +0.5	YEARS OLDER +1.0	YEARS OLDER +1.5	YEARS OLDER +2.0	YEARS OLDER +2.5	YEARS OLDER +3.0	TALLY
					60: 1 minute, 30 seconds or more	minute, 30 seconds to 1 minute, 44 seconds; over age 60: 1 minute, 15 seconds to 1 minute, 29 seconds	minute, 15 seconds to 1 minute, 29 seconds; over age 60: 1 minute to 1 minute 14 seconds.	minute to 1 minute, 14 seconds; over age 60: 45 to 59 seconds	60: less than 45 seconds					
Have someone take 2 pictures of you standing up, from both the front and side of your body. Draw a straight line on the photo (if you have a digital camera, you can do this on your computer, or just draw it on the photo with a ruler). In the frontal photo, it should be straight from your nose through the center of your body. In the side view, the line should be straight from the hole in your ear to the tip of your shoulder to your hip to your inner foot.		Everything aligned		One feature out of alignment			Two features out of alignment			Three features out of alignment		Four features out of alignment		

HEALTH FACTOR	YEARS YOUNGER -3.0	YEARS YOUNGER -2.5	YEARS YOUNGER -2.0	YEARS YOUNGER -1.5	YEARS YOUNGER -1.0	YEARS YOUNGER -0.5	NO CHANGE	YEARS OLDER +0.5	YEARS OLDER +1.0	YEARS OLDER +1.5	YEARS OLDER +2.0	YEARS OLDER +2.5	YEARS OLDER +3.0	TALLY
Blood pressure (systolic/diastolic, mm Hg)	90/65 to 120/81		Less than 90/65; no heart disease		121/82 to 129/85 or less than 90/65 with risk factors for or overt heart disease		130/86		131/87 to 140/90	Women, 141/91 to 150/95	Men, 141/19 to 150/95		Higher than 151/96	
Patrolling Your Own Health:														
My health status, compared with that of others					Excellent		Very good or fair						Poor or bad	
Immunization status						Current including flu, and I know flu vaccination decreases inflammation in my arteries	Current save for flu	Not current for flu and at least one of diphtheria and tetanus, hepatitis B, measles, pneumococcal disease						
Cigarette smoking (in pack-years)***	Smoked fewer than 5 cigarettes in life		Ex-smoker; no cigarettes for more than 5 yr		Ex-smoker; no cigarettes for 3 to 5 yr		Ex-smoker; no cigarettes for 1 to 3 yr		Ex-smoker; no cigarettes for 5 mos. to a year	Ex-smoker; no cigarettes for 2 to 5 mos.	Smoker; 0 to 20 pack-years		Smoker; more than 20 pack-years	
Exposure to secondhand smoke							None		0 to 1 hr a day		1 to 3 hr a day		More than 3 hr a day	

HEALTH FACTOR	YEARS YOUNGER -3.0	YEARS YOUNGER -2.5	YEARS YOUNGER -2.0	YEARS YOUNGER -1.5	YEARS YOUNGER -1.0	YEARS YOUNGER -0.5	NO CHANGE	YEARS OLDER +0.5	YEARS OLDER +1.0	YEARS OLDER +1.5	YEARS OLDER +2.0	YEARS OLDER +2.5	YEARS OLDER +3.0	TALLY
Cigar smoking							None	Ex-cigar smoker; no cigars for 3 yr	Cigar smoker; fewer than 4/wk	Cigar smoker; 4 to 8/wk	Cigar smoker 9 to 18/wk	Cigar smoker; more than 18/wk		
Pipe smoking							None	Ex-pipe smoker; no p/s for 3 yr	Pipe smoker; fewer than 4 times/wk	Pipe smoker; 4 to 8 times/wk	Pipe smoker; 9 to 18 times/wk	Pipe smoker; more than 18 times/wk		
Use of chewing or other smokeless tobacco							None	Has not used for 3 yr	Has used for 3 yr	Has used for over 3 yr				
Use of aspirin or other NSAIDs such as ibuprofen (Advil, Motrin, etc.)		Women over calendar age 50 and men over age 40 who take a 165 or 325 mg tablet or pill/day, if no contra-indication	Women 40 to 50 calendar years of age, and men 30 to 40 who take a 165 or 325 mg tablet or pill/day, if no contra-indication	Women over calendar age 50 and men over age 40 who take a 82.5 or 100 mg tablet or pill/day, if no contra-indication	Women 40 to 50 calendar years of age, and men 30 to 40 who take a 82.5 or 100 mg tablet or pill/day, if no contra-indication		Take no NSAIDs							
Eating breakfast						More than five times a week	4 or 5 times a week	2 or 3 times a week	Less than two times a week					
No. of days per week snacking occurs between meals other than in late afternoon						Rarely, or snack is nuts and/or fruit only	Occasionally, and not usually nuts and/or fruit	3 to 5 days a week, and snack is usually not nuts or fruit	Almost every day, and snack is usually not nuts or fruit					

HEALTH FACTOR	YEARS YOUNGER -3.0	YEARS YOUNGER -2.5	YEARS YOUNGER -2.0	YEARS YOUNGER -1.5	YEARS YOUNGER -1.0	YEARS YOUNGER -0.5	NO CHANGE	YEARS OLDER +0.5	YEARS OLDER +1.0	YEARS OLDER +1.5	YEARS OLDER +2.0	YEARS OLDER +2.5	YEARS OLDER +3.0	TALLY
Average sleep time per day					Women, 6.5 to 7.4 hr	Men, 7.5 to 8.4 hr	Women, 7.5 to 8.4 hr	Men, 6.5 to 7.4 hr		Less than 6.5 hr	More than 8.4 hr			
Total physical activity performed for *at least the last three years* (give yourself most positive category)				More than 90 min of any exercise (ex. walking) per day, for more than 3 yr	More than 50 min of any physical activity, per day, for more than 3 yr	More than 20 min of any physical activity, per day, for more than 3 yr	More than 10 min of any physical activity, per day, for more than 3 yr	More than 5 min of any physical activity, per day, for more than 3 yr	More than 5 min of any physical activity, per day, for less than 3 yr	None				
Amount of stamina exercise (heart rate over 70% of maximal)****					More than 60 min/wk	40 to 60 min/wk	20 to 40 min/wk	10 to 20 min/wk	Less than 10 min/wk					
Amount of strength-building exercise (must exercise at least 6 of 14 major muscle groups)*****					More than 30 min/wk	20 to 30 min/wk	10 to 20 min/wk	5 to 10 min/wk	Less than 5 min/wk					
Resting heart rate					Lower than 75 beats/min; do less than 30 min of stamina exercise/wk; do not have heart disease		Lower than 75 beats/min; do more than 30 min of stamina exercise/wk; do not have heart disease	76 to 91 beats/min; do less than 30 min of stamina exercise/wk; do not have heart disease	76 to 83 beats/min; and do more than 30 min of stamina exercise/wk	83 to 91 beats/min and do more than 30 min of stamina exercise/wk, OR higher than 91 beats/min and do less than 30 min of stamina exercise/wk	Higher than 91 beats/min; do more than 30 min stamina exercise/wk			

HEALTH FACTOR	YEARS YOUNGER -3.0	YEARS YOUNGER -2.5	YEARS YOUNGER -2.0	YEARS YOUNGER -1.5	YEARS YOUNGER -1.0	YEARS YOUNGER -0.5	NO CHANGE	YEARS OLDER +0.5	YEARS OLDER +1.0	YEARS OLDER +1.5	YEARS OLDER +2.0	YEARS OLDER +2.5	YEARS OLDER +3.0	TALLY
Vehicle driven most often						Large car	Midsize car	Small car		Motorcycle				
Wearing of seat belts and presence of air bags, in last 10 trips in a car					Seat belts were worn 10 of 10 times, AND car had air bags 10 of 10 times		Seat belts were worn 8 or 9 of 10 times, OR car had air bags at least 9 of 10 times		Seat belts worn fewer than 7 of 10 times and car had airbags 10 of 10 times; OR seat belts were worn 7 or 8 of 10 times and car had air bags fewer than 6 of 10 times					
Presence of side air bags, in last 10 trips in a car						Car had side air bags 10 of 10 times	Car had side air bags at least 6 of 10 times	Car had side air bags fewer than 6 of 10 times						
Riding on a motorcycle within the last month							No	Sometimes						
Use of helmet when on motorcycle or bicycle							Always	More than 50% of the time	Some-times (between 25% and 50% of the time)		Never, or less than 25% of the time			

HEALTH FACTOR	YEARS YOUNGER -3.0	YEARS YOUNGER -2.5	YEARS YOUNGER -2.0	YEARS YOUNGER -1.5	YEARS YOUNGER -1.0	YEARS YOUNGER -0.5	NO CHANGE	YEARS OLDER +0.5	YEARS OLDER +1.0	YEARS OLDER +1.5	YEARS OLDER +2.0	YEARS OLDER +2.5	YEARS OLDER +3.0	TALLY
Miles driven per year							Less than 30,000	More than 30,000						
Usual speed driven							Less than 5 mph over speed limit	5 to 14 mph over speed limit		More than 14 mph over speed limit				
Use of cellular phone while driving							Fewer than two calls a day	More than four calls a day						
Driving after drinking alcohol							Never	Less than once a month			More than once a month	More than twice a month		
Alcohol consumption on average day (one drink is 5 oz wine, 12 oz beer, or 1.5 oz spirits)					Men over calendar age 35: 1 to 2 drinks a day	Men over calendar age 35 and women over age 40: 1/2 to 1 drink a day	Men over calendar age 35: none to 1/2 drink OR more than 2 but less than 3 drinks a day; women over 40: none to 1/2 OR more than 1 but less than 3 drinks a day		Men under calendar age 35: none to 1/2 drink OR more than 2 but less than 3 drinks a day; women under age 40: none to 1/2 OR more than 1 but less than 3 drinks a day	More than 3 drinks a day				

HEALTH FACTOR	YEARS YOUNGER -3.0	YEARS YOUNGER -2.5	YEARS YOUNGER -2.0	YEARS YOUNGER -1.5	YEARS YOUNGER -1.0	YEARS YOUNGER -0.5	NO CHANGE	YEARS OLDER +0.5	YEARS OLDER +1.0	YEARS OLDER +1.5	YEARS OLDER +2.0	YEARS OLDER +2.5	YEARS OLDER +3.0	TALLY
Highest alcohol consumption in one day within the last year							3 drinks or less	4 drinks or less	5 drinks or less	More than 5 drinks				
Educational level of spouse						Higher than 12th grade		12th grade or lower						
Total cholesterol level					Under calendar age 70: lower, than 130 mg/dl, if no chronic disease	Calendar age 70 or older: lower, than 130 mg/dl	Under calendar age 70, 131 to 160 mg/dl; OR age 70 or older 131 to 240 mg/dl	Calendar age 70 or older: 241 to 280 mg/dl	Under calendar age 70: 161 to 240 mg/dl	Over calendar age 70: higher than 280 mg/dl	Under calendar age 70: 241 to 280 mg/dl		Under calendar age 70: higher than 280 mg/dl	
HDL (healthy) cholesterol					Men or women calendar age 50 or over: higher than 55 mg/dl	Women under calendar age 50: higher than 55 mg/dl	Either gender, any age: 45 to 54 mg/dl	Women under calendar age 50: 40 to 44 mg/dl	Men or women calendar age 50 or older: 40 to 44 mg/dl	Women under calendar age 50: 30 to 39 mg/dl	Men or women calendar age 50 or older: 30 to 39 mg/dl	Women under calendar age 50: lower than 30	Men or women over calendar age 50: lower than 30 mg/dl	
Fasting triglyceride levels (milligrams/deciliter)						Lower than 89.3	89.3 to 208.8	Higher than 208.8						
hs C-reactive protein******					Low					Elevated			Very elevated	
Diet:														
Do you own and use as your main set of dishes plates that are 9 inches in diameter?					Yes		No							

HEALTH FACTOR	YEARS YOUNGER -3.0	YEARS YOUNGER -2.5	YEARS YOUNGER -2.0	YEARS YOUNGER -1.5	YEARS YOUNGER -1.0	YEARS YOUNGER -0.5	NO CHANGE	YEARS OLDER +0.5	YEARS OLDER +1.0	YEARS OLDER +1.5	YEARS OLDER +2.0	YEARS OLDER +2.5	YEARS OLDER +3.0	TALLY
Do you enjoy healthy fat first in each meal?					Yes			No						
Do you eat fiber early in the day?						Yes		No						
Do you avoid simple sugars?			Yes, almost always or always			Most of the time	Sometimes			Never				
Do you take charge of your food every time you eat out?					Yes, always	Most of the time	No							
Have you increased the IQ of your kitchen? *******	By 31 or more IQ points		By 15 to 30 IQ points		By 5 to 14 IQ points		No							
Nuts eaten per week	5 ounces or more		3 to 4 ounces		1 to 2.9 ounces			Some, but less than 1 ounce		None				
Choice of chocolate (1 oz per day)					Always cocoa butter-based		Usually cocoa butter-based		Usually milk fat- or trans fat-based	Always milk fat- or trans fat-based				
Percentage of fat in diet						20% to 30%	31% to 40%, OR less than 20%		More than 40%					
Amount of saturated and trans fat in diet	Less than 20 gm a day									20 to 40 gm a day	41 to 60 gm a day		More than 60 gm a day	
Percentage of polyunsaturated fat in diet					More than 5.85%		4.26% to 5.85%		Less than 4.25%					
Fruits (servings/day)					4 or more				None					

HEALTH FACTOR	YEARS YOUNGER -3.0	YEARS YOUNGER -2.5	YEARS YOUNGER -2.0	YEARS YOUNGER -1.5	YEARS YOUNGER -1.0	YEARS YOUNGER -0.5	NO CHANGE	YEARS OLDER +0.5	YEARS OLDER +1.0	YEARS OLDER +1.5	YEARS OLDER +2.0	YEARS OLDER +2.5	YEARS OLDER +3.0	TALLY
Vegetables (servings/day)					5 or more				None					
Flavonoids (milligrams/day) (see chart 8.2)					High amount: more than 30 mg/day	Moderate amount: 19 to 29.9 mg/day			Low amount: less than 19 mg/day					
Diversity of diet: How many different food groups does your daily diet usually contain? Food groups = milk and milk products and milk substitutes such as soy or rice milk; protein—meat, fish, poultry, or plant protein; fruits; grains; and vegetables.							More than two varieties, on average		Two or fewer varieties, on average					
Do you choose whole grains rather than processed grains?				Women: almost always or always	Men: almost always or always		Sometimes	Never						
Do you wash your hands and your food frequently?			Yes, almost always or always		Most of the time		Sometimes		Never					
Do you use RealAge Cooking Techniques?*******			Yes, almost always or always		Most of the time		Sometimes			Never				
Is there variety in where you shop for food?					Yes			A little			No			
Fiber in diet (grams/day)				Over 21.1	15.2 to 21.1		9.2 to 15.1		3.2 to 9.1		Less than 3.2			

HEALTH FACTOR	YEARS YOUNGER -3.0	YEARS YOUNGER -2.5	YEARS YOUNGER -2.0	YEARS YOUNGER -1.5	YEARS YOUNGER -1.0	YEARS YOUNGER -0.5	NO CHANGE	YEARS OLDER +0.5	YEARS OLDER +1.0	YEARS OLDER +1.5	YEARS OLDER +2.0	YEARS OLDER +2.5	YEARS OLDER +3.0	TALLY
Nutrients in Diet or Taken as Supplements:														
Vitamin C (amount in food and supplements) if not taking a statin drug like Lipitor, Zocor, or Crestor					Men over calendar age 40 and women over age 50: 1,000 to 2000 mg/day*	Men calendar age 40 and under, and women age 50 and under: 1,000 to 2000 mg/day	160 to 1,000 mg/day or more than 2000 mg/day in supplements	Less than 160 mg/day						
Vitamin C (amount in supplements) if taking a statin like Lipitor, Zocor, or Crestor						160 to 200 mg/day as supplements		Less than 160 mg/day as food and supplements	More than 200 mg/day as supplements*					
Vitamin E (amount per day in food and supplements) if not taking a statin drug like Lipitor, Zocor, or Crestor						Women over calendar age 50 and men over age 40: more than 400 IU/day as a supplement	Women under calendar age 50 and men under age 40: more than 400 IU/day as a supplement	No supplement taken every day						
Vitamin E (amount per day in supplements) if taking a statin like Lipitor, Zocor, or Crestor						60 to 100 IU/day as a supplement	No supplement of vitamin E taken every day		More than 100 IU per day taken as a supplement					

HEALTH FACTOR	YEARS YOUNGER -3.0	YEARS YOUNGER -2.5	YEARS YOUNGER -2.0	YEARS YOUNGER -1.5	YEARS YOUNGER -1.0	YEARS YOUNGER -0.5	NO CHANGE	YEARS OLDER +0.5	YEARS OLDER +1.0	YEARS OLDER +1.5	YEARS OLDER +2.0	YEARS OLDER +2.5	YEARS OLDER +3.0	TALLY
Vitamin D (amount in food and supplements)					400 to 2,000 IU or 10 min of sun a day			Less than 400 IU and less than 5 min of sun a day						
Folate or folic acid, a B vitamin (amount in food and supplements)		More than 700 µg/day			401 to 700 µg/day		224 to 400 µg/day			Less than 224 µg/day				
Vitamin B₆ (amount in food and supplements)						More than 6 mg/day	1.5 to 6 mg/day	Less than 1 mg/day						
Fish, excluding shellfish (servings per week)			More than 2 servings			Some fish eaten, but less than 2 servings				None				
Percentage of food prepared without fat or sauces containing a lot of fat, or food that is not fried							No known RealAge effects other than those for saturated fat or fat in diet							
Coffee (4-ounce cups per day)						6 cups or more	1 to 5 cups	None						
Brewed tea (4-ounce cups per day)				6 or more	3 to 5	1 to 3		None						
Iron (amount in supplements)								Any amount of iron as a supplement if you are not iron-deficient						

HEALTH FACTOR	YEARS YOUNGER -3.0	YEARS YOUNGER -2.5	YEARS YOUNGER -2.0	YEARS YOUNGER -1.5	YEARS YOUNGER -1.0	YEARS YOUNGER -0.5	NO CHANGE	YEARS OLDER +0.5	YEARS OLDER +1.0	YEARS OLDER +1.5	YEARS OLDER +2.0	YEARS OLDER +2.5	YEARS OLDER +3.0	TALLY
Vitamin A (amount in supplements)								More than 2,500 IU/day	More than 10,000 IU/day	More than 25,000 IU/day	More than 4,000 IU/day if a smoker or user of tobacco products			
Calcium (amount in food and supplements)				More than 1,200 mg/day		800 to 1,200 mg/day	500 to 800 mg/day		Less than 500 mg/day					
Magnesium (amount in food and supplements)						More than 400 mg/day	300 to 400 mg/day	200 to 300 mg/day	Less than 200 mg/day					
Vitamin B₁₂ (amount in food and supplements)						25 micrograms (µg) or more a day as a supplement		If you do not eat meat or get less than 18 µg/wk as a supplement, OR, 175 µg/wk if you have gastritis or are over age 64						
Multivitamins if without iron and with less than 2500 IU of vitamin A					3 or more a week if you do not eat a diverse diet		1 to 2 a week if you do not eat a diverse diet	None						

HEALTH FACTOR	YEARS YOUNGER -3.0	YEARS YOUNGER -2.5	YEARS YOUNGER -2.0	YEARS YOUNGER -1.5	YEARS YOUNGER -1.0	YEARS YOUNGER -0.5	NO CHANGE	YEARS OLDER +0.5	YEARS OLDER +1.0	YEARS OLDER +1.5	YEARS OLDER +2.0	YEARS OLDER +2.5	YEARS OLDER +3.0	TALLY
Selenium (amount in food and supplements)					176 to 450 µg per day	150 to 175 µg per day			Less than 150 µg per day					
Eating of meat					Never, or less than once a week		Once a week	More than once a week						
Potassium in diet					More than 3000 mg/day			2400 to 3000 mg/day	Less than 2400 mg/day					
Servings of cooked tomatoes (ex: tomato sauce, pizza, spaghetti with marinara sauce) eaten per week			Men, more than 10 servings/ wk		Men, 7 to 10 servings/ per wk; women, more than 10 servings per week	Women, 7 to 10 servings/ wk	2 to 6 servings per week	Women, fewer than 2 servings/ wk	Men, fewer than 2 servings/ wk					
Green tea consumption							No known RealAge effect separate from tea in general; men, may retard aging from prostate cancer							

HEALTH FACTOR	YEARS YOUNGER -3.0	YEARS YOUNGER -2.5	YEARS YOUNGER -2.0	YEARS YOUNGER -1.5	YEARS YOUNGER -1.0	YEARS YOUNGER -0.5	NO CHANGE	YEARS OLDER +0.5	YEARS OLDER +1.0	YEARS OLDER +1.5	YEARS OLDER +2.0	YEARS OLDER +2.5	YEARS OLDER +3.0	TALLY
Weight:														
Body mass index (see Table 8.1)						19.1 to 26.9 kg/m²	In the absence of acute or chronic disease, 19 kg/m² or lower				27 to 31.9 kg/m²		32 kg/m² or higher	
Changes in weight (women)							Weight changes of no more than 5% in any 5-year period		Weight changes of 5% to 10% in any 5-year period		Weight changes of more than 10% in any 5-year period			
Sleep apnea (see Chapters 9 and 12)						None			Treated			Untreated		
Weight gain (since age 18)							Gain of less than 20 lb		Gain of 20 to 40 lb			Gain of more than 40 lb		
DISEASE TRANSITIONS:														
Diabetes and control of blood sugar							None	Type II (adult onset), tight control	Type II (adult onset), average control	Type II (adult onset), poor control	Type I (juvenile onset), tight control		Type I (juvenile onset), average or poor control	

Cardiac Disease:

HEALTH FACTOR	YEARS YOUNGER -3.0	YEARS YOUNGER -2.5	YEARS YOUNGER -2.0	YEARS YOUNGER -1.5	YEARS YOUNGER -1.0	YEARS YOUNGER -0.5	NO CHANGE	YEARS OLDER +0.5	YEARS OLDER +1.0	YEARS OLDER +1.5	YEARS OLDER +2.0	YEARS OLDER +2.5	YEARS OLDER +3.0	TALLY
Coronary artery disease (CAD), but no heart attack yet (as diagnosed by symptoms or scan tests)							None			Has CAD involving 1 vessel, and on active rehab program	Has CAD involving 1 vessel, and not on active rehab program	Has CAD involving 2 or 3 vessels, and on active rehab program	Has CAD involving 2 or 3 vessels, and not on active rehab program	
Coronary artery bypass graft surgery (CABG)							None			Has had CABG involving 1 vessel			Has had CABG involving 2 or more vessels	
Angioplasty (PTCA, balloon dilation of cardiac vessels)							None			PTCA involving 1 vessel	PTCA involving 2 (or unknown no. of) vessels		PTCA involving 3 or more vessels	
Heart attacks							None					Had heart attack involving inferior or posterior part of heart	Had heart attack involving anterior part of heart	
Need for pacemaker							None					Yes, required		
Stroke							None			Ischemic stroke (inadequate blood flow to brain)			Hemorrhagic stroke (bleeding into brain)	

HEALTH FACTOR	YEARS YOUNGER -3.0	YEARS YOUNGER -2.5	YEARS YOUNGER -2.0	YEARS YOUNGER -1.5	YEARS YOUNGER -1.0	YEARS YOUNGER -0.5	NO CHANGE	YEARS OLDER +0.5	YEARS OLDER +1.0	YEARS OLDER +1.5	YEARS OLDER +2.0	YEARS OLDER +2.5	YEARS OLDER +3.0	TALLY
Statin with or without surgery if over age 40			If you have other risks factors for arterial aging and are over age 40		If you need surgery, are over 60, and receive a statin for the 2-week period surrounding surgery		None							
Beta-blocker with surgery if over age 60					If you need surgery and receive a beta-blocker for the 2-week period surrounding surgery		If you do not need surgery OR have calendar age of less than 60							
Pulmonary or lung disease (answer these two topics if you had asthma): Forced expiratory volume as a percent of normal value							Unknown, or higher than 90% of predicted	75% to 90% of predicted		65% to 74% of predicted		Lower than 65% of predicted		
Asthma within 3 yr							None, or rarely and FEV1 100% of predicted or higher	FEV1 80% to 99% of predicted		FEV1 70% to 79% of predicted		FEV1 Lower than 70%		

HEALTH FACTOR	YEARS YOUNGER −3.0	YEARS YOUNGER −2.5	YEARS YOUNGER −2.0	YEARS YOUNGER −1.5	YEARS YOUNGER −1.0	YEARS YOUNGER −0.5	NO CHANGE	YEARS OLDER +0.5	YEARS OLDER +1.0	YEARS OLDER +1.5	YEARS OLDER +2.0	YEARS OLDER +2.5	YEARS OLDER +3.0	TALLY
Mental Disorders:														
Depression (select highest number that pertains)							None	Yes, in past			Yes, a little and not severe		Yes, often or severe	
Panic disorders							None	Present but controlled			Uncontrolled			
Do you react to stress with anger?					Never			Sometimes				Always or almost always		
Suicide attempts							None				Yes, but not within last 5 yr		Yes, and within last 5 yr	
Musculoskeletal Disorders:														
Low back pain							No Real-Age effect proven by itself							
Osteoarthritis						Absent		Present						
Osteoporosis						Absent		Present						
Tests for kidney function							None			Creatinine 1.5 to 1.69 mg/dl	Creatinine 1.70 to 1.99 mg/dl		Creatinine higher than 2 mg/dl	
Pills & tablets of all sizes and kinds taken a day, with or without a prescription; do not include vitamins						0 to 4	5 to 7	More than 7						

HEALTH FACTOR	YEARS YOUNGER -3.0	YEARS YOUNGER -2.5	YEARS YOUNGER -2.0	YEARS YOUNGER -1.5	YEARS YOUNGER -1.0	YEARS YOUNGER -0.5	NO CHANGE	YEARS OLDER +0.5	YEARS OLDER +1.0	YEARS OLDER +1.5	YEARS OLDER +2.0	YEARS OLDER +2.5	YEARS OLDER +3.0	TALLY
Adherence to instructions regarding taking of medications							Perfect or near perfect adherence to instructions	Not perfect nor near perfect adherence to instructions						
Dental disease			None					Gingivitis only					Periodontitis	
Do you see a dental professional every 6 months or whenever he/she suggests you do?				Yes						No				
Air Pollution (use *one* of the next two items): Level of sulfate in the atmosphere (mg/m³) at usual residence						Less than 5 mg/m³	5 to 14.9 mg/m³	15 mg/m³ or more						
or Level (in mg/m³) of fine particulates (smaller than 2.5 μm in diameter) in atmosphere at usual residence						Less than 10 mg/m³	10 to 24.4 mg/m³	More than 24.4 mg/m³						
Level of radon in atmosphere at usual residence						Low or undetectable	Around acceptable EPA level		Above EPA acceptable level					
Sun exposure							Less than 20 min/day, no blisters before age 20	More than 20 min/per day and/or blisters before age 20						

HEALTH FACTOR	YEARS YOUNGER -3.0	YEARS YOUNGER -2.5	YEARS YOUNGER -2.0	YEARS YOUNGER -1.5	YEARS YOUNGER -1.0	YEARS YOUNGER -0.5	NO CHANGE	YEARS OLDER +0.5	YEARS OLDER +1.0	YEARS OLDER +1.5	YEARS OLDER +2.0	YEARS OLDER +2.5	YEARS OLDER +3.0	TALLY
Presence of firearms in home							Women: no history of family violence				Women: in an abusive relation-ship			
Presence of smoke detectors in home							If no one smokes in the home			If device is not installed for each floor and tested, and smoking occurs in the home				
Presence of carbon monoxide detectors in home							If no one smokes in the home	If device is not installed for each floor and tested, and smoking occurs in the home						
Heredity and Other Factors:														
Use of hormone replacement therapy (HRT) for postmenopausal women with no history of breast cancer and no 1st-degree relative who had breast cancer before age 50							None, or if aspirin is used every day and HRT is used for less than 20 years	If aspirin is not used prior to initiating HRT, and HRT used for less than 20 years	If HRT is used for more than 20 years					
HRT for Men (testosterone, HGH, etc.)						Testos-terone use if shaving	None							

HEALTH FACTOR	YEARS YOUNGER -3.0	YEARS YOUNGER -2.5	YEARS YOUNGER -2.0	YEARS YOUNGER -1.5	YEARS YOUNGER -1.0	YEARS YOUNGER -0.5	NO CHANGE	YEARS OLDER +0.5	YEARS OLDER +1.0	YEARS OLDER +1.5	YEARS OLDER +2.0	YEARS OLDER +2.5	YEARS OLDER +3.0	TALLY
						frequency is less than once per day								
Age of parents at time of death		Both lived past age 85		Both lived past age 75	Only mother lived past age 75	Only father lived past age 75							Neither lived past age 75	
Age of grandparents at time of death					All four lived past age 75	Three lived past age 75	One or two lived past age 75			None lived past age 75				
Divorce of parents						Not divorced prior to your 21st birthday			Separated but not divorced prior to your 21st birthday				Divorced prior to your 21st birthday	
Parental / Immediate Family (Brothers, Sisters, Parents, Grandparents, Children):														
Colon cancer							If one or fewer 1st-degree relative had prior to age 40, if an aspirin per day is taken, or if colon-oscopy is performed regularly.			Not getting yearly colon-oscopy, and two or more 1st-degree relatives had prior to age 40				

HEALTH FACTOR	YEARS YOUNGER -3.0	YEARS YOUNGER -2.5	YEARS YOUNGER -2.0	YEARS YOUNGER -1.5	YEARS YOUNGER -1.0	YEARS YOUNGER -0.5	NO CHANGE	YEARS OLDER +0.5	YEARS OLDER +1.0	YEARS OLDER +1.5	YEARS OLDER +2.0	YEARS OLDER +2.5	YEARS OLDER +3.0	TALLY
History of heart disease before age 50							If one or fewer 1st-degree relatives had prior to age 50						Two or more 1st-degree relatives had heart disease before age 50	
Stress, Social Connections, Relaxation Therapy:														
Major disruptive life events in the last 12 mos.							None		1		2		3	
Social groups, friends, relatives seen more than once a month*******				6	3, 4, or 5	2	1				None			
Do you practice relaxation or other stress-relieving therapy?					Yes, regularly	Occasionally		Never						
Use of cell or other phone to call friends regularly			Yes							No				
Do you (or others) think you have a sense of humor, and do you often try to see the funny side of events?			Yes					No						
Do you have a positive outlook on life?			Optimist				Average				Pessimist			
Do you let little tasks accumulate (ex: do you delay in fixing the toilet seat; see Chapter 7)?					No						Yes			

HEALTH FACTOR	YEARS YOUNGER -3.0	YEARS YOUNGER -2.5	YEARS YOUNGER -2.0	YEARS YOUNGER -1.5	YEARS YOUNGER -1.0	YEARS YOUNGER -0.5	NO CHANGE	YEARS OLDER +0.5	YEARS OLDER +1.0	YEARS OLDER +1.5	YEARS OLDER +2.0	YEARS OLDER +2.5	YEARS OLDER +3.0	TALLY
Decision latitude in your job	Great; can prioritize and choose own tasks				Some				Very little				None	
Marriage status				Happily married man		Happily married woman	Single woman or widowed man		Divorced man or widowed woman		Divorced woman		Single man	
Highest educational level completed						Grade 16 (college grad) or higher	Grades 12 through 15	Grade 5 through 11	Grade 4 or lower					
Current intellectual activity	Keep mind active by learning new things every week in formal or informal ways				Active in book group or other learning group once every three weeks or less often			NBC or Fox TV is most stimulating thing I do			This chart is the only intellectually stimulating thing I have done in two months			
Do you play intellectual games and keep your mind active?				Yes					No					
Yearly income					Higher than $150,000	$60,001 to $150,000	$30,001 to $60,000	$15,000 to $30,000	Less than $15,000					

HEALTH FACTOR	YEARS YOUNGER -3.0	YEARS YOUNGER -2.5	YEARS YOUNGER -2.0	YEARS YOUNGER -1.5	YEARS YOUNGER -1.0	YEARS YOUNGER -0.5	NO CHANGE	YEARS OLDER +0.5	YEARS OLDER +1.0	YEARS OLDER +1.5	YEARS OLDER +2.0	YEARS OLDER +2.5	YEARS OLDER +3.0	TALLY
Sexual Practices:														
Mutually monogamous relationship of more than 10 years, and partner is of opposite sex							Yes				No			
Orgasms (per year)	Men, 300 or more		Men, 200 to 300	Women, satisfied with quantity and happy with quality	Men, 100 to 200	Women, satisfied with quantity or quality	Men, 40 to 100	Women, unsatisfied with quality and/or quantity	Men, 25 to 40		Men, 5 to 25	Men, fewer than 5		
Regular use of condoms (for those not in a mutually monogamous relationship)							Yes		No					
Sex partner uses intravenous drugs, trades sex for drugs or money, is an ex-prisoner, or has a sexually transmitted disease							No				Unknown		Yes	
Use of marijuana							Use one time a week or less	Use more than once a week but less than daily	Use every day	Sometimes use more than three times a day				
Use of Ecstasy of any type							Never			Have used, but not in last 10 years		Have used within last 10 years	Yes, current use	
Use of cocaine, LSD, heroin, or intravenous drugs of any type							Never			Have used, but not in last 10 years		Have used within last 10 years	Yes, current use	

HEALTH FACTOR	YEARS YOUNGER -3.0	YEARS YOUNGER -2.5	YEARS YOUNGER -2.0	YEARS YOUNGER -1.5	YEARS YOUNGER -1.0	YEARS YOUNGER -0.5	NO CHANGE	YEARS OLDER +0.5	YEARS OLDER +1.0	YEARS OLDER +1.5	YEARS OLDER +2.0	YEARS OLDER +2.5	YEARS OLDER +3.0	TALLY
People in household (do not count pets)						4 to 6	3	2 or 7	8	1 (you), or 9 or more				
Pet ownership						Dog	None, or other than a dog							
TOTAL:														

PUT TOTAL IN BOX AND IN SUMMARY CHART NEXT PAGE

* Only do an exercise you usually do. If you have not done any strenuous exercise in a while, first read Chapter 9 and then seek a supervised setting to do your first maximum exercise.

**Your maximum heart rate is 220 minus your calendar age.

***A "pack-year" is one pack of cigarettes a day for one year. NSAIDs, nonsteroidal anti-inflammatory drugs.

****Aerobic exercise that increases your heart rate to at least 70% of the maximal heart rate. The maximal heart rate (in beats per minute) is calculated by subtracting your calendar age from 220.

*****Examples of strength-building exercises are lifting weights, resistance exercises, and treadmill on an incline. Major muscle groups are defined in Chapter 9.

******Since various numbers and standards exist for hs-CRP at this time, please ask your doctor if your number is low, normal, elevated, or very elevated.

*******See Cooking the RealAge® Way or the www.realage.com website for RealAge cooking techniques, and for calculation of your Kitchen IQ and suggestions of how to increase it. Flavonoids are found in onions, tea, celery, and cranberries. Mg/day is milligrams a day. IU is international units. A portion of fish is about the size of a pack of cards, approximately 3 oz. BMI is the ratio of weight to height, expressed in units of kilograms per meter squared. PTCA, percutaneous transluminal coronary angioplasty. FEV 1 is the Forced Expiratory Volume in one second. LSD is lysergic acid diethylamide. Major life events include death of a family member, job change, relocation, divorce, lawsuit, financial insolvency.

********People who offer support through major life events (applicable only when two or more such events have occurred in one year).

Total Tally Summary
from Table

×

Multiplier

=

Net **RealAge** Change:

+

Calendar Age:

=

Your RealAge:

(Add positive Net RealAge Change to or subtract negative from calendar age to compute your RealAge)

Calendar Age	Multiplier
<40	0.1
40 to 50	0.15
50 to 60	0.175
60 to 70	0.2
70 to 80	0.175
80 to 90	0.15
90 to 100	0.1

Get Younger Every Day

Plan and Commit to Be as Young as You Want to Be

I f you are new to the RealAge program, this is your chance to join the Revolution, to take charge of your health. If you have already been following the RealAge program, now is your chance to plan and commit to be even younger by using the new health information I've gathered since publication of *RealAge®: Are You as Young as You Can Be?* The test you just took had many more questions (about twice as many) than the original test, so your RealAge is more accurate. Similarly, you now have numerous new choices based on more up-to-date, accurate scientific information to help you make your RealAge even younger.

Now that you know your RealAge, the next step in your RealAge Makeover is to develop a step-by-step Age-Reduction Plan. If you took the test on the computer, look at the list of suggestions you were given. Or look at what you marked on the chart. You have many options—which would you feel most comfortable trying? Start by picking a few quick fixes to jump-start your Makeover, since you'll be younger almost immediately. But don't go too easy on yourself—we all love a challenge—also pick a few more difficult options, so that you can feel the pride of accomplishment when you reach your goal.

It may be that you already practice good lifestyle choices, like daily 30-minute walks. Perhaps you've never smoked at all. That's great. These factors have helped to keep you young. But what else could you be doing? I'm often surprised by what people are and aren't willing to do for the sake of their health. For example, I thought reducing driving speed would be easy when people learn how much it increased their risk of a disabling accident. Nothing could be farther from the truth. Of the first 5 million people taking the RealAge test on-line, fewer than 1,000—a tiny fraction—said they would change their driving speed!

Some of the changes really are easy, such as taking the right vitamins and avoiding the wrong ones, taking an aspirin a day, wearing a helmet when you go biking, and having 10 tablespoons of tomato sauce a week. They're so simple there's no reason not to adopt them. They save five to eight years of aging with almost no effort. Start with the easy ones, then work your way down the list, adding Age-Reduction behaviors as you see fit. Always check with your physician before initiating or stopping any Age Reduction strategy.

Chart 3.1

Seventy-Eight Things You Can Do to Make Your RealAge Younger

QUICK FIXES

With these RealAge age-busters, you can become 5 to 8 years younger with hardly any effort.

I do   I will   1) Take an aspirin a day.
it: do it:

☐   ☐   ■ Take one 325-milligram (mg) tablet of aspirin a day if you
                    are a man over 35 or a woman over 40. This is not only for
                    arterial health: aspirin decreases your risk of immune aging
                    as well. That means you'll have more energy and less
                    chance of developing breast and rectal, colon, and other di-
                    gestive tract cancers. Before you start, check with your doc-
                    tor to make sure you are aspirin-tolerant.
                    RealAge benefit: 0.9 years younger in 90 days
                                        2.2 years younger in 3 years

I do   I will   2) Take folate daily to reduce artery-aging levels of homo-
it: do it: cysteine and decrease your risk of arterial aging, and of colon
☐   ☐   and breast cancer.

                    ■ Consume 800 micrograms (µg) of folate (folic acid) a day in
                    diet or supplement. (Normally we get only 200 to 300 µg
                    from our diet, so you'll want to get at least 600 µg a day
                    through a supplement. Folate has no known toxicity, so you
                    can take the entire 800 µg in a supplement if you want.)
                    RealAge benefit: 1.2 years younger

I do   I will   3) Take vitamin B_6 daily.
it: do it:

☐   ☐   ■ Consume 6 mg of vitamin B_6 a day in food or supplements.
                    RealAge benefit: 0.4 years younger

I do   I will   4) Consume 25 µg of vitamin B_{12} as a supplement.
it: do it:

☐   ☐   ■ Even though food contains B_{12}, a substance secreted by the
                   stomach—active intrinsic factor—must be present if B_{12}
                   from food is to be absorbed. Unfortunately, production of
                   this factor decreases with age. Crystalline B_{12} in supple-
                   ments does not require this intrinsic factor for absorbtion.
                   Therefore, if you take B_{12} as a supplement, you won't be
                   reliant on the presence of intrinsic factor.
                   RealAge benefit: 0.6 years younger

I do   I will   5) Take calcium to keep your bones young.
it: do it:

☐   ☐   ■ Consume 1,200 mg of calcium daily in food or supplements
                   if you are a woman or 1,000 mg daily if you are a man. Take
                   an additional 400 mg if your calendar age is over 60, and 20
                   mg for each 12 ounces of caffeinated soda and 4 ounces of
                   coffee you drink. However, do not take more than 600 mg
                   of calcium at one time, as the body's ability to absorb cal-
                   cium optimally decreases when the dose is higher than this.
                   RealAge benefit: 0.5 years younger

I do   I will   6) Take vitamin D daily to keep bones young.
it: do it:

☐   ☐   ■ Consume 400 International Units (IU) of vitamin D in
                   food or supplements, (600 IU if your are older than 60) or
                   get 10 minutes of sun a day.
                   RealAge benefit: 1.1 years younger

I do   I will   7) Make sure you get enough magnesium.
it: do it:

☐   ☐   ■ Getting 400 mg or so (one-third of the amount of calcium
                   you take) of magnesium a day from supplements or from a
                   magnesium-rich diet reduces your complications from
                   cardiovascular-related problems by decreasing abnormal
                   heart beats and decreasing nerve dysfunction.
                   RealAge benefit: 0.9 years younger

I do I will   8) Don't take unnecessary vitamins and supplements.
it: do it:

☐   ☐   ■ Take a multivitamin that contains all the vitamins and min-
                    erals you need (especially C, D, E, folate, calcium, and
                    magnesium) but no iron, in the correct daily amount. Un-
                    less you are a woman of child-bearing age, do not take vita-
                    min A as an individual (one-ingredient) supplement, and
                    make sure your multivitamin contains less than 2,500 IU of
                    vitamin A. Do not take iron as a supplement except under
                    the supervision of a doctor.
                    RealAge loss: 1.7 years older for taking unnecessary
                    vitamins or supplements

I do I will   9) Floss and brush daily.
it: do it:

☐   ☐   ■ Gingivitis and periodontal disease cause aging of the im-
                    mune and arterial systems. We do not know exactly why
                    gum disease causes aging, but we do know with certainty
                    that it does. For example, a 55-year-old man free of peri-
                    odontal disease has a RealAge that is 2 years younger than
                    his peer who has gingivitis, and 4 years younger than his
                    peer who has full-blown periodontal disease.
                    RealAge benefit: As much as 6.4 years younger

I do I will   10) See a dental professional every six months, or more often if
it: do it: advised to do so, to have your gums checked and cared for.
☐   ☐

                 ■ Regular professional dental care is also necessary to pre-
                    vent gingivitis and periodontal disease
                    RealAge benefit: As much as 6.4 years younger

I do I will   11) Take vitamins C and E daily for their antioxidant and
it: do it: antiaging power.
☐   ☐

                 ■ Consume food containing vitamin C three times a day.
                    Unless you're taking a statin drug, get more than 1,200 mg
                    a day of vitamin C in diet or supplements; spread them out
                    so that you get at least 400 mg in any 12-hour period. How-
                    ever, if you're taking a statin drug for control of cholesterol,
                    such as simvastatin (Zocor), atorvastatin (Lipitor), or rosu-

vastatin (Crestor), take only 200 mg of vitamin C and 100 IU of vitamin E as a supplement, as these vitamins inhibit the ability of statins to keep your arteries young.
RealAge benefit: Up to 1 year younger

I do it: ☐   I will do it: ☐   12) Take proper safety precautions when driving.

■ Buckle your seat belt every time you ride in a car, and drive within 5 miles per hour of the speed limit. Never use a cell phone while driving. When buying a car, buy one that is midsize or larger and make sure it has front and side air bags. Dismantle the front air bags only if you are under 5 feet 2 inches tall or sit close to the steering wheel.
RealAge benefit: 0.6 to 3.4 years younger, depending on your current age

I do it: ☐   I will do it: ☐   13) Wear a helmet when riding a bike.

■ Wear a helmet every time you ride a bike, and you will be protected from needless head injuries. You can reduce your risk of head injury and related aging by as much as 80 percent.
RealAge benefit: 1 year younger if you ride a bike 5 times a month

I do it: ☐   I will do it: ☐   14) Keep immunizations current.

■ This may not save you many years of aging, but it might, and it's simple to do: keep your immunizations current. By making sure you have an annual flu shot and tetanus, measles, mumps, rubella, hepatitis B, and pneumonia vaccinations, you help prevent illnesses that cause you to age. Also, recent data indicate that the flu shot may prevent inflammation (and aging) of your arteries.
RealAge benefit: 0.3 years younger

I do it: ☐   I will do it: ☐   15) Enjoy coffee if you like it and it likes you.

■ Do you love coffee and caffeinated beverages as much as I do? If so, you're in luck. A cup of joe (prepared with a paper filter) can make you younger. (Granted, of course, that you don't have any of the negative side effects of coffee such as migraine headaches, abnormal heartbeats, or gastrointestinal upset.) Further, studies consistently show that coffee reduces the risk of Parkinson's disease and Alzheimer's. So go ahead and have that espresso or latte. Just be sure to use skim milk, don't add sugar, and take a little extra calcium and B vitamins.

RealAge benefit: 0.3 years younger

I do it: ☐
I will do it: ☐

16) Develop an Age-Reduction Plan.

■ Age-Reduction planning is the quickest and easiest yet most important step for keeping you young. It can make the RealAge of a 75-year-old as much as 29 years younger. Obtaining the first 5 to 8 years of age reduction is relatively easy. Achieving more than that requires some work. But isn't having a RealAge of 46 to 48 at a calendar age of 75 worth some work?

RealAge benefit: As much as 29 years younger

MODERATELY EASY CHANGES

These choices will make you younger fast, and they require only a little more effort than the quick fixes. Some, such as eating tomato or spaghetti sauce, are as easy as the quick fixes but require more thought before you decide to adopt them. These changes can help you be 10 to 12 years younger.

I do it: ☐
I will do it: ☐

17) Don't take hormones or so-called "hormone releasers" just because of advertising come-ons.

■ Previously we thought the most powerful antiaging agent for postmenopausal women was estrogen-based hormone replacement therapy (HRT). Now we are told this isn't the case. However, neither of those positions may be correct. We don't know for sure. Nevertheless, there are a lot of hormone come-ons, for everything from dehydroepiandrosterone (DHEA) for men to human growth hormone (HGH). We don't know yet if any of these has a RealAge benefit. Testosterone does have a benefit for specific populations. Remember, there is a substantial RealAge benefit for avoiding the wrong HRT.

RealAge benefit: 2 years younger for avoiding unnecessary hormone therapy come-ons by age 70

I do
it: ☐

I will
do it: ☐

18) Get enough sun, but not too much.

- Some sun (10 to 20 minutes every day) makes your Real-Age 0.9 years younger by producing active vitamin D. You get extra benefit for avoiding too much sun. Wearing sunscreen when you are in the sun longer than 20 minutes, avoiding tanning salons, and taking precautions to avoid excessive sun exposure help prevent aging.
RealAge benefit: 1.7 years younger

I do
it: ☐

I will
do it: ☐

19) Eat tomato or spaghetti sauce and drink tea.

- Tomatoes, when eaten in conjunction with a bit of oil, provides an immune-strengthening antioxidant that has been shown to reduce prostate cancers and breast cancer. It may be the carotenoid in tomatoes, lycopene—also found in guava, watermelon, and pink grapefruit—that is the beneficial component. Lycopene may also prevent arterial aging. In addition, drinking tea may help prevent prostate cancer.
RealAge benefit: 1.9 years younger for men
0.8 years younger for women

I do
it: ☐

I will
do it: ☐

20) Avoid "passive smoking."

- Don't tolerate working, living, or playing in a smoke-filled environment. An hour of passive smoking causes the same amount of aging as smoking four cigarettes yourself.
RealAge loss: 6.9 years older for those exposed to 4 hours a day or more of passive smoking

I do
it: ☐

I will
do it: ☐

21) Have sex.

- The more and the higher quality orgasms you have a year, the younger you are. The average American has sex 58 times a year. Increasing the number to 116 through mutually monogamous, high quality, and safe sex is associated with a RealAge as much as 1.6 years younger. (More sex is associated with a RealAge as much as 8 years younger, depending on frequency and the individual.) We do not have enough data on masturbation to know if that practice produces a RealAge benefit for those who do not have partners.

RealAge benefit: 1.6 to 8 years younger

I do I will   22) Have safe sex.
it: do it:
☐   ☐

- The major risks for consenting adults who have sex outside mutually monogamous relationships are both psychological and physical. One in five sexually active Americans has a sexually transmitted disease, which can increase the rate of aging. Avoid casual sex with high-risk partners and always use condoms correctly.

  RealAge loss: 5 to 8 years older for unprotected sex

I do I will   23) Drink alcohol in moderation.
it: do it:
☐   ☐

- Women who have one-half to one alcoholic drink a day and men who have one or two drinks a day have a younger RealAge. People who are at risk of alcohol abuse or addiction, or who have a family history of alcohol or drug abuse or addiction should not drink alcohol at all.

  RealAge benefit: 1.9 years younger

I do I will   24) Take all necessary (and *only* necessary) medicines, and
it: do it: take them correctly.
☐   ☐

- Discuss your medication with your doctor and pharmacist, and always disclose all prescriptions, over-the-counter drugs, vitamins, and supplements that you take both regularly and occasionally. Adhering to medication regimens as prescribed by your doctor makes your RealAge 0.9 years younger. Avoiding drug interactions makes your RealAge 0.7 years younger.

  RealAge loss: 1.6 years older for taking medicines
          incorrectly

I do   I will   25) Eat breakfast daily.
it: do it:

☐   ☐   ■ No one is sure why, but eating breakfast makes you
                    younger (see Chapter 11).
                    RealAge benefit: 1.1 years younger

I do   I will   26) Laugh a lot.
it: do it:

☐   ☐   ■ Laughter is a whole-body stress-reducer. It helps open lines
                    of communication with others and reduces anxiety, tension,
                    and stress. Laughter makes your immune system younger.
                    RealAge benefit: 1.7 to 8 years younger

MODERATELY DIFFICULT CHANGES

These Age-Reduction strategies require a little more work and commitment, but once you've made the effort, you'll love watching those needless years fade away.

I do   I will   27) Eat a balanced diet that is low in calories and high in
it: do it: nutrients.
☐   ☐

                 ■ Eating a diverse diet that includes four or five servings of
                    fruit a day, four or five servings of vegetables a day, and only
                    whole grains will help keep you feeling young. Eat fish
                    three times a week and do not eat red meat more than once
                    a week.
                    RealAge benefit: 4 years younger

I do   I will   28) Eat only healthy fat.
it: do it:

☐   ☐   ■ A certain amount of fat is essential to your health. Get 25
                    percent of your calories from healthy fat: mainly mono-
                    unsaturated and polyunsaturated fats, which are found in
                    olive oil, canola oil, avocados, flaxseed, fish, and nuts.
                    RealAge benefit: 3.4 years younger

I do   I will   29) Avoid saturated and trans fats.
it: do it:

☐   ☐   ■ Trans fat, which has been called "the hidden fat" because it
                    wasn't listed on food labels, will be listed on food labels

starting in 2005. If one of the first five ingredients on a label is milk fat, fat from a four-legged animal, saturated fat, or partially hydrogenated vegetable oil, don't buy that product. Saturated and trans fats turn on genes that increase production of a specific protein, and this in turn causes or contributes to inflammation of your arteries. Inflammation of your arteries is one of the major causes of aging to avoid. This increased aging of the arteries and immune system makes you slower today and more likely to experience impotence, wrinkling of the skin, heart disease, stroke, memory loss, serious infections, and cancer.

RealAge benefit: More than 4 years younger

I do it: □
I will do it: □

30) Train your taste buds to love food that makes you younger.

- Love of fat is not a genetically inherited taste. It's a taste we acquire. If you switch from whole milk to skim milk, in about eight weeks the whole milk won't taste very good, and the skim milk will taste great. Similarly, when switching from unhealthy fat to healthy fat it will take about eight weeks for you to retrain your palate. Yes, the first time you have Baked Lay's potato chips, they will taste like cardboard if you're used to full-fat Fritos. However, if you keep eating the baked version, in eight weeks you'll love them, and the full-fat Fritos will taste greasy. Learn how to convert a high-saturated-fat diet like Atkins into a healthy-fat diet.

RealAge benefit: At least 3 years younger

I do it: □
I will do it: □

31) Enjoy healthy fat first in each meal.

- Having fat first in a meal will slow emptying of the stomach. To get this effect, you need to eat about seventy calories of fat, which is approximately a half tablespoon of olive oil, six walnuts, twelve almonds, or twenty peanuts. Having fat first is important because slowing the emptying of your stomach means you'll feel full with less food, and you'll eat less. It also helps keep the amount of sugar in the blood at a lower consistent level, because sugar is absorbed in the intestine, which comes after the stomach. Having fat first also helps the absorption of fat-soluble nutrients such as

lycopene in tomatoes and lutein in leafy vegetables, as well
as the fat-soluble vitamins in nutritional supplements.
RealAge benefit: 1.8 years younger

I do   I will   32) Make your kitchen part of your RealAge Makeover.
it: do it:

□   □   ■ Many kitchens have a bewildering array of implements and
pots and pans that have accumulated over the years but make
little difference to your RealAge. The key to a great kitchen is
to stock only the equipment that helps you cook in a
nutrient-rich, calorie-poor, and fabulously tasty way. Here
are some of the things that will make your kitchen more
RealAge-friendly: a sauce pan with a heavy bottom, two
heavy-bottom baking sheets, a blender with a substantial
motor and an extra blender container, three colanders, a
heavy square or rectangular pan for roasting or baking, a
sauté pan, a cutting board for produce and another for fish
and meats, a food chopper, a food mill, a garlic press, a grater,
a food processor, kitchen shears, and a great cutting knife.
RealAge benefit: Up to 4 years younger

I do   I will   33) Learn a new RealAge cooking technique every month.
it: do it:

□   □   ■ There are only six cooking techniques you need to learn to
make fabulous-tasting RealAge-smart food easily. One of
those is sautéing. When you sauté, you put a few vegetables
in a hot pan with just a little healthy fat, which brings out
the flavor of the vegetables. In contrast, when you pan fry
with lots of fat, you lose the flavor of the vegetables and just
taste the fat. Thus, learning to sauté can help reduce your
RealAge, as would learning to pan roast, grill on a stove top,
or use the microwave to make a great-tasting risotto. (All of
these techniques can be found in *Cooking the RealAge® Way*
and are listed in Chapter 8 in this book.)
RealAge benefit: Up to six years younger

I do   I will   34) Wash your hands and food frequently and well.
it: do it:

□   □   ■ Although serious food-borne illness doesn't occur very often, it can be devastating. More than 40 million Americans

suffer from food poisoning every year, and most of this is just a version of *"turista."* However, several thousand Americans die each year from food-borne illness they didn't even know they had. The easiest way to prevent disease is to wash your hands frequently. Replace your kitchen sponge with inexpensive kitchen towels. After you use each towel, wash it with a solution of sodium hydroxide or bleach. You are less likely to transfer and allow propagation of single germs in the kitchen into disease-causing groups of germs.
RealAge benefit: 0.4 years younger

I do   I will   35) Buy and use 9-inch plates.
it: do it:

☐   ☐

- One of the most important ways to minimize arterial and immune aging is to reduce portion sizes that sap your energy. The key is using 9-inch plates rather than the usual 11- or 13-inch plates. Remember to leave space between each portion and to stop eating when you first feel full.
RealAge benefit: 3.1 years younger

I do   I will   36) Eat five servings of fruit a day.
it: do it:

☐   ☐

- If you think five servings sounds like a lot to eat every day, remember that a serving is the size of a small fist. Add half of a banana to cereal in the morning for one serving, or drink a smoothie to get three of four servings at once. Before you know it, you'll have had your five servings, deliciously. Remember to wash the fruit well but keep the peel. If you peel an apple, a pear, or a tomato, you're tossing most of the fiber and active ingredients. For example, in the tomato, more than 90 percent of the beneficial substances are within 3 millimeters of the skin. Have fruit attractively displayed every day in a bowl in your house; you'll reach for it first.
RealAge benefit: 1.4 years younger

I do   I will   37) Eat four or five servings of delicious vegetables a day.
it: do it:

☐   ☐

- If you're not much for vegetables now, an important part of eating more vegetables is retraining your digestive tract. Slowly increase your intake so your digestive system can adjust. Have veggies that are great tasting and substitute them for other foods.

RealAge benefit: 2 to 5 years younger

I do it: ☐   I will do it: ☐   38) Eat nonfried fish three times a week.

■ Fish oils and fish protein can make you younger. You don't have to worry about the mercury content if you eat a variety of fish (such as salmon, bass, or tilapia) harvested from different sources. It may not be just the fish oil that provides the benefit. A number of studies have shown that fish protein has a separate benefit from the fish oil. Nevertheless, it is fish oil (the omega-3 oils) that seems to have a great benefit in reducing the amount of inflammatory proteins your genes produce.

RealAge benefit: Up to 3 years younger

I do it: ☐   I will do it: ☐   39) Enjoy flavonoids.

■ Only approximately sixteen choices in nutrition have been shown to make a difference in mortality rates; consumption of flavonoids is one. Flavonoids decrease the rate of arterial and immune aging. These substances are similar to vitamins, but unlike vitamins are not essential for life. Thirty-one milligrams a day is the ideal. The richest sources of flavonoids (given as approximations) are onions (4 mg in one small onion), green tea, cranberries (8 mg per cup or per 8 ounces) broccoli (4.2 mg per cup), celery, tomatoes (2.6 mg for one medium tomato), apples (4.2 mg for one medium apple), garlic, strawberries (4.2 mg for one cup), oats (3 mg for one cup), one 5-ounce glass of red wine, or a 5-ounce glass of grape juice (3 mg).

RealAge benefit: 3.2 years younger for getting 31 mg of flavonoids a day

I do it: ☐   I will do it: ☐   40) Choose whole grains rather than processed grains.

■ Whole grains have also been shown to make a difference in aging of the arteries and immune system. Instead of enriched flour, processed flour, or semolina, choose breads and pastas made from whole-grain wheat. It may take a little retraining of your cooking processes and palate, but it's worth the benefit.

RealAge benefit: 1.2 years younger for men
2.3 years younger for women

I do   I will
it: do it:
☐   ☐

41) Eat fiber early in the day.

■ Fiber helps prevent high peaks in glucose levels that accelerate arterial aging. Insoluble fiber is found in many foods: grapefruit, oranges, grapes, raisins, dried fruit, sweet potatoes, peas, and zucchini, but especially in whole-wheat bread. Soluble fiber is the stuff found in cereal. Any breakfast fiber, soluble or insoluble, slows your stomach from emptying, so you don't get as hungry later in the day.
RealAge benefit: 0.6 years younger

I do   I will
it: do it:
☐   ☐

42) Take charge every time you eat out.

■ When you eat out, why pay for something that ages you? Learn to ask questions of your servers, and learn to ask for healthy, great-tasting choices: "Could you ask the chef to substitute marinara sauce for the Alfredo sauce?"
RealAge benefit: 2 to 14 years younger, depending on how frequently you eat out

I do   I will
it: do it:
☐   ☐

43) Learn to read labels and avoid foods having saturated and trans fats, simple sugars, or processed grain as one of the first five ingredients.

■ One of the keys to making yourself radically younger is to choose foods that don't contain too much of these unhealthy ingredients. It's as easy as reading the label. For each food you choose, read the label to determine

1) the portion size,
2) the calorie content,
3) the fat content,

4) the simple sugar content, and

5) the processed grain content.

RealAge benefit: 3.6 years younger

I do
it:
□

I will
do it:
□

44) Make healthy substitutions when cooking.

■ Use substitutions to make a big difference in your rate of aging. You can do this and still have great tasting food. For baked goods, try this switch for four weeks: If a recipe calls for 3 tablespoons of butter, try 2 tablespoons of butter and 1 tablespoon of an oil substitute (drained applesauce or prune puree). For the next four weeks, try 1 tablespoon of butter and 2 tablespoons of the oil substitute. In eight weeks you and your family will love the taste, and your RealAge will be 3 to 12 years younger.

RealAge benefit: 3 to 12 years younger

I do
it:
□

I will
do it:
□

45) Get a good night's sleep on a regular basis.

■ Sleeping regular hours can help you stay young. That means 7 hours a night for women and 8 hours a night for men.

RealAge benefit: 3 years younger

I do
it:
□

I will
do it:
□

46) Get your potassium.

■ Another of the 16 factors in nutrition consistently shown to decrease the rate of aging of the arteries is getting enough potassium in the diet. You need at least 3,000 mg a day. What foods contain potassium? Half a cup of tomato paste has 1,340 mg. Dried peaches, baked potatoes, sole, salmon, and sardines have 600 to 800 mg per serving. Watermelon, dried apricots, steamed scallops, and bananas have 400 to 600 mg per serving. Chestnuts, milk, and artichokes have 300 to 400 mg per serving. So it shouldn't be that hard to get your potassium.

RealAge benefit: 2.3 years younger

I do
it:
□

I will
do it:
□

47) Become a lifelong learner.

▪ People with higher levels of education and those who continue to be involved in activities that stimulate the mind undergo less mental aging. The person who graduates from college and continues to learn in a formal educational setting or in informal ways has a RealAge that is 2.5 years younger than that of the high school dropout.
RealAge benefit: 2.5 years younger

I do
it:
□

I will
do it:
□

48) Learn a new game that requires intelligence.

▪ Keeping your mind active is key, and we are never too old to learn new games. Whether it's a card game, a new move in chess, an Internet game, or a crossword puzzle, each one helps keep arterial aging, immune aging, and even accidents at bay.
RealAge benefit: 1.3 years younger

I do
it:
□

I will
do it:
□

49) Identify your genetic risks and use Age-Reduction strategies to mitigate them.

▪ If, for example, cardiovascular disease runs in your family, take extra precautions to prevent arterial aging. Your RealAge will be 4 years younger if both your parents (or grandparents, if your parents aren't that old yet) lived past the age of 75. If no first-degree relative (parent, brother, sister) had breast, colon, or ovarian cancer diagnosed early, you are an additional 0.2 to 11 years younger than if a first-degree relative had those diagnoses.
RealAge benefit: 2 years younger if your dad lived past 75;
4 years younger if both parents lived past 75;
and 1 additional year younger for every 5 years longer either parent lived past 80.

MORE DIFFICULT CHANGES

These Age-Reduction steps require commitment and work, but the payoff is huge in "years younger."

I do   I will   50) Lower your bad (LDL) cholesterol.
it: do it:

□   □   ■ Try to keep your total cholesterol level below 200 mg/dl
                        (milligrams of cholesterol per deciliter of blood), and aim
                        to have your LDL (remember "lousy") cholesterol level at
                        100 mg/dl or below.
                        RealAge benefit: 3.3 years younger for men
                                             0.6 years younger for women

I do   I will   51) Raise your good (HDL) cholesterol.
it: do it:

□   □   ■ Try to keep your HDL (remember "healthy") cholesterol
                        at 60 mg/dl or above, but in no case let it go below 45
                        mg/dl. A little alcohol, more exercise, healthy fats, or even
                        medication may be necessary, but the RealAge benefit is
                        substantial.
                        RealAge benefit: 2.5 years younger for men
                                             4.7 years younger for women

I do   I will   52) Control your triglycerides.
it: do it:

□   □   ■ Triglycerides are substances produced from simple sugars.
                        These substances turn into plaque in your arteries. Learn
                        how to keep your triglyceride levels below 100 mg/dl by
                        avoiding simple carbohydrates and by keeping portion
                        sizes reasonable.
                        RealAge benefit: 1.3 years younger

I do   I will   53) Keep your high-sensitivity C-reactive protein level in the
it: do it: normal range.

□   □   ■ C-reactive protein, a substance released by the body in re-
                        sponse to injury, is a marker of inflammation in the arteries.
                        Keep your high-sensitivity C-reactive protein (hs-CRP)
                        level in the normal range by avoiding chronic infections

and by getting treatment for chronic infections if you do get them. Chronic infections arise from conditions such as gum or tooth disease. Preventing or treating many other low-grade chronic infections, such as urinary tract infections or prostatitis, is a key to keeping your immune system and arteries younger. I explain methods for controlling your hs-CRP in Chapters 4 and 5.
RealAge benefit: 4 years younger

I do   I will   54) Exercise regularly, expending at least 3,500 kilocalories of
it: do it: energy a week.
☐   ☐

- Walking 110 minutes a day or doing the equivalent of other activities such as gardening, or doing more vigorous exercise for a shorter time, can bring your level of physical activity up to the optimal Age-Reduction range. But any physical activity done with regularity has benefit: walking just half an hour a day gives you half of the "years younger" that optimal amounts of general physical activity provides.
  RealAge benefit: 3.4 years younger

I do   I will   55) Make yourself strong.
it: do it:
☐   ☐

- Do strength-building exercises, such as weight lifting, three times a week for at least 10 minutes each time. These exercises are particularly important for women because they help maintain bone density.
  RealAge benefit: 1.7 years younger

I do   I will   56) Build stamina.
it: do it:
☐   ☐

- Do stamina-building exercises that boost your heart rate and aerobic intake for at least 20 minutes, three times a week. You should exercise vigorously enough to raise your heart rate to 70 percent of the maximum for your age group, or to break a sweat.
  RealAge benefit: As much as 6.4 years younger

I do   I will   57) Avoid air pollution and environmental toxins.
it: do it:

☐   ☐   ■ Avoid jobs that expose you to pollutants or toxins.
                      RealAge loss: 2.8 years older

I do   I will   58) Choose to live where pollution rates are low.
it: do it:

☐   ☐   ■ When you're selecting a place to live or work, check the web-
                      site for the Environmental Protection Agency (see Chapter
                      6). Its pollution ratings show the areas and cities that have
                      excellent records for having the fewest very small (0.01 to 2.5
                      microns in size) particles in the air. This is important be-
                      cause it's the smallest particles that get farthest in your lungs
                      and disable your immune system, increasing your risk of in-
                      flammation and subsequent cancer and arterial aging.
                      RealAge benefit: 2.2 years younger

I do   I will   59) Patrol your own health.
it: do it:

☐   ☐   ■ Seek quality medical care and be alert to any early warning
                      signs of developing conditions. Do what you can to ensure
                      feeling healthy and do not ignore any indications that
                      something is wrong.
                      RealAge benefit: As much as 12 years younger

I do   I will   60) Manage chronic diseases.
it: do it:

☐   ☐   ■ Learning how to manage diseases such as diabetes, cardio-
                      vascular disease, arthritis, sleep apnea, and many others can
                      dramatically decrease the impact they can have on aging.
                      RealAge benefit: Depending on the disease, with
                                proper disease management the effect on
                                aging can be diminished considerably,
                                sometimes to almost indiscernible rates.

I do   I will   61) Build social networks.
it: do it:

☐   ☐   ■ Having a network of close friends and/or family can help
                      prevent aging from excessive stress.
                      RealAge benefit: 2 to 30 years younger

I do   I will   62) Call friends daily.
it: do it:

☐   ☐   ▪ Calling friends and discussing things with them is a Real-
                      Age trick that all of us can choose. Whether it's a phone call
                      at home or, even better, while walking, all have great bene-
                      fits.
                      RealAge benefit: 8 years younger

I do   I will   63) Visit friends at times of stress.
it: do it:

☐   ☐   ▪ When your friends are stressed, they become older and
                      may even clam up and not talk to you. That makes both
                      you and your friend older.
                      RealAge loss: 8 years older if you avoid friends at time of
                                      their stress
                      RealAge benefit: 8 years younger if you visit them in times
                                      of their stress

I do   I will   64) Eat food that comes from a variety of sources.
it: do it:

☐   ☐   ▪ None of us can predict what contamination will occur in
                      the food chain. It isn't only pesticides. Farm-raised fish
                      have been contaminated, as have native soy and corn crops.
                      The best protection is to vary your food sources: buy from
                      more than one grocery store, go to more than one fish
                      seller, purchase from different stalls at a farmers' market,
                      and dine out at more than one restaurant.
                      RealAge benefit: 1 year younger

I do   I will   65) Manage your finances and live within your means.
it: do it:

☐   ☐   ▪ Feeling out of control financially (particularly, undergoing a
                      bankruptcy) can cause unnecessary aging.
                      RealAge loss: 8 years older

THE MOST DIFFICULT CHANGES

*These are the conditions that age you the most and are the hardest to fix. Working to over-
come these obstacles is one of the most important things you can do toward keeping your
RealAge young.*

I do   I will   66) Keep your blood pressure low.
it: do it:

☐   ☐   ■ Blood pressure of 120 to 130/80 to 85 mm Hg is considered
                  normal but not ideal. Keeping your blood pressure at
                  115/76 mm Hg or less makes you 9 years younger than if
                  your blood pressure were 130/86. It also makes you over 25
                  years younger than someone with blood pressure of 160/90
                  or more. Reducing your blood pressure from 130/86 to
                  115/76 makes you 4.5 years younger in 6 months, and 9
                  years younger in 3 years, provided you reduce your blood
                  pressure before any permanent structural damage occurs in
                  the arteries.
                  RealAge benefit: 10 to 15 years younger for blood pressure
                                   of 115/76 mm Hg
                  RealAge loss: 10 to 15 years older for blood pressure of
                                140/90 mm Hg

I do   I will   67) Stop smoking.
it: do it:

☐   ☐   ■ Smoking one pack of cigarettes a day makes you over 8
                  years older than the nonsmoker. Cessation of smoking can
                  make you 1 year younger in 2 months, and 7 years younger
                  in 5 years.
                  RealAge benefit: If you quit, you can regain 7 of the 8 years
                                   you lost from smoking.
                  RealAge loss: 8 years older for smokers

I do   I will   68) Own a dog, and walk it!
it: do it:

☐   ☐   ■ Dog owners stay young longer, presumably because they
                  get exercise caring for their dog. (It may be that other pets,
                  such as cats or birds, help decrease stress too, but we don't
                  yet have the data to prove it.)
                  RealAge benefit: 1 year younger

I do   I will   69) Maintain a constant, desirable weight.
it: do it:

☐   ☐   ■ Reduce your weight gradually to what you were when you
                  were 18 (women) or 21 (men) years of age. Lose weight
                  slowly and consistently, avoiding yo-yo dieting, because rapid

gains and losses also cause aging. Your goal should be to reduce your body mass index to less than 23 (see Chapter 8).
RealAge benefit: 6 years younger

I do   I will   70) Reduce stress.
it: do it:

☐   ☐   ■ Having three or more major life events in a one-year period
                  can create more than 30 years of aging. Having lots of
                  friends, strong support networks, and strategies for coping
                  with stress can minimize the effect.
                  RealAge loss: During high-stress times, 30 to 32 years
                              older for people without strategies for stress
                              reduction.
                              During high-stress times, as little as 2 years
                              older for people with effective strategies for
                              stress reduction.

I do   I will   71) Complete nagging unfinished tasks (NUTs).
it: do it:

☐   ☐   ■ Recent data indicates the small, nagging, recurrent prob-
                  lems (such as the broken toilet seat that shifts when you sit
                  on it) add up to the effect of one major event. So deal with
                  these NUTs as they occur to keep your RealAge younger.
                  RealAge loss: 8 years older if you do not deal with these.

I do   I will   72) Have a backup stress-reduction technique on hand.
it: do it:

☐   ☐   ■ You can never have enough techniques to reduce or man-
                  age stress. If one of them fails you—you've pulled a muscle
                  and can't exercise—you can try another, such as medita-
                  tion. (Even an act as simple as scrunching up your face as
                  tightly as you can for 15 seconds and then releasing it is a
                  quick, effective stress-releaser we can all use.)
                  RealAge benefit: 6 years younger for being able to reduce
                              stress when you can't do it otherwise.

I do   I will   73) Cut back on excessive consumption of alcohol.
it: do it:

☐   ☐   ■ Alcohol addiction and abuse can cause severe aging, bring-
                  ing about liver failure and triggering cancers. Drinking

more than three drinks a day causes you to age needlessly.
RealAge loss: 3 years older

I do   I will   74) Overcome a drug addiction.
it: do it:

☐   ☐   ■ Illicit drugs such as cocaine and amphetamines rapidly in-
                  crease your rate of arterial aging. Others, such as heroin,
                  can result in death from an overdose. A drug addiction can
                  seem almost impossible to overcome, but it is not. Seek
                  professional help today.
                  RealAge loss: 8 years older for drug use

I do   I will   75) Recover from a severe emotional trauma.
it: do it:

☐   ☐   ■ Whether you have suffered the death of a loved one or have
                  been the victim of a violent crime—whatever the trauma—
                  you owe it to yourself to seek help in your recovery. Thera-
                  pists, support groups, and even just time alone with loved
                  ones can all help aid you in your recovery.
                  RealAge benefit: 8 to 16 years younger

I do   I will   76) Keep a positive attitude.
it: do it:

☐   ☐   ■ If you see the glass as half-full rather than half-empty,
                  you'll be happier, live with less disability and pain, and be
                  more likely to adopt other behaviors that make your Real-
                  Age younger. Many techniques such as completing a
                  nightly gratitude journal can help you reframe situations,
                  and learn to enjoy a positive attitude.
                  RealAge benefit: At least 6 years younger

I do   I will   77) Stick to your RealAge plan!
it: do it:

☐   ☐   ■ This is not so difficult but very important.
                  RealAge benefit: Up to 29 years younger

I do   I will   78) Celebrate success when you get a year younger.
it: do it:

☐   ☐   ■ It is important for all of us to make sure we celebrate our
                  successes. Buy a new outfit, buy a new kitchen pot, buy a

colorful plate or pan. Throw a "year-younger" party. You deserve it: you have made yourself over from the inside out—the best and most lasting Makeover!

RealAge benefit: Many years younger

Your Personal RealAge Makeover Plan

The test you took to ascertain your RealAge has many more questions than the original test (about twice as many), so your RealAge is now more accurate. Also, we offer lots of new options for your Makeover. Now that you have a sense of some of the suggested lifestyle changes, you will discover as you continue reading exactly how and why these changes will benefit you.

Try to keep an open mind, even if your first reaction to a choice is that it's one you're just not willing to make. Readers have consistently reported reconsidering their decision not to adopt an Age-Reduction strategy once they've seen the kind of impact on their Makeover it can have. For example, you may be averse to taking pills of any kind. But when you see the important cancer-preventive benefit of daily folate, and learn how much younger it will make you, you may change your mind. The chapters that follow allow you to weigh the merits of everything from completing unfinished tasks, to taking a 30-minute walk every day, to making sure your vitamin has less than 2500 IU of vitamin A. Don't try to do everything at once. Begin by adopting just two or three strategies, and watch your Makeover kick into gear and the years start to fade away.

A RealAge Makeover Success Story: Tom M.

Tom M. is what he calls a kibitzer. He gets paid an awful lot of money for advising hospital executives on strategic plans and specific actions. One day Tom came to me for medical care. He had borderline elevated blood pressure, an LDL cholesterol level of 160 mg/dl, and HDL of 36. However, Tom didn't want to take blood pressure pills or cholesterol-lowering drugs.

I gave him a list of seven things he could do to lower his levels without medication. He had seen this list before, but being a type A personality, he'd tried to do them all at once, failed, and become discouraged. This time, I urged him to pick just one or two.

He started with the same one that many people do—walking thirty minutes a day. He also cut down on red meat, to less than four ounces a week. After four weeks of walking, he added ten minutes of strength-building exercise a day, and learned several different techniques for stress reduction. He started avoiding all trans fat. Over a three-month period Tom transformed himself from a fifty-seven-year-old with a RealAge of sixty-eight to a fifty-eight-year-old with a RealAge of fifty-two. He looked more than ten years younger. He had lost eighteen pounds, and his blood pressure was now in the 120 to 125 over 75 to 85 mm Hg range—not perfect, but a lot better than the 130 to 160 over 90 or so that it had been before he started this program. His LDL cholesterol is now 96 mg/dl, and his HDL cholesterol is 49. The change in his health, while dramatic, was relatively quick and easy. He had given himself a RealAge Makeover: he looked, felt, and was many years younger. He had started with just two things from his list and had added more with time.

If you have enough discipline to do even one of those things, such as walking thirty minutes a day, then you have the discipline to get younger. Are you willing to walk thirty minutes a day? Not just some days but every day, come rain or shine—in a mall or through the corridors of a store or a business or a hospital. Every day. No excuses! It's the one decision I've seen that differentiates those patients who are successful from those who are not. If you try to do seven things at once, as Tom had before, you will decrease your odds of success. Trying to do too much at once can be overwhelming. It's far too easy to throw oneself into a new program with gusto, only to burn out and go right back to the old way of doing things. When it comes to your RealAge Makeover, as it comes to so many things in life, moderation is the key. Time and time again, I have seen that the people who have been the most successful at making themselves over have begun by choosing only two or three strategies. They took several months to become completely comfortable with these new strategies, so that they seemed like a normal part of their lifestyles, and rewarded themselves for doing so. Only then would they add two or three more. They would frequently check their RealAges, and modify and update their Makeover plans.

One patient calls me every Monday morning. "Mike, I've done such-and-such. What's my RealAge now?" Over four years she has gradually and consistently given herself a RealAge Makeover. She feels fifteen years younger, and she is. She's dropped twenty-six pounds, and it all started with a commitment to take a thirty-minute walk everyday. Then she added other choices.

A method many of my patients have found helpful is to adopt some steps from the Quick Fixes category first. Just seeing the concrete changes they have already made in their RealAges by doing so motivates them to do more. Of course, many of the other RealAge choices require more resolve. But don't the most important things in life—like having a family, or a career—always require a little effort? And doesn't making an effort toward a goal make you feel all the more pride when you achieve it? The key is in a combination of self-motivation and self-reward (or better yet, if you can get some friends to join you, mutual motivation and reward). Besides, most of the choices are not that difficult; you just need to leave your comfort zone and try something new. But isn't it worth it, when the result is that you've added quality years to your life?

Granted, some of the goals that may be a part of your RealAge Makeover are downright difficult. No one would deny that losing weight, adopting a three-tiered physical activity program, quitting smoking, managing stress, managing a chronic disease, and controlling blood pressure require serious commitment. But while the commitment required is big, the payoff is far bigger. The RealAge difference between two people who have the same calendar age but different blood pressure (above 140/90 mm Hg versus 115/76) can be as much as twenty-five years (see Chapter 4). Likewise, a person who has developed strategies for stress management—including a strong support network of friends and family—can have, in times of crisis, a RealAge as much as thirty years younger than a similar person in a similar situation who does not have a support network (see Chapter 7). Remember to prioritize your plan. Which steps are easy? Which steps are difficult but important? Which are less important? Deciding that you will floss your teeth every night requires only that you buy dental floss and use it. Other decisions involve more work.

Decide what load you can handle. If you have two Age-Reduction goals that are in the Most Difficult category, you probably won't want to initiate both at the same time. Pick one Age-Reduction strategy and follow it, and then, once you have the hang of it, start another. Don't, for example, try to quit smoking and lose weight at the same time. Choose one and once you have succeeded with that, adopt the other. Take the case of Elaine T. She started with thirty minutes a day of walking. Then she was able to lift weights. Finally, she quit smoking—a tough one. But succeeding with the smaller tasks made it easier.

Some people cannot handle a very big load now but can adopt one choice and then add more later, even much later. A patient and close personal friend of mine realized the importance of his RealAge when I told him that failing to take his blood pressure pills exactly as prescribed was making him five years older. He was astounded. "I thought my blood pressure pill-taking habits or lack thereof would just make me die a year or two early. I didn't realize it made me live with less energy and less vitality today. Five years less is a pretty big effect for just skipping a pill every other day." For my friend, just taking the first step of taking the pills and aspirin made all the difference. In fact, it kept him alive until he was motivated to adopt many additional age-reducing choices ten to fifteen years later. Yes, it took him a while, but it was better late than never. The more choices he made, the younger his RealAge eventually became.

The easiest way to make an overwhelming task seem manageable is to break it into smaller parts. If you're trying to lose weight, begin like Elaine or Tom did by walking thirty minutes a day. They've lost over twenty-five and eighteen pounds, respectively, in just six months. When you've walked every day for thirty days in a row, reward yourself by buying beautiful new nine-inch plates and eating a diet rich in fruits, vegetables, and fibers. At the start of meals, substitute cut-up vegetables for bread. Then work on cutting back the amount of saturated and trans fats in your diet (see Chapter 8). Don't worry about losing pounds right away; start by developing healthy eating habits. You might be surprised that the pounds come off on their own. Once you have eating under control, start to cut back on calories or begin to integrate more exercise into your life. Adding a new lifestyle choice to your RealAge Makeover is good, but what's really important is that you continue it over the long run. The greatest stress-reduction plan involving yoga and meditation does you no good if you abandon it after a couple of weeks or months and go back to feeling stressed. To get the RealAge benefit of a stress-reduction plan, you have to practice it consistently over the long run.

Photocopy the pages of Chart 3.2 and write out your plan. Just putting something down in black and white will help bolster your sense of commitment. Post your RealAge Makeover Plan where you can easily see it. Tape it to the refrigerator door, or leave it on your nightstand so you can commit to the next day's plan before you go to sleep. Look at it often and remember what you can do to get younger. Recalculate your RealAge every few months, or whenever you adopt a new Age-Reduction strategy. That way you'll know how much younger your RealAge Makeover has made you.

Chart 3.2

Personal RealAge Makeover Plan

My RealAge is: _____.

I want my RealAge to be: _____.

Now that I have calculated my RealAge, what behaviors *could* I adopt to make myself over?

1. _____.
2. _____.
3. _____.
4. _____.
5. _____.
6. _____.
7. _____.
8. _____.

Which behaviors am I willing to change?

1. _____.
2. _____.
3. _____.
4. _____.
5. _____.
6. _____.

Which three are the most important?

1. _____.
2. _____.
3. _____.

Which three are the easiest?

1. _____.
2. _____.
3. _____.

Dates: _____ to _____.
In the next 3 months, I will adopt the following three Age-Reduction behaviors:

1. _____.
2. _____.
3. _____.

Dates: _____ to _____.
After 3 months, I will add the following three Age-Reduction behaviors to my Makeover program:

1. _____.
2. _____.
3. _____.

In 3 months, my RealAge will be: _____.

In 1 year, my RealAge will be: _____.

In 3 years, my RealAge will be: _____.

The Difference Between RealAge Maximums and RealAge Interactions: The Impact on You and Your RealAge Makeover

Keep in mind, as you read this book and review the choices that will help make your RealAge younger, that the RealAge numbers presented in these chapters are the maximum possible effects. They presume only that a single behavior is affecting age reduction and do not take into account the interactions between the effects of several behaviors. Therefore, the numbers are not cumulative. This method has the benefit of allowing you to compare the relative value of health choices, but also the drawback of not accounting for multiple interactions. Therefore, you can't just add up the benefits to calculate your new Real-Age. That's why you need the computer or the chart (in Chapter 2).

Take the effect of moderate and regular alcohol consumption. In Chapter 11, we will explore how one-half to one drink a day (for women) and one to two a day (for men) can make you more than two years younger, if you are not at risk for alcohol abuse. This benefit is astounding. Is it true? Yes. Is it true for you? Not necessarily. Although a person who does nothing else to protect himself or herself from aging may well have a RealAge benefit of more than two years simply by having a little wine or beer with dinner, most of us make many other health decisions as well. The alcohol choice is affected by other choices, such as walking, smoking, eating vegetables and fruits, taking aspirin, and statin therapy.

Indeed, none of us has only one factor affecting his or her rate of aging. We all have multiple factors. You cannot simply add up all the years of benefit that certain behaviors provide and subtract those from your calender age. Let's say you floss your teeth and see a dental professional regularly (6.4 years younger), have low blood pressure (twelve years younger), own a dog (one year younger), do all three components of physical activity (nine years younger), and have the weight you had at age 18 or 21 (eight years younger). You cannot simply total these years, subtract them from your calender age, and say you are 36.4 years younger. The RealAge concept would be meaningless, as you worked your way back into childhood, even into negative years! Rather, the beauty of the RealAge calculation process on the Internet, and to a lesser extent in Chart 2.1, is that it considers the interrelationship between the range of behaviors, and determines the impact of these interactions for you.

Therefore, when it comes to your RealAge Makeover, the effect of any one behavior will depend on the other health behaviors and choices you follow. This involves complex equations and mathematics, which is why computers are required. These complex calculations can inform you of the relative and absolute values of your choices. This is what makes RealAge so revolutionary: it gives us the ability to calculate the effect of complex and multiple behaviors on aging all at once. It places a value on the effects different behaviors will have on you, and provides the information you need to make informed choices about the way in which you are going to age.

RealAge Means Better Lifestyle Choices

As you keep reading the book, you will learn about good lifestyles choices that will fuel your RealAge Makeover. You will learn why and how behaviors as diverse as taking folate and buckling your seatbelt can help you make your RealAge younger. I will go over the studies and discuss the biologic impact of the seventy-eight health and behavior choices. I will show you which ones help keep you young longer, and will provide suggestions and strategies for incorporating these changes into your life. I begin with the big three: aging of the arteries, aging of the immune system, and aging from environmental factors—and show how each one contributes to the overall aging equation. Then I will discuss healthy lifestyle choices such as staying physically and mentally active, avoiding secondhand smoke, eating a traditional Mediterranean diet, reducing stress by staying in touch with friends, getting good dental care, and many others that will help you make your RealAge younger.

When you give yourself a RealAge Makeover, you help to keep your calendar age from making you feel "old." Why would you not want to live like a person who is ten, twenty, even twenty-five years younger? In the chapters that follow, I will give you the tools to do just that; to be healthier and younger in both mind and body. Join all the other folks who have made themselves healthier through the RealAge program. You have nothing to lose but needless aging.

Keep the Blood Pumping

Reverse Arterial Aging: The Easiest, Fastest Way to Gain Energy

Simply stated, keeping your arteries healthy and young is the single best thing you can do for your health and your RealAge Makeover. Keeping your arteries young helps you guard against heart attack, stroke, memory loss, vascular disease, and impotence; improves the quality of orgasm; and helps prevent wrinkles. Not taking care of your cardiovascular system can make your RealAge as much as twenty years older. Luckily, it's easy to measurably slow the aging of your arteries through good RealAge lifestyle choices.

The following are the major factors in arterial aging:

- Your blood pressure is the most important indicator of arterial aging. By keeping your blood pressure at the ideal level of 115/76 mm Hg (millimeters of mercury), you can make your RealAge as much as ten years younger than if your blood pressure were at the national median of 130/86, and as much as twenty-five years younger than if you had high blood pressure (140/90 or more). Almost all of us can attain the ideal blood pressure of 115/76.
  Difficulty rating: Most difficult
- Atherosclerosis (the buildup of fats along the arterial wall) is the second leading cause of aging of the arteries, right behind high blood pressure. The two conditions reinforce one another. Reducing the amount of lipid plaques along the walls of your arteries will help keep them young. Diet, exercise, vitamins, and even statin drugs have been documented to improve and lengthen life by reducing aging of the arteries.
  Difficulty rating: Most difficult

- Knowing your high-sensitivity C-reactive protein (hs-CRP) value and reducing it into the normal range can make your RealAge 3.2 years younger. This blood test lets you know the amount of inflammation in your body. Inflammation can affect the arteries and immune system. Chronic infections are common and often cause elevated hs-CRP levels. When no chronic infection is identifiable, some physicians recommend taking an aspirin, exercise, trying an antibiotic for two weeks (based on the most likely pathogen and your gender, predispositions to infections, and age), and eating healthy fats. If none of these measures reduces hs-CRP to normal levels, starting a statin drug (such as Lipitor, Zocor, or Crestor) may keep inflammation in your arteries at bay.
  Difficulty Rating: Moderately difficult
- Taking an aspirin (325 mg [milligrams]) a day can make your RealAge 2.2 years younger by the time you reach fifty, and 2.9 years younger by the time you hit seventy. Aspirin helps keep your arteries free of lipid buildup and has other bonuses in preventing aging of the immune system and in preventing specific cancers.
  Difficulty rating: Quick fix
- Hormone replacement therapy in the form of estrogen and progesterone for women had great promise, and still does. However, this combination has not yet been the magic antiaging potion it first promised to be. Why have the randomized controlled trials come out differently from the older risk-factor epidemiology studies? What do we think will prove to be true in the long run? DHEA (dehydroepiandosterone), advertised as the "hormone replacement therapy for men," and HGH (human growth hormone and its releasing-factor substitutes) have not yet been effective, nor has testosterone, except for specific groups. Are hormones the answer for our arteries? We don't know now and won't for sure until we have better data. At present, avoid hormone come-ons.
  Difficulty rating: Moderately easy

It's this simple: nothing ages you faster than mistreating your heart and arteries. Conversely, nothing keeps you younger than taking care of your cardiovascular system. More Americans die from cardiovascular disease than from any other cause. In addition, more Americans are disabled by arterial disease than by any other condition. Cardiovascular disease will seriously afflict half of us, and will kill more than 40 percent of us. It's not fun skipping physical activities you like because you're in pain, or because your arteries aren't working. It's also not fun when malfunctioning arteries take a toll on your sex life.

Most of the premature aging your arterial system undergoes is a result of your lifestyle. You age yourself by not taking proper care of your body. The good news is that you can start reversing the process right now. The scientific data indicate that you can overcome years of bad choices and aging and make your arteries significantly younger.

Simon's story in Chapter 1 is pertinent. He was a man of forty-nine who was unable to walk more than half a block because of arterial disease. However, it was reversible, and he took action to make his RealAge younger. He made himself over. Now, at age sixty-eight, he walks a hilly golf course almost every day, sometimes twice a day, plays squash vigorously, and enjoys wine, sex, and a lot of other things in life. His quality of life has improved dramatically. His need for surgery at age forty-nine may very well have been a lucky wake-up call, but it was a drastic and risky one. But you do not have to wait for such a wake-up call.

Because our arteries are what tie the body together, and in fact connect to every cell, it's easy to see why they affect our health to such an overwhelming extent. While most of us think of heart attacks and strokes when we think of arterial aging, these are just the most dramatic results, by which time a person's arteries have been severely damaged.

Imagine your arteries as being like the streets in a city. We use the streets of a city to get from place to place. Similarly, your blood uses the arteries as a means to get from one place to another. It uses the vessels to carry nutrients and oxygen to the cells, and then carry carbon dioxide and other by-products of metabolism away from the cells. But the arteries, just like streets and highways, eventually wear down. They become clogged with fatty buildup called plaque, or narrowed from swelling and inflammation. The arteries also develop "potholes." That's what inflammation really does: it causes swelling and erosions, and potholes where plaque can insert itself. Clots can then form in the potholes. Clots can grow, break off, and be carried away by blood flow into the small arteries of the heart or brain, or to the arteries of the sex organs, kidneys, or other vital organs. The older and more congested arteries get, the more subject they are to blood clots, the body's version of traffic jams. Just as a traffic jam can affect a part of the city or the entire city, so can congested arteries affect one organ or the entire body. When arteries are congested, the cells do not get the nutrients they need and can suffer from a buildup of metabolic by-products.

Blood is made up of water, nutrients, hormones and other signaling agents, and several cellular elements—red cells, white cells, and platelets. Platelets (and sometimes white cells) are the cells we have to watch out for when it comes to cardiovascular disease. Platelets are covered by an enzyme that, when activated, causes them to stick to each other and form a clot.

The fact that blood can clot is a very good thing. Clotting is what stops us from bleeding excessively when we get injured. But as we age, we can develop blood clots where we don't want them—on the walls of the arteries. And fat eventually builds in the walls of the arteries, slowing the flow of blood and causing platelet pileups—blood vessel traffic jams—that slow the flow of blood even more. These platelet pileups can form small clots in the arteries. If a clot gets too big, it can fill the entire artery, and blood can't get through at all, putting the tissue supplied by that artery at risk of dying. When the arterial system becomes inflamed, the walls of the arteries can become swollen, also closing off the flow of blood. In this case, oxygen and essential nutrients don't get to the organs as they should, causing them to age more rapidly. The heart has to work harder to push the blood where it's supposed to go, increasing blood pressure and stressing the arteries even more. Indeed, just as a major traffic jam can affect a whole city, cardiovascular disease can stress your whole body.

You probably already know some of the things you can do to prevent this from happening to your system. Eating a diet low in saturated and trans fats, doing all three forms of physical activity (any strength-building exercise and stamina-building exercise), avoiding or managing stress, and even taking aspirin, are all good lifestyle habits that can help keep the arteries young. You also probably know some of the things that age your arteries: not being physically active, and eating food high in saturated and trans fats. Bad habits tend to snowball. A diet rich in unhealthy fats makes us feel tired, which makes us less likely to exercise. And even mild forms of cardiovascular disease can make us feel old and tired, further adding to the snowball effect.

A key to your RealAge Makeover—and your overall health and well-being—is to take special care of your arteries and heart. That is why discussion of the arterial health comes up in almost every chapter of this book. In this chapter, we discuss the fundamentals of how to care for your arteries, and explain why you should see arterial health as it pertains to every aspect of your life. You will understand how everything you do contributes to or detracts from it, and learn to safeguard your arterial health through a multitude of small, healthy lifestyle decisions. Taking an aspirin a day, drinking a glass of wine with dinner, and taking the right vitamins, minerals, and micronutrients in the proper amounts—and avoiding the wrong ones—are all quick, easy, and painless ways to make your cardiovascular system healthier.

The Importance of Lowering Your Blood Pressure

When starting your RealAge Makeover, the best place to begin is by learning your blood pressure numbers. Since the difference between having a low blood pressure and high blood pressure can mean a RealAge difference of more than twenty-five years, knowing what yours is, and getting it lower if it's too high, should be your number one priority as you launch your new program.

Don't be surprised if you get your blood pressure checked and it's too high. Eighty-nine percent of all Americans have blood pressure higher than the ideal for preventing aging, 115/76 mm Hg. About one quarter of all adult Americans (50 million) have blood pressure above the American Heart Association's danger zone of 140/90. Even the old standard that many consider ideal—120 to 130 mm Hg for systolic and 80 to 85 for diastolic—is too high for optimal health (and youth). More to the point, high blood pressure (hypertension) is one of the leading causes of heart attack, stroke, heart failure, impotence, and kidney failure.

While it can be unsettling to discover that you have high blood pressure, you are then in a position to do something about it and to give yourself more energy every day. This is far better than the most common scenario, which is to do nothing. Since high blood pressure has no symptoms, most people who have it feel fine, and do not realize that the loss of energy they feel as they get older is accelerated by their high blood pressure. Therefore, the temptation is to let it slide, instead of seeing it as the indicator of an opportunity to make yourself younger by taking actions to make it lower.

In the Veterans Administration system, even when pills are given free to patients with hypertension, only 37 percent take the pills the way they are prescribed, and more than 70 percent do not even achieve "good" blood pressure readings. Yet control of blood pressure is an important and easy way to keep your RealAge younger. If you don't like pills, there are many other things to do.

Even though my patients know about the devastating effects of high blood pressure, some of them will do almost anything to avoid taking their medication. Roger V., a longtime associate at the University of Chicago, called me about his father-in-law, Jake. Jake had just retired from a long career as an aircraft engineer. A World War II veteran and proud of the fact he had never been sick, Jake never went to doctors. His retirement physical was the first time he had seen a doctor in forty years. Reportedly, his doctor had told Jake he had a "touch" of high blood pressure—160/90, more than a "touch" by anyone's standards. Nevertheless, Jake steadfastly refused to take any medicine, return to the doctor, or do anything at all to lower his blood pressure.

Jake and his wife, Sara, brought a motor home. For three years they took trips, went to art museums and cultural events, and meandered around the country just enjoying their free time. After forty years of working hard, they were finally reaping the benefits. Jake called it "the great life." He told his daughter, Joyce, and Roger, "Don't worry about my blood pressure. Now that I'm not working, I'm not under any stress. My blood pressure's sure to have dropped."

Since nothing seemed wrong, no one paid too much attention. Then it happened. Jake had a stroke. It left him partially paralyzed and impaired his speech. He needed a walker to get around. In a matter of minutes, he had lost "the great life" he had worked all his life to enjoy. What needless aging!

Despite all the medical care Jake received after the stroke, he still refused to take his blood pressure medication. Finally, his kidneys started to fail, a side effect of hypertension. Roger and Joyce brought him to see me.

Giving him the "cold, hard, facts on aging," I finally convinced Jake to accept blood pressure treatment. With medication, his blood pressure dropped and his kidney function improved. Indeed, he managed to live a fairly good life, remaining relatively independent for another decade, until his kidneys finally gave out entirely. Although his post-stroke life was adequate and he made the best of it, it was not the life he had dreamed about.

That's not the end of the story. Several years ago, Joyce was also diagnosed as having high blood pressure. Just like her father, she refused to go on medication. Roger pushed her to take the medicine, but she refused.

"Joyce," I asked her, "are you *nuts*?"

She replied, "I just don't like taking medications."

"Joyce," I told her, "you just watched what happened to your father. Think how hard it was on him and your mother. It broke your heart to watch him suffer. It broke all of our hearts. Now you're telling me that you are going to risk exactly the same thing?"

I explained how and why high blood pressure is a silent killer—and a silent ager. After I showed her that lowering her blood pressure could make a twenty-year difference in her RealAge, she was convinced of the importance of taking blood pressure medicine. Even so, her resistance remained strong. She was concerned about side effects. I told her that although blood pressure medication could have side effects, most of them varied according to the individual. I explained that if this happened, we'd work together to find a blood pressure medication that would not only reduce her blood pressure but also maintain her quality of life.

For example, when taking some blood pressure medications, some people feel dizzy when they exercise, which is a symptom of dehydration. If this happened to Joyce, she could drink plenty of fluids. Also, a small percentage of people have lower potassium levels, but most only need to add a banana a day to their diets. In rare cases, side effects can include gout as well as impotence for men, and a change in sexual pleasure for women. With a little adjustment of the medication and dosages, those side effects can usually be eliminated. A number of different blood pressure drugs are available, and some of them work better for some people than others. Sometimes side effects are the most important clues for figuring out what's going on in your body.

Luckily, Joyce was finally convinced. By taking the medication, she reduced her blood pressure to 125/85 mm Hg, making her RealAge eight years younger, and she experienced only minimal side effects.

Many of my patients can stop using blood pressure pills after they start exercising and eating properly because they lose weight, and the physical activity lets their arteries get years younger, just as appropriate medications do. A crucial step in taking medications is not to alter the way you're taking the medications without your physician's knowledge and consent. Quitting any medication abruptly can put enormous stress on your body and cause unnecessary aging.

When a condition—such as arthritis, for example—has a symptom like chronic pain, the patient is motivated to monitor that condition. But because high blood pressure has no such overt symptoms, it can be difficult to focus on keeping blood pressure low. But keeping it at 115/76 can make your RealAge as much as ten years younger than if your blood pressure were the national median of 129/86. In contrast, having blood pressure 140/90 or higher can make your RealAge six to ten years older than if you were at the national average (see Table 4.1). In certain groups of people (African-Americans, among others), the aging effect of high blood pressure is even greater. And keeping it down is a key way to keep your energy up and make a substantial difference to your RealAge Makeover.

What Is Blood Pressure and How Is It Measured?

You're probably familiar with having your blood pressure checked; it's a routine part of every visit to the doctor. But not everyone is clear on exactly what that blood pressure reading actually means. What exactly is the doctor measuring with that inflatable cuff?

What is being measured is the amount of force your blood is putting on the arteries as it flows through them. Blood pressure is always presented as a fraction. For example, 129/86 mm Hg is the median blood pressure for Americans in their mid-to-late forties and early fifties. The top number in the fraction is the systolic pressure, the pressure exerted on the artery walls when the heart beats. The bottom number, the diastolic pressure, is the pressure exerted when the heart is at rest, between beats. The higher your blood pressure, the more stress and strain you put on your body, and the more bumps and potholes you create in your arteries. Reducing your blood pressure means that you'll stop burning away years needlessly.

Blood pressure is measure with a quick painless test using an instrument called a sphygmomanometer: that rubber cuff that gets tight on your upper arm as it's inflated. Now that you're in the process of a RealAge Makeover, be sure to ask what your blood pressure is, and write it down. And when you get it lower through healthier lifestyle choices—such as increased physical activity—be sure to celebrate your success.

Don't just get your blood pressure checked once; keep track of it, and how it varies, over time. Blood pressure is often elevated when you are anxious, upset, or in a hurry. Just being in a doctor's office can raise your blood pressure. This "white-coat hypertension" does increase your risk of coronary artery disease but not as much as continually high blood pressure. In fact, any time your blood pressure is elevated, even if it is during a period of stress, you are at higher risk of arterial aging. So when you have your blood pressure measured, make sure you've had enough time to calm down, have not eaten recently, are seated and relaxed, and aren't talking to someone about an issue you are passionate about. If your blood pressure is high, or higher than you would like it to be, go to your local pharmacist and buy a sphygmomanometer or even simpler blood pressure measuring device. Your doctor or the pharmacist can show you how to use it. Sometimes your doctor will ask you to undergo continuous twenty-four to seventy-two-hour "ambulatory blood pressure monitoring." This produces the most accurate blood pressure reading for the purpose of predicting aging of the arteries. That measurement is the one that should average about 115/76 mm Hg. You don't have to pay much in terms of aging if your blood pressure is lower than that.

Monitor your blood pressure regularly, keeping track of any fluctuations. You can be far more vigilant than anyone else. After all, it's your body, and you have the most to lose—or gain. As a general guideline, every increase of two points in the systolic number and three points in the diastolic number increases your RealAge about one year. That is a huge effect and often a huge opportunity to make yourself younger and to improve your quality of life for a long time.

It's common for your systolic blood pressure (and sometimes diastolic, too) to increase as you age. As you get older, the walls of the arteries become less elastic and clogged with buildup from fats and lipids. Your heart is forced to work harder, becoming enlarged, and the arteries become scarred and damaged. This process is common, but not inevitable. Unfortunately, once it begins, it snowballs: with damaged arteries, the heart has to work harder, which causes even more scarring. Arterial plaques can form, then enlarge, and heart attacks and strokes are more likely to occur. More than one and a half million Americans suffer heart attacks every year, and approximately 700,000 Americans die from heart disease and its consequences yearly. Seven hundred thousand Americans have strokes every year, and 167,000 die from these strokes and their side effects.

In rare cases of high blood pressure (less than 5 percent) the elevation is caused by an underlying medical condition. When this underlying condition is discovered and corrected, blood pressure returns to normal. However, in most cases, high blood pressure isn't caused by an unknown condition. The good news is that for most people, there are lifestyle choices you can make that will change your blood pressure to a more ideal and less aging value.

How Do You Achieve Ideal Blood Pressure?

What should you do if your blood pressure is higher than the ideal of 115/76 mm Hg?

- Eat a more nutritious diet with less than 20 grams of saturated and trans fat a day.
- Eat nine (yes, nine! it isn't that hard) servings of fruits and vegetables a day, including more than one serving of tomato sauce.
- Get more physical activity.
- Lose weight. Even ten pounds makes a big difference in your blood pressure and RealAge.
- Stop smoking.
- Consider cutting your sodium intake to less than 1,600 mg a day. This choice should be made with your doctor. Most patients find this choice very difficult, and in my experience, it is not very effective for most patients.
- Increase your intake of potassium, calcium, and magnesium.
- Prevent inflammation by doing things such as preventing gum disease and enjoying olive oil.
- Avoid stress and consider strategies to reduce stress, such as increasing social connections or using relaxation therapy, biofeedback methods, cognitive therapy, exercise, or yoga.
- If your blood pressure is close to or higher than 130/84 mm Hg (my interpretation of where the aging "danger zone" starts) talk to your doctor about taking medicine to reduce hypertension, at least until the other non-drug techniques reduce your blood pressure to under 130/84 mm Hg all on their own.

Table 4.1

The RealAge Effect of Combinations of Diastolic and Systolic Blood Pressure Readings

FOR MEN:

DIASTOLIC BLOOD PRESSURE (mm Hg)	SYSTOLIC BLOOD PRESSURE (MILLIMETERS OF MERCURY mm Hg)				
less than 80	less than 120	120 to 129	130 to 139	140 to 159	greater than 160
CALENDAR AGE			REALAGE		
35	30.2	32.2	33.9	35.6	40.4
55	47.3	50.4	53.1	58.8	62.4
70	60.2	63.9	67.0	71.0	78.8

DIASTOLIC BLOOD PRESSURE mm Hg	SYSTOLIC BLOOD PRESSURE mm Hg				
80–84	less than 120	120 to 129	130 to 139	140 to 159	greater than 160
CALENDAR AGE			REALAGE		
35	30.6	33.6	35.0	36.3	40.6
55	49.4	52.7	54.7	56.8	62.8
70	62.8	67	69.1	72.2	79.3

DIASTOLIC BLOOD PRESSURE mm Hg	SYSTOLIC BLOOD PRESSURE mm Hg				
85–89	less than 120	120 to 129	130 to 139	140 to 159	greater than 160
CALENDAR AGE			REALAGE		
35	33.0	35.0	36.0	37.1	41.0
55	51.6	55.0	56.4	57.8	63.2
70	65.5	70.0	71.6	73.3	79.9

DIASTOLIC BLOOD PRESSURE mm Hg	SYSTOLIC BLOOD PRESSURE mm Hg				
90–99	less than 120	120 to 129	130 to 139	140 to 159	greater than 160
CALENDAR AGE			REALAGE		
35	35.8	36.7	38.6	40.5	44.6
55	56.0	57.3	59.6	62.5	68.6
70	71.2	72.7	75.8	79.0	86.6

DIASTOLIC BLOOD PRESSURE mm Hg	SYSTOLIC BLOOD PRESSURE mm Hg				
100 or greater	less than 120	120 to 129	130 to 139	140 to 159	greater than 160
CALENDAR AGE	REALAGE				
35	39.2	40.1	42.5	45.5	50.0
55	60.6	62.1	66.1	70.1	77.2
70	76.7	78.5	83.5	88.5	97.7

FOR WOMEN:

DIASTOLIC BLOOD PRESSURE mm Hg	SYSTOLIC BLOOD PRESSURE mm Hg				
Less than 80	less than 120	120 to 129	130 to 139	140 to 159	greater than 160
CALENDAR AGE	REALAGE				
35	30.3	32.3	34.0	35.5	40.3
55	47.4	50.5	53.2	55.7	62.3
70	60.4	64.1	67.3	70.8	78.6

DIASTOLIC BLOOD PRESSURE mm Hg	SYSTOLIC BLOOD PRESSURE mm Hg				
80–84	less than 120	120 to 129	130 to 139	140 to 159	greater than 160
CALENDAR AGE	REALAGE				
35	30.7	33.7	35.0	36.2	40.4
55	49.6	52.8	54.8	56.6	62.6
70	63.1	67.3	69.3	72.0	79.0

DIASTOLIC BLOOD PRESSURE mm Hg	SYSTOLIC BLOOD PRESSURE mm Hg				
85–89	less than 120	120 to 129	130 to 139	140 to 159	greater than 160
CALENDAR AGE	REALAGE				
35	33.1	35.0	36.0	37.0	40.8
55	51.7	55	56.3	57.6	63.0
70	65.7	70	71.4	73.0	79.6

| DIASTOLIC BLOOD PRESSURE mm Hg | SYSTOLIC BLOOD PRESSURE mm Hg | | | | |
90–99	less than 120	120 to 129	130 to 139	140 to 159	greater than 160
CALENDAR AGE	REALAGE				
35	35.6	36.8	38.4	40.2	44.1
55	56.0	57.0	58.9	62.1	68.0
70	70.9	72.3	75.4	78.5	86.0

| DIASTOLIC BLOOD PRESSURE mm Hg | SYSTOLIC BLOOD PRESSURE mm Hg | | | | |
100 or greater	less than 120	120 to 129	130 to 139	140 to 159	greater than 160
CALENDAR AGE	REALAGE				
35	38.9	39.7	42.1	45.1	47.6
55	60.3	61.6	65.5	69.4	73.2
70	77.1	78.0	82.9	87.9	95.1

mm Hg is the abbreviation for millimeters of mercury.

If you have higher-than-ideal blood pressure, pay special attention to the recommendations in Chapters 7, 8, and 9 on stress reduction, great nutrition, and exercise. If your family has a history of cardiovascular disease, pay even more attention. These chapters show how easy it is to make small changes in food and physical activity that incorporate artery-healthy habits into your life. Lowering your blood pressure is not an impossible task.

Talk to your doctor to formulate a blood pressure reduction plan that takes your particular needs and concerns into consideration. Your doctor can help you decide if you should be on medicine for hypertension and, if so, which medication would work best for you. Because several kinds of treatments are available and some may suit you better than others, you should ask about all of them. If you experience side effects or don't feel as good as you think you should, don't discontinue your medicine without talking to your doctor first. Doing so can provoke a severe aging event, such as a heart attack or stroke. Talk to your doctor about how to withdraw and switch to other treatments.

Sometimes people hesitate to set up a blood pressure reduction plan with their physicians because they think that once they start taking medication, they'll be on it for a lifetime. Happily, that's very often not true. I've seen many patients start with pills, but then wean themselves off as other lifestyle choices make that possible. My patient Linda is a great example of one such success story.

A RealAge Makeover Success Story: Linda

Linda came to me to control her hypertension and aging. She was a sixty-year-old head of household whose husband worked one hundred hours a week as a chief executive officer of a Fortune 100 company. Linda worried a lot, and she had recently developed hypertension. She hadn't exercised in three years except for leisurely one- to two-hour strolls with her husband once a week. She was quite stressed about one daughter who was divorced and had a young child, and about another daughter with whom she had a difficult relationship. She spent a fair bit of time managing two homes. Over the last year, Linda's blood pressure had risen from 125 to 135 over 80 to 85 mm Hg, to 150 to 160 over 85 to 95 mm Hg. Her bad (LDL) cholesterol was 180 mg/dl (milligrams per deciliter; we want it under 120), and her good (HDL) cholesterol was 36 mg/dl (we want it over 45). In addition, her C-reactive protein level (a marker of inflammation) was above normal.

We set a goal for her to walk thirty minutes a day. After a month, she started doing resistance exercises with a trainer, and then stamina exercises. I hoped that exercise and cutting the trans fat from her diet would enable her to lose fifteen pounds. I also hoped that her blood pressure would be in the 120/80 range, her HDL cholesterol would increase to over 45 mg/dl, and her LDL cholesterol would fall to under 120 mg/dl.

Linda started working hard at this, diligently walking thirty minutes a day and even calling a friend daily to report on her walks. We agreed she would start taking low doses of both a lipid-management drug and a blood pressure-controlling diuretic ("water pill"). She used a blood pressure machine at home to monitor her status. To keep her blood pressure readings to less than 125/85 mm Hg on a consistent basis, she had to increase her diuretic pill to 25 mg twice a day. When this was done, her blood pressure was usually in the 110 to 125 over 80 to 85 mm Hg range.

After eight weeks of walking and four weeks of resistance exercise, Linda's heart rate decreased and her arteries got younger. Her blood pressure went down to 105 to 110 over 70 to 75 mm Hg. We then cut the diuretic to once a day, and over the next two months, she was able to eliminate the diuretic altogether. Her lipids normalized, and we were able to eliminate that pill, too, over the next two months.

After six months Linda had lost twelve pounds, was exercising regularly, and was eating more fruits and vegetables. She had eliminated most saturated and trans fat from her diet. Her HDL cholesterol had increased to 63 mg/dl, and her LDL cholesterol had dropped to 114 mg/dl. Her C-reactive protein level became normal. Through a regimen carefully managed by her physician, she was able to transform her health and wean herself off medication.

Although it is possible for many people to eliminate their need for drugs, this process should only be done under the care of a physician. With regard to my own patients, I believe that controlling blood pressure is so important that they should start with the pills. We can gradually reduce or eliminate the medicines once blood pressure, lipid values, and inflammation markers have become normal.

Your doctor can also tell if your high blood pressure is "sodium-sensitive." A small minority of people are sensitive to sodium. That is, their blood pressure responds to the amount of sodium they ingest. If you think that you are salt-sensitive, you should cut back on foods containing salt (see Chapter 10). However, if you think that getting rid of the salt shaker will be enough, think again. Most of the sodium we ingest comes from processed packaged foods, not from salt we add ourselves. Everything from soda pop to most breakfast cereals contains high levels of sodium. Learn to be a label reader. To avoid major sodium loads, eat fresh fruits and vegetables instead of processed food.

Reducing blood pressure requires more commitment than most of the Age-Reduction strategies we talk about in this book. If you start to think it's too much work, remember that your RealAge will become about one year younger for every three-point drop in systolic blood pressure and for every five-point drop in diastolic blood pressure. What could be better than that?

Stopping Atherosclerosis: Open Up Your Arteries!

The second most significant sign of arterial aging is atherosclerosis—the buildup of fats and lipids (plaque) in the walls of the arteries. The resulting narrowing of the artery's diameter increases blood pressure. Also, irregularities and inflammation at the tip of the plaques and in the arteries can produce an irregular surface on which clots can form.

One of the effects that makes high blood pressure so bad is that it increases the turbulence of blood flow. That is, blood flow becomes less smooth. This encourages even more fatty buildup in the artery walls. Also, clots may be disturbed or knocked off by turbulent blood flow. If the clots do break off, they can travel to smaller vessels in the heart or brain and produce heart attacks or strokes.

It's a vicious cycle. Atherosclerosis is a primary cause of high blood pressure. (Hypertension is often the first sign that the arteries are starting to harden.) In turn, the higher blood pressure rises, the more quickly fats build up, causing even more atherosclerotic aging, and a positive feedback system feeds on itself to make you feel, look, and be older and less energetic.

What causes fats to build up? What allows fats to seep into the arterial wall? We're not sure. Scientists postulate that either inflammation of the blood vessel walls or an excessive and accelerated bombardment of blood against the arterial walls (the very same conditions high blood pressure causes) causes micro-holes, triggering this process. Moreover, the higher your total blood cholesterol, and specifically, the higher your LDL cholesterol, the worse the problem becomes.

There are two common types of cholesterol, low-density lipoproteins (LDL), and high-density lipoproteins (HDL). I always think of "L" for "lousy" and "H" for "healthy," because LDL cholesterol accelerates fatty buildup in the arteries, whereas HDL cholesterol actually helps inhibit such buildup. That's why you want to have a low lousy (LDL) reading and a high healthy (HDL) reading. A high total cholesterol reading can be misleading, because one of the two components is healthy and the other is harmful. (See Chapter 8.)

Men are likely to suffer from arterial aging at an earlier age than women. Women usually don't undergo arterial aging until after menopause. Also, some population groups and families are more prone to arterial aging than others. For example, if you are male and a number of close relatives (a father, a brother, or an uncle) have had heart attacks or strokes, especially under the age of sixty-five, you too could be at risk of atherosclerosis at an early age. You need to pay particular attention to arterial aging. The same would be true of people who are significantly overweight, those who have high LDL cholesterol readings or a high hs-CRP level (discussed next), and, of course, those who have high blood pressure.

Know Your hs-CRP:
Preventing Potholes in Your Arteries
and Disturbances in Your DNA

Hs-CRP is the high-sensitivity assay (measurement) of C-reactive protein. This value is elevated when inflammation of virtually any type exists in the body. At three different times, the RealAge scientific advisory team considered adding hs-CRP to the RealAge program. However, only one of us felt strongly that the data were clear enough to do so. For one thing, the importance of hs-CRP to the rate of aging had not been shown to be an independent factor—that is, a factor not related to any of the other factors the RealAge program already took into account. Also, at those three times, we did not know how to lower hs-CRP and make it normal. This is a consideration because the RealAge program consists of actions that you can take to make your RealAge younger. As of late 2003, we know that hs-CRP is an independent factor, and equally important, we now know how you can reduce your hs-CRP. So the scientific advisory team considered hs-CRP once again and voted unanimously to include it in the RealAge program.

Why exactly is hs-CRP important? Many scientists now consider arterial aging primarily an inflammatory disease, and not only related to lipids. This hypothesis has not been an easy one for cardiologists to accept. We know that most heart attacks and strokes occur in patients with normal LDL cholesterol values. That does not mean that LDL cholesterol is unimportant, but it does indicate that other factors may also be important. Inflammation may be the most important of all factors other than hypertension. We now know that inflammation (elevated hs-CRP) is at least twice as important to control as a too-high level of LDL cholesterol or a total cholesterol of 280 mg/dl. The data are clear. Infection and inflammation are two major causes of aging of both the arteries and immune system.

In the U.S. government's Women's Health Initiative, which studied approximately 28,000 women, the cardiovascular mortality rate was 3.1 times higher for those with elevated hs-CRP than for those with the lowest levels. In a Danish study, the mortality rate was 2.1 times higher for those with elevated hs-CRP than for those with the lowest levels; and in the World Health Organization's MONICA Study on monitoring cardiovascular disease, the mortality rate was 2.6 times higher. In studies in other countries, the rate of a cardiovascular event such as a heart attack was 1.87 to 3.6 times higher with elevated hs-CRP. The mortality rate from all causes was 1.4 to 2.3 times higher for those in the highest 20 or 25 percentile of hs-CRP values than for those with the lowest levels.

We now know you can reduce your hs-CRP level with a two-week course of antibiotics to eradicate low-grade nonspecific bacterial infections, such as inflammation of the gums, prostate, or urinary tract. In addition, exercise, aspirin and aspirin-related drugs, and statin drugs all help decrease hs-CRP. The statin class of anticholesterol medications (Zocor, Lipitor, Crestor) also have major anti-inflammatory effects on arteries. In fact, many physician-scientists now believe the major benefit of these statin drugs in decreasing arterial aging is their anti-inflammatory effect. Having a normal C-reactive protein level—meaning one that is normal in your doctor's office and on three different occasions over a two-year period—will make your RealAge four years younger.

Table 4.2 shows the effect of various levels of C-reactive protein on your RealAge.

An Aspirin a Day Keeps the Doctor Away

Why Not Make Yourself Younger Today?

Chances are you've got a true wonder drug in your medicine cabinet—aspirin. I would go so far as to say it's the most useful drug of the twentieth century, and may still prove the most useful of the twenty-first century. It's a truly remarkable medicine that can kill pain, reduce fever and swelling, and, we now believe, make you younger.

It's doubtless not news to you that aspirin can get rid of a headache or a fever, but its antiaging properties might be. The fact is that taking an aspirin or even half an aspirin a day will help keep your arteries free of plaque buildup. Moreover, an aspirin a day reduces the incidence of breast cancer, colon and rectal cancer, and other cancers in the gastrointestinal tract. Taking 325 mg of aspirin a day can have the long-term benefit of making your RealAge as much as 2.2 years younger when you're fifty-five, and as much as 2.9 years younger by the time you're seventy.

We don't really know how aspirin produces its age-reducing effects. We think it helps keep the arteries free of clots in two ways. First, aspirin decreases inflammation in the arteries. Second, it inhibits the prostaglandin system, an enzyme system that causes platelets to stick together. Also, aspirin may help the body build auxiliary blood vessels, so that if and when clots do break off, enlarge, and clog blood vessels, the body has alternate routes for blood flow around the clogged vessel. Aspirin may help decrease inflammation in the walls of the blood vessels that are caused by infections elsewhere in the body (or those caused when particles such as homocysteine attack blood vessel walls), and thus prevent the turbulent blood flow that can lead to fatty buildup.

Perhaps even more encouraging, aspirin decreases aging of all arteries (to the brain, the heart, the legs, the skin, etc.) studied. The most recent studies on aspirin and aspirin-related drugs show a decrease in the incidence of strokes, especially the practically undetectable small-scale strokes that are often associated with memory loss. Aspirin and chemically similar drugs such as ibuprofen (for example, Motrin and Advil) are called *nonsteroidal anti-inflammatory drugs*, or NSAIDs. All NSAIDs appear to have this antistroke effect. Best of all, the sustained use of aspirin or other NSAIDs reduces the incidence of Alzheimer's disease, presumably because it helps keep the arteries in the brain young. Although we don't know all the ways aspirin may help our blood vessels, we do know that it has a significant impact.

Many studies have documented the benefits of aspirin in preventing cardio-vascular disease. Some have been small-scale studies and some have been large-

Table 4.2	The RealAge Effect of High-Sensitivity C-Reactive Protein (hs-CRP)*			

FOR MEN:

	hs-CRP LEVEL			
	LOW	NORMAL	ELEVATED	VERY ELEVATED
CALENDAR AGE	REALAGE			
35	33.9	35.0	36.3	37.2
55	53.7	55.0	57.2	58.1
70	68.3	70.0	72.4	73.3

FOR WOMEN:

	hs-CRP LEVEL			
	LOW	NORMAL	ELEVATED	VERY ELEVATED
CALENDAR AGE	REALAGE			
35	34.1	35.0	36.1	37.0
55	53.9	55.0	57.0	57.9
70	68.6	70.0	72.2	73.0

*Since different standards for measurement of hs-CRP now exist across laboratories or countries, I use low, normal, elevated, and very elevated, lacking standard numerical measurements. Please ask your physician if your hs-CRP value is low, normal, elevated, or very elevated, according to the laboratory used.

scale, but all of them indicated that aspirin helps reduce the incidence of heart attacks. In one rigorously controlled study, the effect of aspirin was quite dramatic: aspirin reduced the incidence of heart attack by 44 percent. Approximately 10,000 physicians were recruited for this research. All these doctors regularly took pills supplied to them by the study coordinators. Some of the participants were given real aspirin and the others were given placebos. In the more than five years of the study, the physicians who took aspirin had 44 percent fewer heart attacks than those who took the placebo. In fact, the results were so dramatic that the National Institutes of Health panel overseeing the study halted it midstream, deciding that study participants who had not been taking aspirin but were at risk of heart attack should also receive the benefits of aspirin.

As with so many other RealAge lifestyle choices, the benefits of aspirin are achieved after consistent practice over a long period of time, and are only kept as long as you continue taking aspirin regularly. The risk factors in these studies are calculated presuming at least a ten-year period of aspirin therapy. I estimate that a patient would need to be on this therapy for at least three years to get the full benefit. So, if you are a man over forty or a woman starting menopause, you should consider taking an aspirin a day for the rest of your life. (See page 112 for exactly when to start. It might be earlier or later for you, depending on certain factors. Also, remember to check with your physician before starting or stopping any Age-Reduction strategy.)

When it comes to aspirin therapy, there are differences between the genders. Women benefit a little less in their forties and fifties from aspirin than men, because woman usually don't develop cardiovascular disease until menopause. Unfortunately, most of the aspirin studies don't provide specific data on women. Since the cardiovascular systems of men and women do not differ significantly, and on the basis of what we know about women's health and aging in general, I feel comfortable recommending that women start taking an aspirin a day around the time of menopause.

An Added Benefit: Aspirin Reduces the Risk of Cancer

It's wonderful that taking aspirin on a regular, daily basis may help our arterial health. But now there's even more good news—it can also prevent some of the most common kinds of cancer: colon cancer, rectal cancer (which causes the second most disability and death in both men and women), and stomach cancer. The data are pretty conclusive, as they consist of both epidemiologic studies and, now, randomized controlled trials.

This discovery was made quite by accident by researchers who were conducting a study on people at high risk of a hereditary kind of colon cancer called familial polyposis. They were surprised to notice that patients who took aspirin or other NSAIDs had significantly lower rates of colon cancer than their family histories would have predicted. Further studies confirmed this decreased risk. Then a major study coordinated by the American Cancer Society involving 635,000 people found that those who took aspirin or other NSAIDs reduced their risk of colon cancer by approximately 40 percent compared with those who did not routinely take aspirin. In study of 121,000 nurses, those who took aspirin regularly over a ten-year period had a 44 percent lower incidence of colon cancer. In fact, in seven epidemiologic studies, individuals who took at least one aspirin a day had a 40 percent (on average) reduction in the frequency of colon and rectal cancers compare with their peers who did not use aspirin regularly. These epidemiologic results stimulated two randomized controlled trials. In one of these trials, 636 patients with prior colon and rectal cancer, and thus at risk of recurrence, were given either 325 mg of aspirin a day, or a placebo. The aspirin group had a 36 percent lower recurrence rate of cancer. In a second study, 1,285 people with precancerous colon polyps were given either a placebo or aspirin (81 or 325 mg a day). The aspirin groups had a 41 percent lower rate of colon cancer. Thus, aspirin can help prevent colon and rectal cancer.

Taking an aspirin every day can also help reduce breast cancer, again by 20 to 45 percent. Currently, these data come only from epidemiologic studies, but there are enough such studies to make it very likely that the data will be confirmed by randomized controlled trials in the future. From an ethical standpoint, it is becoming difficult to perform randomized controlled trials with aspirin in the risk group, however, as most people at risk of cancer should already be taking an aspirin a day for its beneficial effect on arterial aging. The more aspirin proves itself to be such a wonder drug, the more difficult it is to give a placebo to a group of people who really should be taking aspirin. The final word on aspirin therapy is that we still don't know exactly how aspirin decreases cancer risks; we just know that it does.

Aspirin: An Herbal Remedy Turned Mainstream, But It Still Has Side Effects

Aspirin is one of the oldest and safest drugs we have. Its main ingredient, acetylsalicylic acid, is found in willow bark, which has been used as a home remedy for headaches for more than three hundred years. Aspirin, as we now know it, was discovered more than a hundred years ago by the German scientist Hermann Dressler, who isolated it in its chemical form. Since then, those powdery white pills have been a staple of the family medicine cabinet.

So aspirin really began as an herbal remedy. It seems every herbal remedy or bit of folk wisdom has a kernel of truth in it, and it is the job of physician scientists to find that kernel. In Chapter 10, we talk about how a physician can discover the kernel of truth in an herbal remedy when we discuss the ginseng story.

The Dietary Supplement Health and Education Act (DSHEA) allows herbal remedies to be sold in the United States. However, the remedies aren't necessarily available in the form known to be most effective. This is not the case with aspirin. It was tested and sold widely before the DSHEA of the early 1990s. As a result, aspirin is provided in a much more consistently regulated fashion. Furthermore, it is not true that natural remedies do not have side effects. Aspirin has some significant side effects.

Aspirin is good for the arteries because it inhibits the enzyme system that causes clotting. However, for the same reason, and also because it is acidic, aspirin can exacerbate ulcers. It's even possible for aspirin to cause ulcers. The majority of these negative side effects result from the acidity of the aspirin and how it affects the stomach's lining. Luckily, there are ways to reduce those effects. Your doctor may recommend a coated aspirin, which will not be as irritating to your stomach, or that you avoid aspirin. A way for most of us to reduce the possibility of stomach ulcers is to take the aspirin with a half glass of warm water before and another half glass of warm water after taking the aspirin. And take the aspirin one or two hours after eating. The food acts as a protective barrier for the stomach lining, and the water helps dissolve the aspirin and dilute its acidity. Alka-Seltzer is another way to get your aspirin without stomach problems, but the downside is that Alka-Seltzer has a high sodium content.

Do you have to worry about thinning the blood too much by regularly taking aspirin? Probably not. Aspirin disarms the clotting function of a platelet for the life of that platelet. Platelets regenerate every seven to ten days, and you need to constrain six-sevenths of the platelets to receive the benefit to the arteries. The one-a-day dosage keeps the clotting of platelets at a constant, low functioning level. However, if you're facing surgery, let your doctor know about your aspirin therapy. He or she might recommend discontinuing aspirin two or three days before the surgery, just to make sure your platelet system will be adequate for clotting. However, most data now suggest a lower risk of adverse effects after surgery if you continue to take aspirin even the morning of surgery, even heart surgery. Aspirin seems to diminish many of the adverse postsurgical effects associated with inflammation. These data are new in the last several years, so many physicians may not yet accept this use of aspirin.

Make sure you take enough water when you take aspirin or any other NSAID, particularly before exercise. These drugs can cause kidney problems if you get dehydrated. That's especially true if you take an anti-inflammatory drug such as ibuprofen before you exercise: make sure you continually hydrate when exercising.

You shouldn't take aspirin while you have either chicken pox or the flu, because of the very rare possibility of getting Reye's syndrome, a toxic reaction to aspirin that affects children almost exclusively but can occasionally affect an adult. In addition, if you have a medical condition such as diabetes, asthma, kidney problems, or blood pressure that is either too high or too low, or are involved in a sport that causes traumatic injuries frequently, be sure to talk to your doctor before starting an aspirin regimen. Aspirin seems to lower blood pressure and can inhibit kidney function in individuals with diabetes or kidney problems. It's also possible for aspirin to trigger an asthmatic effect. However, the chances of any problems occurring from taking just one aspirin a day for Age Reduction are slim. If you do fall into any of the categories mentioned, talk to your doctor to see if there are possible alternatives.

Most of us have a favorite painkiller, and there can be a lot of brand loyalty among consumers. Since both aspirin and other NSAIDs are advantageous, does it matter which NSAID you take? Should you take the same one you take for pain, or should you switch to aspirin for this therapy? I'd suggest you switch to aspirin, since we know much more about it than the other NSAIDs, particularly about how safe it is. And aspirin has clearly been shown to have a significant age-reducing effect.

Aspirin was the first NSAID we ever had; it is the prototype. Because some people couldn't or didn't want to take aspirin, chemists invented drugs that were similar to aspirin. The best known is ibuprofen, but there are many others. All of these drugs reduce pain and swelling, but have different benefits and side effects. For example, for many people ibuprofen provides better pain relief than aspirin. However, when it comes to deactivating the enzyme system that causes blood platelets to stick together, aspirin is the most effective drug to take; aspirin deactivates the system for the life of the platelet, whereas most other NSAIDs produce only a temporary effect. However, the effectiveness of aspirin and some other NSAIDS in reducing the risk of cancer seems to be the same. We think some "designer aspirins"—the so-called "COX-2 inhibitors" (discussed below)—have the promise of also reducing cancer, with fewer side effects. So far, though, the antiaging benefits haven't been as substantial as those for aspirin.

Never take aspirin and other NSAIDS together, except under supervision of a doctor. Remember to talk to your doctor before starting treatment with aspirin or any other NSAID.

When to Start Taking Aspirin

We don't know the proper time to start taking aspirin, but it appears that the benefits outweigh the side effects for men over forty and women over fifty. That's when arterial aging begins to be a serious risk factor for both. However, the anticancer effects now appear to be strong enough and substantial enough to outweigh the risk in the general population, so that we can say that men should start taking an aspirin a day around age thirty-five and women around age forty.

"Designer Aspirin" and Other NSAIDS
Can Aspirin Really Be Improved?

Aspirin is clearly a wonder drug, but even a wonder drug can have a downside. In addition to reducing pain, aspirin and all of the NSAIDs can also eat away at the stomach lining (causing bleeding and ulcers), inhibit clotting, and in rare cases damage the kidneys.

The problem with aspirin and its cousins, such as ibuprofen, is that they aren't "specific." That is, their effects aren't targeted—limited to just one thing—and so they have many effects, some desirable and some perhaps undesirable. Their beneficial effects come from their ability to block cyclooxygenase-2 (COX-2), an enzyme that promotes inflammation, pain, and fever. Unfortunately, the drugs are even more effective at inhibiting COX-1, a related enzyme essential for the health of the stomach lining and kidneys. It might be very beneficial to create compounds that selectively inhibit COX-2 but have no effect on COX-1. At least three drugs do exactly that, including rofecoxib (Vioxx) and celecoxib (Celebrex). Newer, possibly even more selective COX-2s are under development.

Over the past decade, epidemiologic data have indicated that aspirin and other NSAIDs can protect against certain cancers, Alzheimer's disease, and arterial aging. Inhibition of COX-2 seems to be the key to the ability of these drugs to reduce aging. Thus, designer aspirin may really be a better aspirin, providing youth-promoting benefits for the arterial and immune systems without the aging side effects. So far, however, data have not shown that these more expensive alternatives are clearly superior for most people for antiaging. As of now, what would I do? If I had an upset stomach, I would try Celebrex or Vioxx. If not, I would stay with the 325-mg tablet of aspirin a day with a glass of warm water. For now, that is—I'm going to keep my eye on the new products that are developed.

There are other factors that can affect when you should start taking aspirin. If your family has a history of arterial aging or cancer—breast, colon, rectal, or other cancers of the gastrointestinal tract—you might talk with your physician and consider taking an aspirin with a glass of warm water every day from age twenty-five. However, we really don't have good enough data to make that a firm recommendation. Conversely, if you do not have a history of colon, rectal, or breast cancer or arterial aging events in your family until very late, you might hold off on the aspirin until age fifty if you're a man, or until age sixty if you're a woman. Again, talk with your physician about what's right for you.

Hormone Replacement Therapy: What Happened?

We usually associate hormones with the onset of puberty. They are responsible for turning our sweet children into temperamental teenagers. Many think that as we grow older, a decrease in hormone levels, especially the sex hormones, causes our arteries to age. And we hypothesized that reversing that process of hormone decline with supplemental hormones might be one of the mainstays of preventing arterial aging. Before the 1990s, estrogen and other HRT (hormone replacement therapy) was prescribed and taken for menopausal symptoms such as insomnia and hot flashes; in the 1990s HRT started to be widely used for its presumptive benefit in slowing arterial aging and heart disease. Even though estrogen was the first and best hope, we now hear a clear "no" to its benefits. However, I still believe there is hope that hormones really do make your Real-Age younger.

Hormones have a huge effect on our bodies and their development. Hormones make us able to flee in the face of danger, rather than freeze in panic. In addition, they help us metabolize food. Hormones are produced by glands such as the adrenal and the thyroid, and are largely directed by signals from the hypothalamus, a neural control center at the base of the brain. Hormones are released into the bloodstream and stimulate various physiologic activities. Epinephrine, released during fear or excitement, is a hormone. So is cortisol. So is insulin. Of course, the most well-known hormones are the sex hormones—testosterone for men, and estrogen and progesterone for women.

During puberty, our bodies release hormones into our bloodstreams that allow us to become physically mature and sexually reproductive. During our peak reproductive years (early to mid-adulthood), these hormones remain at a high level in our systems. However, as we reach our fifties and sixties, production of these hormones decreases substantially. By our eighties and nineties, they are almost nonexistent in our bloodstream. Since there is a clear relation between our calendar age and the level of hormones in our blood, it's logical to wonder if we could keep ourselves younger by keeping our hormone levels high.

The Epidemiologic Data

The question is not an easy one to answer. I believe that a decrease in hormone levels is one of the factors that make us age. Correspondingly, we used to think—and may one day think again—that hormone replacement therapy

(HRT) makes us younger. What went wrong between the prior studies and the current randomized controlled trials?

The problem with hormone treatments is that many of the hormones that might be used as supplements—with the exception of estrogen and progesterone—either have not been very well studied, or are known to have serious side effects. For example, anabolic (tissue-building) steroids, the kind of hormones athletes are barred from taking, do add muscle mass but also cause all kinds of problems, from skeletal deterioration to aggressive "killer" psychosis. Some hormone replacement therapies can even cause cancer. Hormone systems are "level-sensitive," so taking more than your body is designed to handle is unhealthy for you. In fact, for most hormone systems there's a disease that comes from having too much in the bloodstream, as well as disease from having too little.

No matter what you think about aging, it is best not to put something into your body that might be harmful. Hormone replacement therapy is an evolving treatment. Studies will show us more over time. As of this printing, HRT cannot be recommended.

To review, epidemiologic studies examine people and see what happens without any intervention. The science team doesn't control any factors; people behave as they would normally, and scientists see what happens. In randomized controlled trials, more factors are controlled, so these types of studies are more definitive. In the risk-factor epidemiologic studies prior to 2001, there was evidence that HRT was a benefit. Women normally have arterial aging events seven years later than men. The benefit or delay in arterial aging prior to menopause was thought to be due to estrogens. After menopause, women caught up with men in arterial aging, presumably because estrogens aren't present in enough quantity to protect women.

Many epidemiologic studies showed that women who took estrogen replacement therapy had lower incidences of heart attacks, strokes, Alzheimer's disease, and fractures of the spine and hip than similar women who were not taking such therapy. These benefits were plausible, as estrogens in test tubes increase arterial elasticity. That is, estrogens allow arteries to dilate, a sign that arteries are staying youthful. Also, estrogens increase beneficial HDL cholesterol. So women on estrogen replacement therapy had fewer heart attacks, strokes, and less memory loss. Thus, it was reasonable to think that this form of HRT was a benefit.

What the Randomized Controlled Studies Showed: No
Benefit, and Possibly Harm? Or Is There Harm?

Then the Women's Health Initiative and another series of randomized controlled studies came along. These randomized controlled trials looked at large numbers of women. Women were randomly enrolled into one of two groups. One group received HRT, and one group received a placebo. The two groups were then observed for differences in aging events.

In the Women's Health Initiative, the group being given HRT consisting of estrogen plus progestin was terminated before the end of the study. Not only was the combination HRT harmful to some, but even worse, no benefit could be found *and* HRT was found to be harmful. The risk of breast cancer was higher in the patients undergoing estrogen and progestin (a progesterone) replacement therapy: four more breast cancers every 5,200 years of treatment. That is to say, if 5,200 people were treated for one year, there would be an increase of four breast cancers. (Perhaps it's more relevant to say that if 225 people were treated for twenty years, four more would develop breast cancer.) There was also an increase in heart attacks of four in 5,200 and an increase in strokes of four in 5,200, but no difference in mortality (deaths) between the women given HRT and those not given HRT.

Why were the results of this study so different from the many earlier epidemiologic studies? There are two possible factors. First, the new study may not have been designed optimally. We all know that estrogen promotes blood to form a clot: we say it has a procoagulant effect. In fact, we've known since the mid-1970s that people who take estrogen have an increase in clotting, and should therefore take an aspirin or some equivalent anticlotting agent each day. In the Women's Health Initiative, that precaution wasn't prescribed as part of the study. Therefore, some of the increase in stroke and heart attacks—maybe even all of the increase—might have been eliminated if the women had been given aspirin.

Second, all the randomized controlled trials I know of use Prempro, a combination estrogen–progestin therapy. The selection of this particular HRT for study was logical, as Prempro is the most common HRT used by women worldwide. I have been told the Prempro for the study was donated by its manufacturer, saving the National Institutes of Health several million dollars a year, each year, for the duration of the studies. However, after the studies started, it was learned that the progestin in Prempro antagonizes (counteracts) the effect of estrogen on the arteries (at least in test-tube studies). Thus Prempro may not be an optimal HRT for either study or use.

Hormone Replacement Therapy and the Risk of Cancer

Both epidemiologic studies and randomized controlled trials have specifically implicated HRT in breast, ovarian, and uterine cancers. The explanation why HRT seems to promote cancer lies in the fact that hormones work as chemical signals. The body produces them in a gland and sends them out in the bloodstream to give instructions to other parts of the body. In order for these other parts of the body to "hear" the signal, they must have a specifically attuned place—a *receptor*—where the chemical signal is able to attach and deliver its message. Just as important as estrogen are the estrogen receptors. Without them, the body wouldn't be able to respond to the signal.

The subject of estrogen and estrogen receptors is a complicated one, and many types of estrogen receptors that have been identified so far. There are three that I consider important to understand. For simplicity's sake I will call them estrogen-1 (E1), estrogen-2 (E2), and estrogen-3 (E3) receptors. Let's assume that E1 receptors are located in breast and uterine tissue and are linked to the development of female traits such as breast enlargement, menstruation, and a high-pitched voice. The interaction between estrogen and the E1 receptors appears to promote breast, ovarian, and uterine cancers, apparently by initiating tissue growth. Estrogen-2 receptors are linked to the cardiovascular system, and in test-tube studies (but not the randomized controlled studies referred to above), these receptors have made it possible for estrogen to have a protective cardiovascular effect. Finally, E3 receptors allow bones to strengthen. Each receptor type (E1, E2, and E3) has a slightly different structure from the others, like a series of slightly different locks. While native estrogen is like a master key that fits into all the locks, each substitute may fit into only one or another lock.

When a woman takes estrogen supplements after her body has stopped producing high levels of estrogen, she is extending the period of her body's exposure to estrogen, and this increases her risk of E1 receptor stimulation, and of breast and uterine cancer. However, even though estrogen replacement therapy does increase the risk of breast and uterine cancer, that increase in risk is still low except in high-risk groups. Members of higher-risk categories for breast and uterine cancers include women who are overweight by forty pounds or more; women who are either childless or were over twenty-nine at the time of their first childbirth; and women with one or two first-degree family members (mother, sister, daughter) who developed breast cancer before the age of forty.

On the other hand, a new study shows that estrogen therapy is associated with a 35 percent reduction in colon and rectal cancers. Therefore, estrogen appears to be able to protect you from certain types of cancer. As with any complicated medical or health issue that seems to have both pros and cons, the first place to start when considering HRT therapy is with a discussion with your doctor.

Scientists are attempting to design better estrogens—ones that have benefits without the side effects. Your doctor and the news media will let you know when any of the new "designer" estrogen replacement drugs becomes available, and which might be appropriate for you. These are estrogen-like compounds that promise to retard bone loss and arterial aging but not pose a risk of uterine or breast cancer. These new drugs will be designed to target the E2 and E3 receptors, providing both cardiovascular and bone-strengthening benefits, while at the same time overlooking the E1 receptors and preventing the kind of overexposure to estrogen that increases the risk of cancer. Since these drugs will not cause the development of breast tissue or have other "feminizing" effects, men may also be able to take them.

Like naturally occurring estrogens, synthetic estrogens interact and bind with specific receptors. However, they don't do so in the same way. The difference between how naturally occurring and synthetic estrogens interact with receptors is the basis for one of the great promises of modern biotechnology. Within it lies the possibility of a synthetic "designer" estrogen that would antagonize E1 receptors—stopping the development or growth of breast cancer—and not cause feminization, but would stimulate E2 and E3 receptors and thus retard arterial aging while strengthening bones. It's a very exciting concept that may soon be a reality.

The first several of these so called designer estrogens has been released: one, raloxifene (Evista) by Eli Lilly, looks very promising. At present, raloxifene (Evista) seems to decrease the risk of breast cancer and retard skeletal aging by stengthening bones. Many readers know of tamoxifen (Nolvadex) as a treatment to reduce breast cancer recurrence. Tamoxifen can also be called a designer estrogen like Evista, that antagonizs or blocks the estrogen effect on breast tissue receptors. Do these drugs affect other estrogen receptors? Yes. Does Evista delay arterial aging? Early studies indicate this potential. (Tomoxifen does not decrease arterial aging in early studies.) But that is a great potential for this class of drugs—to delay or reverse arterial aging, strengthen bones, and decrease breast and uterine cancer rates. Will Evista or another drug in this designer estrogen group work to keep men younger, too? Only further research will answer these questions clearly, and a breakthrough with this drug or an alternate designer estrogen will probably occur in the near future.

Until we have such a drug, make sure you get annual gynecologic exams, mammograms, and Pap smears so that precancerous conditions and early cancers can be detected and stopped. The randomized studies on HRT continue to investigate the use of estrogen alone—without progestin—in a select group of women. Because a woman needs to take a progestin with the estrogen if she still has a uterus, only women who have had hysterectomies and don't need progestin are still being studied. So far there has been no harm, at least from the estrogen therapy, that is greater than the benefits. We'll learn more as the study continues.

In the Meantime, What Can You Do About Insomnia and Hot Flashes?

I think it is possible that the Women's Health Initiative or other studies will show that estrogen replacement therapy administered without progestin or with a different type of progestin does have beneficial effects, because the epidemiologic data seem too strong to think otherwise. The estrogen therapy may prove to be a benefit when we learn how to administer it correctly, and when it's given from the beginning with a drug that inhibits clotting, such as aspirin.

Until then, what can a woman do if she has hot flashes or insomnia or wants to protect her arteries or bones? First, to protect your arteries, do all the other things we mention in this book, such as taking aspirin, taking the right vitamins in the right amounts and avoiding the wrong ones, getting your flavonoids, taking lycopene (the red stuff in tomato sauce), flossing your teeth, managing your blood pressure, learning stress-control techniques, and doing all three kinds of physical activity. If you have insomnia, alternatives to estrogen are soy, the herbal extracts red clover and black cohosh, and small doses of drugs called "selective serotonin-reuptake inhibitors" (SSRIs), such as citalopram (Celexa), paroxitine (Paxil), fluoxetine (Prozac), and sertraline (Zoloft). Soy, red clover, and black cohosh all contain estrogen-like substances that affect some estrogen receptors. However, test-tube experiments report a wide variation from batch to batch in the ways and extent these substances affect estrogen receptors. The variation is to be expected, since the average soy preparation tested in one study consisted of one hundred twenty-four different isoflavones, the substances in soy that affect estrogen receptors. (I am careful to state *affect*, as some isoflavones "turn on" specific receptors while others block the very same receptors from being "turned on," just as some keys turn a lock, while others fit into the lock but do not turn it. The randomized controlled studies that have tested soy on women with menopausal symptoms have shown no consistent effect of soy on night sweats and insomnia. Similarly, when the placebo effect was taken into account, the studies on red clover and its isoflavones also show no effect on hot flashes or night sweats. It is interesting to note that the placebo produced a benefit of approximately 35 percent in the studies with both soy and red clover. Black cohosh seems to be slightly more effective. Thus, any one of these supplements may work (each works in about 35 percent of all tested women), but I can't say definitively what will work for you.

For the patient who doesn't get relief from any of these supplements and is really suffering from hot flashes and night sweats, I recommend trying the selective serotonin-reuptake inhibitors, or returning to estrogen replacement therapy. (She should work with her physician to make a rational choice.) If she decides to restart estrogen therapy, in my opinion she should start taking a daily aspirin two or three days in advance, and choose a preparation using micronized progestin. The fact that insomnia and hot flashes are so disturbing to the patient's lifestyle probably means that relief from those symptoms would make her RealAge younger (see the RealAge benefit of sleep in Chapter 11). So, perhaps for this particular patient, the optimal therapy would be the combination of aspirin and estrogen plus a micronized progestin, as in FemHRT.

Some new but highly controversial evidence shows that there might be a benefit for several HRTs in men. There has even been discussion of making some of these male hormones available to women. The benefit of doing so has not been proven yet, but I will review them next.

Men, Hormone Replacement, and the Case for DHEA

Dehydroepiandrosterone (DHEA), a hormone secreted by the adrenal cortex, has received a lot of attention in the media and among the public. It has been hailed as the hormone treatment for men. Unfortunately, the data have not backed up the claims. DHEA has not been proven to improve arterial health—or any other kind of health, for that matter. It even has potential risks. But let's look at exactly what we know.

Around 1994, we began hearing news stories that DHEA made men feel great. But this shouldn't really have been such big news. DHEA is a steroid, and all steroids make you feel great . . . for the short term. However, over the long term, they can do a lot of harm. In fact, certain steroids can cause serious health problems such as cancer, and can weaken the immune system.

Food supplements are not regulated as prescription drugs. Since DHEA is considered a food supplement, its manufacture is not governed as tightly by FDA regulations, and the dosage levels in different brands can vary widely. No rigorous medical studies have been conducted on the long-term efficacy of taking DHEA. More important, almost all of the studies that have monitored DHEA for more than a year have evaluated the effects of variation in *naturally occurring* levels of the hormone in the bloodstream, and have not considered the role of supplements. Therefore, we currently have no means to predict the effects on your health of taking DHEA over the long term.

DHEA is a hormone that is a precursor to (forms the basis of) androgens and estrogen. The body breaks DHEA down into the sex hormones. Men who take DHEA report feeling more youthful, with increased energy and revived libido. "I feel like I'm twenty again," says one sixty-year-old convert. "My wife has that sparkle back in her eyes," says another. Unfortunately, a feeling of vigor and well-being does not mean that DHEA can't cause real damage. There is a multitude of drugs (including cocaine and heroin) that make you feel good, but are actually bad for your health. DHEA might make you feel younger now, but we just don't know how it might affect your RealAge in the long run. It may well make you older.

In the Rancho Bernardo study (conducted in Rancho Bernardo, California), which has been the most significant study on the effect of DHEA on aging to date, researchers found that over a twelve-year period, men whose naturally occurring DHEA levels remained high had a 40 percent lower risk of heart disease and arterial aging. This was initially very promising. However, the follow-up study that covered nineteen years reported a much reduced benefit for having an elevated DHEA level. In this study, the risk was only lower by 14 percent. In RealAge terms, that means the benefit of DHEA, at most, might be only 1.5 years. Subsequent randomized studies have found no definite benefit. With regard to arterial aging, some of the studies found a benefit; some, a harm; and most, no effect at all.

There has also been speculation that DHEA might strengthen the immune response. While some studies in humans have backed up this theory, others have indicated that DHEA might help blunt immune responses: the opposite effect. In fact, some studies on women with autoimmune disease (see Chapter 5) have used DHEA to suppress the immune system. We just don't yet know for sure whether DHEA can strengthen or weaken immune responses, and to what degree. The studies that have shown significant benefits to the immune response were conducted mostly on rodents, who do not produce DHEA naturally. Therefore, we can't assume this data applies to humans. So we don't yet know the effect of DHEA on the immune system.

There may be some possible benefits to DHEA. But let's look at the possible drawbacks. In the two largest randomized studies on whether use of DHEA would reduce the dose of other steroids needed to treat lupus (an autoimmune disease), the need for other steroids was in fact reduced, but some worrisome problems also occurred. In this study, women were given DHEA or Prasterone (one specific brand of DHEA) and observed for one year. Because some of the DHEA is metabolized to testosterone, 41 percent of these women had acne, whereas only 19 percent taking placebo had acne. Abdominal discomfort was commonly reported, but was successfully treated with a medication that decreases stomach acid. Another study reported that higher DHEA levels correlated with a higher incidence of breast cancer in postmenopausal women. A study at Johns Hopkins Medical School found that women who had high levels of male hormones (androgens) such as DHEA and its derivatives had higher incidences of ovarian cancer. That raised a red flag. Doctors worried that DHEA might be tied to other kinds of cancers as well.

DHEA is the precursor to androgens, and high levels of androgens have been linked to prostate cancer in men. DHEA may also increase pituitary gland tumors in the brain. Since DHEA functions as a growth hormone under certain conditions, it may cause isolated precancerous cells to transform into rapidly growing tumors. Higher androgen levels can also increase the problem of male pattern baldness—certainly not a dangerous condition but one that might make you look, if not feel, older.

A 1998 study published in the Journal of the American Medical Association tested sixteen products. The amount of DHEA in the products ranged from none to 150 percent of the amount claimed on the label. Only seven products met the standards required of all drugs: 90 to 110 percent of the amount on the label.

If you decide to take DHEA, you first need a complete physical, including measurement of your current DHEA levels. You might already have a naturally high level. You will also need screenings every six months for prostate cancer, as well as regular checks of your DHEA levels to make sure they're in the right range. That's a lot of hassle for a drug that has no proven powers of age reduction.

DHEA seems to play no role in heart disease. It doesn't seem to retard aging of the blood vessels, although long-term studies haven't been done yet. As for the sexual powers attributed to DHEA, the one controlled study on the use of this supplement showed no indication that DHEA improved libido or sexual desire. As for other claims that DHEA increases muscle mass, helps one lose weight, and improves one's mood, these seem to be more wishful thinking than proven scientific results.

Many more studies are being done on DHEA right now. In the next five years, we should know if it has any benefits or serious risks. We will have a much better sense of what the proper dosage should be and if there really are Age Reduction effects. Until then, I recommend the use of other Age Reduction methods and avoidance of DHEA.

What About Testosterone?

Testosterone is *the* male hormone. One of its effects is to increase aggressiveness. In some instances, this aggressiveness has led to crimes of rage, and death. But recently, low does have been given to men who have low levels of natural testosterone. What happened?

Two randomized controlled trials studied the effects of these doses. Arterial aging events—stroke and heart disease—did decrease, and substantially. Disability and overall mortality also decreased, and quality of life increased.

However, these were small investigations that studied only men who showed clinical signs of testosterone deficiency (for example, they did not need to shave) and a low level of free testosterone (the amount not attached to protein in the blood and therefore able to travel into the tissues). In addition, one controlled trial indicated a benefit in quality of life and mortality rates for combining low doses of human growth hormone (HGH) with low doses of testosterone for men deficient in testosterone. These studies do not yet convey a RealAge effect for those with normal testosterone levels, especially since several of the studies show that even a small dose of testosterone can result in rage and aggressiveness problems in some patients. (I also suspect that testosterone may increase the growth of dormant prostate cancers.) Nevertheless, the data look good that testosterone, when given in proper doses, may end up producing a RealAge benefit for those who really need it. We may also be able to use testosterone for both men and women. Even though testosterone is a male hormone and causes some undesirable body characteristics in women, it also seems to have some beneficial effect in increasing female libido and enjoyment of sex.

Under no conditions should you take anabolic steroids unless they are specifically prescribed by a doctor. These powerful synthetic drugs mimic testosterone and are therefore used to build body tissue and muscle mass. They are extremely dangerous in some people, causing a wide variety of conditions ranging from cancer to extreme psychosis. If you take Age-Reduction seriously, you should be especially careful to stay away from steroids, because they can make your RealAge many years older.

What is the current verdict on hormone therapy? We can't yet make a decisive judgment. Unfortunately, that leaves women and men hanging. We'll have more information in the future; in the meantime, many other choices are available to keep your arterial system young.

■ **In Chapter 10, learn how specific vitamins protect your arteries.**
Taking the right group of these substances in the recommended doses

can make your RealAge more than six years younger. Be sure to read the sections on folate, B_6, and B_{12}, because taking these three vitamins regularly can make your RealAge more than three years younger. Also, learn how vitamins C and E taken together help protect your arteries. Remember to take less C and E if you are also taking certain drugs, such as the statins (for control of cholesterol). Taking both vitamins C and E in recommended doses can make your RealAge more than one year younger.

■ **Note the information on aging of the immune system in Chapter 5.** You should be sure to brush and floss your teeth and see a dental professional every six months, or more frequently if needed, to avoid periodontal disease. The bacteria that cause periodontal disease are believed to trigger an immune response that can cause inflammation of the arteries.

■ **When it comes to arterial youth, pay attention to the additional big three: good nutrition, regular physical activities, and stress reduction.** These are so important that an individual chapter is devoted to each. By eating a diet rich in healthy nutrients (including healthy fats, lycopene, and flavonoids), and low in saturated and trans fat and simple sugars, you will be able to make your RealAge more than ten years younger. By doing the three kinds of physical activity regularly (it's really not that hard!), you can make your RealAge more than eight years younger. Eating a healthy diet and getting plenty of exercise will reduce the stress you experience from both everyday and major life events.

■ **Pay particular attention to Chapter 7, which gives tips for managing stress.** Effective management of stress can prevent significant arterial aging and make your RealAge over thirty years younger than it would have been.

To help make arteries younger and to facilitate a RealAge Makeover from the inside (the arteries) out, this memory aid may be useful:

R—Reduce your stress (eliminate nagging unfinished tasks), blood pressure, and inflammation.

E—Eat smart by making good and good-tasting choices.

A—Activity is a must (at least two types a day).

L—Laugh a lot, and learn other stress management techniques that work for you.

A—Age less with aspirin (plus the right vitamins in the right doses, and avoid the wrong ones).

G—Gum and tooth care make you younger.

E—Engage in intellectual pursuits.

By now I'm sure you understand why the health of your arterial system is the most important gauge of your RealAge. For any RealAge Makeover, your arteries are key to keeping yourself as young as you can be from the inside out.

The Immune System

Your Personal Bodyguard Against Disease

If you ask people what they fear the most when it comes to their health, many will say "the Big C"—cancer, the second leading killer in the United States. In fact, cancer may soon pass heart disease and become number one. Cancer is a terrifying prospect, and can be seen as a reflection of the fact that your body—in particular, your immune system—is getting older and not protecting you from disease the way it should. Working proactively to keep your immune system strong and young is the best way to safeguard yourself against a devastating group of diseases. There are many lifestyle choices you can add to your RealAge Makeover plan that will help keep you healthy, young, and cancer-free.

In this chapter we discuss the three-pronged RealAge approach to cancer and cancer prevention. It includes avoiding exposure to substances that cause cancer, preventing the initiation of cancer into your genes, and preventing the growth of cancer once it starts. This chapter also explains how cancer works, and the strategies for prevention, because it is far easier to prevent cancer than it is to cure it. And using good lifestyle choices to prevent cancer makes your Real-Age younger.

- Two of the most anxiety-provoking and prevalent types of cancer are prostate and breast cancer. Combined, these two diseases kill more people than any others except heart disease and lung cancer. Every year in the United States, about 250,000 new cases of prostate cancer are diagnosed, and 40,000 men die from this cancer. An estimated 210,000 new cases of breast cancer occur annually, and 40,000 women die from it. Those are devastating numbers. And yet we have a wonderful new tool to fight against prostate and breast cancer: tomato sauce. Yes, that delicious red sauce you put on pasta can be a powerful weapon in your RealAge Makeover arsenal. And its benefits might not just be against cancer; tomato sauce may also retard or reverse aging of the arteries. A pretty wonderful benefit for something so pleasant as eating spaghetti, wouldn't you agree? In terms of RealAge, eating tomato sauce can make a man as much as 1.9 years younger and a woman as much as 0.9 years younger.

Difficulty rating: Quick fix

▪ Although we now all know that the sun worshipper's habit of sunbathing for hours isn't good for us, we shouldn't avoid the sun altogether. Sunlight helps our bodies produce an adequate amount of vitamin D. Vitamin D appears to strengthen the immune response and helps prevent certain kinds of cancers. Learning how to strike a balance between too much sun and not enough can make your RealAge 1.7 years younger.

Difficulty rating: Moderately easy

▪ Now you have another reason to see your dentist: it's an important part of your RealAge Makeover plan. Not only do you keep your smile white and bright, you help protect yourself against periodontal disease and make your RealAge 6.5 years younger. In contrast, people with acute periodontal disease are as much as 2.7 years older than their calendar age. The bacteria that cause periodontal disease appear to trigger an immune response that causes inflammation throughout the body. A side effect is inflammation of the arteries, a major precursor to heart disease. Other possible results are stroke, impotence, wrinkling of the skin, and even miscarriage. We don't yet understand exactly the full effect of dental care on the overall system, but we do know that those who floss and see a dental professional regularly live longer, and with more energy.

Difficulty rating: Moderately easy

Whenever I give a lecture about RealAge, I am always asked the same question: "If I prevent arterial aging and lower my risk of heart attacks, strokes, and other forms of cardiovascular disease, won't I just die from something worse, like cancer?"

Cancer is a frightening prospect for most people, and with good reason. It's the second leading killer in the United States, accounting for 22 percent of all deaths annually. Each year, more than a million Americans are diagnosed with cancer, and more than half a million die from cancer. Cancer is also a tragic irony, because it's a disease of one's own body gone awry. Cancer begins with one cell that fails to keep in line with the other cells around it and suddenly begins growing, dividing, and dividing again, forming a mass of malignant cells—a tumor. If the tumor gets large enough or spreads (metastasizes), it can be fatal.

The good news is that 80 to 90 percent of cancers are linked to environmental causes, which means that many cancers can potentially be prevented. Making a commitment to keeping your immune system young is an essential part of your RealAge Makeover plan, and the best way to avoid getting cancer. This chapter explores how the immune system works, what cancer is, and how it can be prevented.

The Immune System

When we discussed the cardiovascular system, we used the metaphor of your body being a city, and your arteries being the streets that run through it. Now, as we discuss the immune system, we can say that your immune system is the justice and security systems that remove undesirable characters from your city. The immune system protects the body from outside invasion by locating and destroying potentially harmful bacteria and viruses. It does so through the workings of certain cells and signaling processes that identify and destroy potentially hazardous toxins and invading organisms.

Some of these genes are called *proofreader genes*, and they exist in every cell except red blood cells. Proofreader genes protect the body against insurrection from within by rooting out cells that have become abnormal or malignant. They do this by scanning the rest of your genes and destroying cells that contain an error or a change in your DNA (deoxyribonucleic acid). In this way, the immune system helps keep bad collections of cells (an initial tumor) from growing into a clinical cancer. (A clinical cancer is one that has become apparent in some way; for example, by causing symptoms, or as the result of physical examination or laboratory test.)

Back in the 1960s when I was in medical school, we didn't understand how invading organisms could wreak havoc on our health. We thought that bacteria and infections just caused colds, pneumonia, or tooth abscesses that could be treated with antibiotics. However, there was a small group of people who suspected otherwise, and we freshman medical students at the University of California in San Francisco were extremely fortunate to be exposed to their radical new theories. That group included a young assistant professor of microbiology, Michael Bishop; a graduate student in microbiology, Harold Varmus; and a brilliant biochemist named Herbert Boyer, who later started the biotechnology company Genentech.

We were taking microbiology to learn about bacteria and bacterial infections. In 1967 we knew that antibiotics had transformed the practice of medicine from one of mainly just diagnosis to one of treatments with pills, or so we thought. We soon-to-be physicians looked forward to learning how to prescribe medications to help our patients get rid of infections easily.

One day Bishop overheard us wishing we could drop the discussion of microorganisms and how they multiply in cells and, instead get on to the treatment phase. He said something like, "Understanding infectious diseases is the future of medicine. Someday you'll learn that most mental illnesses, heart disease, strokes, and even cancers are caused by infectious agents that change how your genes and the rest of your body function. You'll see: microbiology will rule the world." Most of us thought that his vision, so radically different from that of the rest of the medical community, was a little weird. Who ever thought an infectious disease caused depression, let alone heart disease or cancer? Not anyone who worked in traditional medicine during the 1960s. We should have listened more closely when he and his colleagues asserted that they were going to discover how DNA repairs itself, which specific genes cause cancer (oncogenes), and how viruses can cause normal genes to turn into oncogenes. Because that is exactly what they did.

To say back in 1967 that cancer was caused by infectious agents was way out there. But that's what Bishop theorized, and that's what he eventually proved to be true. Thanks to Bishop's work, infectious diseases—infectious agents and the inflammation they cause—are now understood to be essential components of age-related diseases, such as the arterial aging that inflammation causes. Bishop and Varmus won a Nobel Prize for this work less than three decades later.

So, although immune diseases and inflammation seem less "glamorous" and are more complex to understand than diseases of the heart and arteries, insight into them is important for all who want to delay aging and prevent age-related disease. Because unfortunately, our immune system begins to fail in two fundamental ways as we age. It can become negligent, allowing abnormal cells—either infectious agents or cancer cells—to grow unchecked. Or it can become overzealous, turning on the body and attacking normal tissues, as occurs in autoimmune diseases. Many forms of arthritis, connective tissue diseases, and allergies are autoimmune diseases. Because the immune system is so complex, it can even be negligent *and* overactive at the same time.

Keeping the immune system in working order is a slightly more complex task than protecting the cardiovascular system. The immune system consists of millions of free-floating cells that roam the body in search of abnormalities. All of these cells need to coordinate with each other in order to provide adequate protection. To obtain such coordination, the body uses chemical signals and signal inhibitors: hormones, neurotransmitters, cytokines, and the substances that oppose their effects. It's not important that you understand the immune system in all its complexity. What is important is that you realize that the ability of your immune system to do its job is directly related to how well you care for it.

You can care for your immune system in several ways. One is by getting regular physical activity. People who exercise have higher functioning of proofreader genes. Another way is by including specific nutrients in your food. We will explore the specific nutrients that help prevent cancer later in this chapter.

Understanding Cancer: What It Is and How It Works

Cancer is a disease of our DNA—the substance in our cells that contains all the information about how we grow and develop. You inherit your initial set of DNA from your parents (half from your mother and half from your father) when the egg and sperm fuse, and that DNA regulates what color eyes you have, how tall you will be, and every other growth and physiologic change from the day you're born until the day you die. Each of our cells contains an identical set of DNA, and as we grow this DNA is duplicated with every single cell division. Each of us starts out as a single cell, but by the time we are adults, our bodies contain 75 trillion cells. That means that trillions and trillions of cell divisions occur during your lifetime.

Simply stated, there are two different types of cells: germ-line cells and somatic cells. Germ-line cells are our reproductive cells: eggs in the female and sperm in the male. All of the other cells in the body are somatic cells, which make up more than 99 percent of the body. The somatic cells are living, changing cells: They grow, divide, and die. As long as you are alive, your body replaces these cells continuously. During your lifetime almost all the somatic cells in your body—except brain and nerve cells—will be replaced thousands, if not hundreds of thousands, of times. Your stomach lining, for example, is in an almost continual state of cell division, making new cells every single day. With so many cell divisions continually occurring throughout the body, it stands to reason that occasionally there will be a mistake—a mutation. Most cancers stem from mutations of somatic cells.

The root of the problem is that DNA can get damaged. Pieces of the instructions on the genes can get knocked out or changed. That can happen when you have a shortage of some substances involved in duplication. For example, a shortage of folate results in uracil being used in the new DNA where thymidine should have been. When this occurs during the process of cell division, when the DNA is being copied to the new cell, a mutation occurs. If the mutation occurs in the wrong place—in an active gene, for instance—it can result in one of two things. It can disrupt the function of the cell, causing it to die. Or it can cause the cell to begin dividing wildly and become a cancer.

Mutations can occur in another way, when the DNA in a cell is damaged by an irritant. Examples of irritants that can damage DNA are radiation, inflammation, or free radicals (unstable molecules that arise from metabolism and can damage cells). If these mutations do not kill the cell, they get passed on when the cell divides. How many of these mutations will you undergo in your lifetime? Probably millions.

Fortunately, not only do most of the mutations not cause cancer, most of them don't affect us at all. They do not occur in sections of the DNA containing active genes, or they do not disturb the action of a gene. Or the body repairs them. In contrast, lethal mutations are so significant that they kill the cell right away, at which point the mutation disappears and is not passed on. Probably 99.9 percent of all the mutations you undergo belong to one of these two classes.

However, there is a third type of mutation. In addition to the harmless mutations and the lethal mutations, there is a tumor-causing type. These are the rare cancer-causing mutations that tell the cell to begin growing and dividing uncontrollably. Your body has a regulatory system that keeps the number of cells in your body at a more or less constant level. The genes that regulate this process are known as cell-cycle genes, because they tell the cell when to divide, to grow, and to divide again. Some of these cell-cycle genes are the proofreader genes I described earlier: they scan the DNA when it replicates, ensuring that no mutations have been acquired. If a mutation has occurred, the proofreaders either fix it or kill the cell. A few of these cell-cycle and proofreader genes are also known as oncogenes (cancer genes), because mutations in these genes are tied to the development of cancers. If a gene that is supposed to tell a cell to stop growing stops working properly—that is, mutates—then the cell grows uncontrollably, dividing faster than it should. Moreover, its daughter cells inherit the mutation and grow out of control themselves. The effect multiplies, and soon there is a mass of rapidly dividing, quickly growing cells, a tumor, the Big C.

Fortunately, your body is usually able to recognize abnormal cells and destroy them before they cause harm. Most abnormal cells are rooted out and excised by the proofreader genes and the immune system. In addition, the general immune system also destroys many precancerous and early cancer cells. We don't understand exactly how this happens, and the immune system is not a perfect system. It is not always able to recognize the differences between cancer cells and normal cells, because the cancer cells send out signals to divert or hide from immune defenses. However, it has long been known that people with healthier immune systems are less likely to develop cancers, and that precancerous cells are often rooted out by the body.

Research is increasingly showing the role that the general immune system plays in cancer prevention. Hence, your body prevents cancer by three mechanisms—one genetic, two immunologic. Sometimes the whole cell isn't destroyed, but your DNA is actually repaired. One of the major discoveries of the last half century was discovery of the mechanism by which the body can repair its DNA (part of the Bishop-Boyer-Varmus set of hypotheses and discoveries). The body can repair a mistake by cutting it out and inserting the right substance, which is called a nucleotide. The body then splices the DNA back together again, restoring the DNA to its original configuration.

Of course, according to the law of averages, the longer you live—that is, the more divisions your cells undergo—the more likely you will undergo a mutation in a cell-cycle gene. And you exponentially increase your rate of mutations or the rate of mistakes in fixing mutations when you expose your body to harmful chemicals, radiation, buildup of free radicals, or inadequate nutrients (especially folate, B_6, and B_{12}). In these cases, the odds that you will undergo a mutation in the wrong place increase dramatically.

As you age, your second line of defense—your immune system—tends to be less vigilant and does not as readily detect and destroy these abnormalities. Luckily, you're not helpless in this process. In fact, the good news is that you can slow and even reverse the rate of aging of the immune system.

For the sake of your long-term health, and your RealAge Makeover plan, you should adopt a three-pronged approach to keeping your immune system young and avoiding cancer. You should adopt behaviors that

1. decrease the likelihood of changes in your DNA,
2. increase the detection of errors in DNA, and
3. strengthen your immune response so you decrease propagation of cancer cells.

Doing these things to keep your immune system youthful can make your RealAge over twenty years younger.

Cancer Genes: What Do They Mean to You?

Despite the recent stir about "cancer genes," fewer than 10 percent of all cancers are linked to genetic inheritance. How do we know that cancer is generally linked to lifestyle rather than heredity? Studies have investigated this topic in sets of Japanese twins and Chinese brothers, in which one person remained in the native country while the other emigrated to the United States. Even though the number of microscopic cancer cells (cancers that were not clinically evident) were the same for both members of each pair, the rates of actual clinical cancer were very different. For example, the brothers who stayed in China had one-seventh the rate of clinical cancer of their brothers who emigrated to America. The twins who stayed in Japan had one-third the rate of prostate cancer of their twins who went to America. Is this inherited genetics? Probably not, since the study subjects were brothers and twins. Something in the environment (possibly, maybe even probably, our food choices) increased the clinical rate of prostate cancer in the United States compared with that in Japan or China.

Although the vast majority of cancers are believed to stem from environmental causes, it is worth considering for a moment those people who have an inherited genetic predisposition to the disease. Almost every week a major news story reports the discovery of a new cancer gene. "Researchers have identified the breast cancer gene." "Scientists announce the discovery of the colon cancer gene." Most of these genes—or, more precisely, genetic mutations—run in families, isolated populations, or ethnic enclaves. They are mutations that lie in the germ-line cells—that is, in the egg and sperm—and are passed down from parent to child. They are often identified in populations that are endogamous (populations in which people marry within the same group). The propensity for these specific genetic mutations occurs in such populations because the more closely related people are, the less variation there is in the gene pool. Because many of these mutations are recessive, appearing only when both parents are carriers, the trait is more likely to show up when both parents have a similar genetic background.

If you belong to a population at risk of a genetically linked cancer, the discovery of a gene can have an immediate impact. You can be tested for the gene to learn whether or not you have inherited it. Although this sounds ominous, and undergoing such tests can be very frightening, there is a more positive way of thinking about it. By getting tested, you will know whether or not you have the gene. If you don't have it, you can quit worrying. If you do have it, you can minimize the risks—*and the aging*—it can cause.

If you do not belong to the group at risk, the news about cancer genes is less immediate but no less important. By identifying mutated forms of a gene, researchers are better able to understand what a gene does when it functions normally, and they are better able to target specific gene pathways that are implicated in specific forms of cancer. By understanding the biochemical processes by which a cancer grows, scientists get closer to understanding how we might prevent and even treat such cancers. Because all cancers are genetic, whether caused by an inherited mutation or an acquired one, the more we learn about the genetics involved in the development of cancers, the better prepared we will be to treat all cancers, and to prevent them.

Inheriting a cancer gene does not mean that you will get cancer. It means you have an increased risk of getting that particular type of cancer. People who inherit the form of a gene that causes cancer in 100 percent of cases rarely survive childhood. When scientists say that they have "found a cancer gene," they mean that they have found a gene which, when mutated, increases a person's risk. For example, even though scientists refer to the recently discovered BRCA-1 gene as the "breast cancer gene," they are not being accurate. No woman really has a "breast cancer gene," a gene whose function is to cause cancer. Instead, she may have inherited a copy of a gene that contains a specific mutation affecting the ability of that gene to function properly. The effect is to increase her predisposition toward breast cancer.

Many of the so-called cancer genes are two-hit genes. Because we inherit DNA from both of our parents, in many instances we have two working copies of a particular gene. If one doesn't work, the other covers for it. In many genetically linked cancers, a person will inherit a working copy of the gene from one parent and a nonworking copy from the other. The odds of that person getting an acquired mutation in the one working copy in a particular cell of the body are much higher than the odds for people who have two working copies of the gene. People with two working copies would need to get two acquired mutations—a mutation in both copies of the gene in the same cell—in order to develop that cancer. Other cancers require two mutations in two different genes, or two in the same copy of a gene. One mutation usually won't cause the cancer, but two mutations will. This is true, for example, with certain eye cancers called retinoblastomas. Because there are millions of cells in the eye, the chances of an acquired mutation occurring in any one cell is relatively high. The chance of two acquired mutations occurring in exactly the right places is relatively low. However, we know that certain people are born with one of the mutations already. Hence, the odds of their developing another mutation over their lifetimes are extremely high, making them genetically predisposed to developing this type of cancer.

Recently, inherited links have been discovered for certain types of breast and colon cancers, allowing us to identify people predisposed to developing these diseases. Such mutations account for a minority of all such cancers. For example, in breast cancer, genetic predisposition is thought to account for less than 4 percent of all cases. However, genetic predisposition is implicated in nearly a third of all breast cancers that develop in women under forty, showing just how much having one of these genes can affect one's risk.

Having a cancer gene can make your RealAge dramatically older, because you would have the same likelihood of developing cancer as a much older person. For example, a thirty-five-year-old woman who tests positive for the BRCA-1 breast cancer gene and whose mother and sister both developed breast cancer before the age forty has a RealAge that is seventeen years older. Her Real-Age would be fifty-two. By knowing she has the gene, she can make other choices that make her RealAge younger again. The dilemmas involved in this scenario are extremely complex, and individual counseling is recommended.

Cancer: Avoiding the Causes Is Better Than a Whole Lot of Cure

Most cancers can be prevented, and they are much easier to prevent than cure. Cancers can have many different causes: radiation, viruses, carcinogens, and random mistakes in the cell cycle. Some may be caused by lack of the right nutrients, such as folate, B_6, and B_{12} in food. Other possible causes are an inherited genetic predisposition, or just plain chance.

In many cases, cancers can develop because of a combination of factors. For example, no one doubts that smoking increases the incidence of lung cancer. Almost 90 percent of lung cancers are linked to cigarette smoking. Nevertheless, some smokers appear to be even more susceptible to cancer than others. Some people appear to produce higher levels of the enzyme that makes smoke carcinogenic. Thus, their genetic predisposition, combined with their behavioral choices, contributes to an even greater risk of lung cancer. This effect is a good example of how cancer can be caused by a combination of environmental factors and inherited tendencies.

The risk posed by smoking can be compounded by other factors as well. For example, asbestos and radon are known carcinogens (cancer-causing agents). Smoking greatly amplifies the risk of either, since smokers are significantly more sensitive to these carcinogens than nonsmokers. Although nonsmokers who are exposed to asbestos are five times more likely to develop lung cancer than nonsmokers who are not exposed to asbestos, smokers exposed to asbestos are ninety times more likely to develop lung cancer! Cigarettes and heavy drinking are another volatile combination, causing more cancers and more aging when together than alone.

Despite the fact that newfound cancer genes have gotten a lot of press, the truth remains that most cancers arise from or are promoted by our lifestyle choices, such as what we eat or don't eat. Of course, smoking cigarettes is a well-known culprit. The shocking fact is that almost one-third of all cancers diagnosed in Europe and the United States can be linked to tobacco use and account for more than 150,000 deaths in the United States each year. But less commonly known is that food choices are thought to contribute to another third of cancers, especially stomach and colon cancers. People who eat diets low in saturated and trans fats, and rich in nutrients and healthy fat, have a significantly lower incidence of cancer. Also, thinner people are at lower risk of breast, prostate, and uterine cancer, perhaps because such cancers are linked—at least some scientists believe—to high exposure to the sex hormones estrogen and testosterone, and these hormones are stored in fat. Heavy alcohol consumption is another lifestyle choice that can have an effect. People who drink excessively have higher levels of mouth, breast, and liver cancers.

Vitamin D is an element that is essential for the functioning of proofreader genes. Many of us are deficient in vitamin D, so taking vitamin D or getting ten to twenty minutes of sun a day would improve functioning of our proofreader genes. Combined with adequate exercise, it's an easy way to strengthen your proofreader gene function and help prevent cancer. Another is keeping an adequate amount of folate, B_6, and B_{12} in your system. These are also necessary for the repair process to proceed normally.

We also know that hazardous chemicals, too much sun, and radioactivity can age your immune system and increase your risk of cancer. Stress clearly weakens the immune response—the death of a loved one, for example, measurably decreases the number of T cells (a kind of white blood cell important for immune defenses) for as long as a year after the event. Even small but chronic nagging stresses weaken the immune response. These nagging stresses and major life event stresses clearly age the immune system. And, of course, there is AIDS (acquired immunodeficiency syndrome), a disease that directly attacks the immune system.

Cancer and Aging Across the Genders

Prostate Cancer

Ask any man what he fears most about aging, and he'll tell you heart attacks or cancer. But in his heart of hearts, what he fears the most is impotence (or erectile dysfunction). Since virility is a sign of youthful manhood, losing the ability to perform is something that makes men feel most acutely that their bodies are failing and they are getting old.

There are four major causes of impotence: arterial disease, stress, psychological issues, and prostate problems. Of the four, prostate cancer is one of the most feared and predictable reasons for loss of sexual function, and clinical prostate cancer is at least 70 percent preventable.

The prostate is a small gland at the base of the penis. As men age, the prostate tends to become enlarged and often cancerous. In fact, most older men show signs of having microscopic cancers in their prostates. The enlargement, from both noncancerous causes (called *benign prostatic hypertrophy*), and from cancers can be highly uncomfortable. A swollen prostate cuts off urine flow, increases the need to urinate, and often makes urination painful. Sexual performance can become limited. And that ages us physiologically and psychologically.

Effective drugs can be given to reduce the size of an enlarged prostate. A finding from New York's Mount Sinai Hospital revealed that the drug Finasteride may decrease the risk of prostate cancer. In that one study of men taking that drug for benign prostatic hypertrophy, the incidence of subsequent prostate cancer decreased by almost 50 percent. Unfortunately, the cancers that did show up were particularly devastating. Thus while Finasteride may effectively decrease the growth of many cancerous cells, really aggressive cancers can still thrive.

Prostate cancer is the most common cancer found in men. Some 250,000 new cases are diagnosed each year, and it causes 40,000 deaths annually, making it second only to lung cancer as the cause of cancer fatalities for men. More than 60 percent of men over the age of eighty will develop cancerous prostate cells. Those of us who plan to live into our eighties—healthily, heartily, vibrantly, and as young as sixty-year-olds—need to be especially careful to protect ourselves from this cancer.

Treatments for prostate cancer, such as surgery, chemotherapy, and radiation, are just as devastating as all cancer treatments are, but they also have an added side effect. Almost all the therapies are associated with a significant loss of sexual function in more than 50 percent of the cases.

Breast Cancer

Ask any women what she fears most about aging and she may tell you memory loss or an inability to care for herself. But what many women tell me they fear most is breast cancer. Like prostate cancer, breast cancer is psychologically and emotionally devastating. Even the least invasive therapies, such as lumpectomy with chronic tamoxifen therapy, are emotionally wrenching and sometimes disfiguring, especially if the cancer has spread.

Breast cancer is the most common cancer of women, but it is not limited to women: for every one hundred women who get it, so does one man. The incidence of breast cancer has been increasing steadily from one in twenty women in 1960 to one in eight today.

Clearly, both men and women owe it to themselves to make avoiding these cancers a priority in their RealAge Makeover plans. So, what can we do to help prevent these devastating diseases? The answer is as near as your kitchen.

Tomato Sauce and Perhaps Green Tea Will Help Keep You Cancer-Free

The good news is that the threat of these cancers we fear so much can be diminished substantially with a delicious and simple weapon: tomato (or spaghetti) sauce. Studies have shown that the risk of developing prostate cancer is as much as one-third lower among men who frequently eat foods containing tomatoes or tomato paste as among men who rarely eat such foods. Men who eat tomato products ten or more times a week have a 34 percent reduction in severe metastatic prostate cancers compared with men who eat tomatoes less than twice a week. Similarly, studies have shown the risk of developing clinical breast cancer is 30 to 50 percent lower among women who frequently eat foods containing tomatoes or tomato paste.

These findings were backed by a study investigating a wide range of men in Hong Kong, Tokyo, Milan, New York, Chicago, and Albuquerque. The incidence of microscopic prostate cancer was the same for all groups, no matter what their geographic location or genetic heritage. The chances that those microscopic cancers would develop into full-blown prostate cancer varied wildly across locations, with the number of fatalities due to prostate cancer differing significantly. The areas of the world having the lowest levels of severe, or metastatic, prostate cancer are Mediterranean, especially Greece and Italy, where tomato-based foods are central to the diet. In areas where tomato-based foods are not common, the risk of cancer increased markedly.

How can the simple tomato be such a wonder drug? The reason appears to be the vegetable's anti-inflammatory and antioxidant power. In particular, the tomato contains a particularly vital ingredient, lycopene.

The Possible Healing Properties of Lycopene

Lycopene apparently helps retard or reverse the aging of cells that can promote cancer growth in both the prostate and the breast. Even though lycopene is one of several carotenoids known for their antioxidant properties, other mechanisms may be responsible for the tomato's powerful benefits (see Chapter 8). Carotenoids (pigments found primarily in yellow, orange, and red fruits or vegetables)—are similar to vitamins: both facilitate specific chemical reactions. Unlike vitamins, though, carotenoids are not required for survival. A key function of carotenoids is to attach to free radicals, packaging them so they can be washed out of the body, and preventing them from damaging our cells and chromosomes.

Tomato paste, raw tomatoes, and cooked tomatoes all contain lots of lycopene. However, our bodies cannot absorb lycopene unless fat is present. Drinking a glass of tomato juice by itself, or eating slices of plain raw tomato does not provide us with much lycopene. Some experts question whether we can absorb lycopene from raw tomatoes even when fat is present. Tomatoes cooked lightly in oil—as in pasta sauces—result in a two- to threefold rise in lycopene concentrations in the bloodstream the day after ingestion. Although slightly cooked tomatoes appear to have the strongest effect, raw tomatoes with a little olive oil, sun-dried tomatoes in oil, or possibly even tomato juice eaten with a few nuts or a bit of cheese may also increase lycopene levels.

Studies have found that most men get their lycopene from tomato sauce on pizza or pasta. Unfortunately, the usual pizza with cheese—not to mention pepperoni and sausage—tends to be extremely high in saturated fats. You can eat tomato products without so much fat by eating tomato or spaghetti sauces on pasta, eating a roasted tomato with a drizzle of olive oil as a salad, trying our quick-to-make healthy pizza from *Cooking the RealAge® Way*, eating tomato-based soups, putting salsa on meats or salads, and even having ketchup more often as a condiment with foods that have just a little fat. (See Table 5.1 which shows how the amount of tomato-rich foods eaten weekly will affect your RealAge.)

If you're not wild about tomatoes, there are other foods that are rich in lycopene. One medium guava, one quarter of a medium watermelon, two cups of fresh red bell peppers, or two cups of red grapefruit will all provide the same amount of lycopene you'd get from a serving of tomatoes. One cautionary note: we do not know it is the lycopene in the tomato that is the cancer-preventing agent, just that tomatoes reduce the risk of cancer. While we're not quite certain it's the lycopene, we think it is likely to be the lycopene that makes the tomato so beneficial.

Table 5.1	The RealAge Effect of Tomatoes

FOR MEN:

Servings of Tomato-Rich Foods Eaten Per Week*

CALENDAR AGE	Less than 1	1 to 3	4 to 7	8 to 10	More than 10
			REALAGE		
35	35.3	35.1	35	34.9	34.7
55	55.8	55.3	55	54.6	54.2
70	70.9	70.4	70	69.3	68.8

FOR WOMEN:

Servings of Tomato-Rich Foods Eaten Per Week*

CALENDAR AGE	Less than 1	1 to 3	4 to 7	8 to 10	More than 10
			REALAGE		
35	35.2	35.1	35	34.9	34.9
55	55.3	55.1	55	54.8	54.4
70	70.4	70.2	70	69.7	69.3

*A serving is one tablespoon or the amount of tomato sauce on one slice of pizza.

Lycopene appears to have other benefits as well. A 1997 reanalysis of the data gathered in the EURAMIC Study (a historic international study on antioxidants and heart disease) found that men and women with the highest levels of lycopene in their bodies had the lowest risk of arterial aging. In a study from Kuopio, Finland, mortality from cardiovascular disease decreased more than 70 percent. In a study from Rotterdam, plaque decreased 45 percent. Although there have been only three studies to date, results have been favorable for those with the highest levels of lycopene compared with those with the lowest levels. Furthermore, in the ARIC study, which looked at the development of atherosclerosis by measuring the thickness of artery walls, artery walls were 19 percent thicker (had greater amounts of plaque, which is bad) in those with the lowest levels of lycopene than in those with the highest levels.

RealAge requires four outcome studies on human beings before we will include a factor in the RealAge program. So the RealAge scientific team needs one more equally rigorous study before we can claim that lycopene produces a Real-Age benefit for arterial aging. If these effects are confirmed in a fourth outcome study, that would translate to a benefit of more than five years younger for the average fifty-five-year-old man.

If you are trying to increase your lycopene levels in your blood, do not eat foods containing the fat substitute olestra, such as potato chips. (The brand name of the substitute is Olean, and brands of the chips include Frito-Lay's WOW, Utz's Yes!, and Fat-Free Pringles.) This "fake fat" removes fat-soluble vitamins from your body and dramatically reduces the amount of lycopene in the body. One study found that eating just six olestra potato chips every day for a month reduced the amount of lycopene in the body by 40 percent, and eating sixteen chips a day can reduce lycopene by as much as 60 percent.

Green Tea: A Cure for Prostate or Breast Cancer?

Another substance that appears promising in the prevention of prostate and breast cancer is green tea. Several studies of East Asian populations found that men who drink large amounts of green tea have lower rates of prostate cancer, and women who consume large amounts of green tea have reduced rates of breast cancer. Studies have isolated individual molecules and flavonoids in green tea that may be responsible. We don't know the mechanism of action of flavonoids, but they are powerful antioxidants, some even more powerful than vitamins C and E combined. Flavonoids also have anti-inflammatory effects. However, it may well be effects other than antioxidant or anti-inflammatory effects that produce the benefit of flavonoids in keeping the immune system young.

Unfortunately, the green tea molecule is notoriously fragile. The freezing and dehydration processes that imported green tea must undergo destroy the chemical compound that is linked to the reduction of the growth of prostate and breast cancer cells. To get any benefit from green tea, a person must drink as much as fifty cups a day. Soon I expect to see tests of commercially available pills containing the green tea extract in its proper form. While doubt remains, green tea extract may well be an aid in preventing prostate and breast cancer. Keep your eyes open for any new information on the subject. Other preliminary research also indicates that green tea—and black tea, too—may have other cancer-fighting abilities.

In both examples of prostate and breast cancer prevention, we have seen how a nutrient in our diet can affect our risk of getting cancer. Eating is one way we interact with our environment, and one way we can lessen the impact of environmental factors on our risk of developing cancer. Another environmental cause of cancer is sunshine. How exactly does the sun promote or reverse aging?

Sunshine and Your Health: How Much Is Too Much?

Everybody loves to be outside on a sunny day. But while being in the sun may make us feel good, we all know that too much time spent in the sun can eventually cause wrinkling and even worse, skin cancer. Wrinkles, which are actually signs of skin damage and aging, make you look and feel older than you are. Skin is one of the most important organs of the body. Wrinkles show that the skin is losing the elastin that keeps it young and healthy. Some forms of skin cancer make your RealAge significantly older very fast.

At the same time, there is also a RealAge benefit to getting a little sun every day. Sunshine is essential for our bodies to turn specific kinds of cholesterols in foods into vitamin D, an important nutrient that helps decrease aging of the cardiovascular and immune systems. The liver and kidneys then convert vitamin D into vitamin D_3, the active form of the vitamin. Just ten to twenty minutes of sunlight a day appears to be the optimal amount that each of us needs; this amount can make your RealAge 0.7 years younger.

Unfortunately, many Americans live in areas where the sun isn't strong enough for them to get this benefit. It takes a fair bit of energy from the sun to convert the cholesterol precursors of vitamin D to vitamin D; just any old sunshine won't do. In fact, anyone who lives north of Raleigh, North Carolina, won't get this benefit of the sun from October 1 to April 15, because the sun does not have enough energy during this period to convert precursor vitamin D to vitamin D. If you live in the North, or live in the South but cannot get some sun every day, you should take 400 IU of vitamin D daily, or 600 IU if you are over sixty years of age (see Chapter 10). Studies on mood elevation show that sunlight and exposure to broad-spectrum light help improve our mood. Seasonal affective disorder (SAD) and other kinds of depression can be improved by exposure to sunlight. So some sun is good. How much is too much?

What about skin cancer? As a general rule, your risk of skin cancer is determined by how much sun exposure you received thirty years ago, not how much sun you are exposed to now, because it takes a while for these cancers to develop into clinically significant events. Those who had severe sunburns as children are at much higher risk of skin cancer than those who never burned. However, just because the sun exposure you got as a child is the most crucial to your risk of skin cancer doesn't mean you can be careless as an adult. If you plan to be in the sun for more than ten or twenty minutes a day, take precautions.

Too much sun ages us because exposure to ultraviolet light destroys elastin and promotes wrinkles. It also damages the chromosomes in skin cells. Chromosomes are the strands of DNA contained in each cell in your body. If you look through a microscope at sun-damaged skin cells, you can see actual breaks in the chromosomes where they have been damaged by solar radiation. Amazingly, the sun can even damage the chromosomes in cells not directly exposed to sunlight. This chromosomal damage can lead to cancers.

The vast majority of skin cancers—90 percent of the roughly 550,000 reported cases of skin cancers each year—are of two types: basal cell cancers, and squamous cell cancers. Even though these skin cancers are rarely fatal and can usually be removed surgically without major aging repercussions, they are often disfiguring. However, there is a third type of skin cancer that is much more insidious. Malignant melanomas are very serious and can be fatal. Approximately 54,000 cases are reported each year.

Although Caucasians have more skin cancers than Asians, Hispanics, or African-Americans, anyone can get skin cancer. More important, skin cancer is the form of cancer increasing most rapidly. Rates have been increasing more than 10 percent a year for the last ten years among all population groups. Perhaps this is because we're living longer. If it takes thirty years for sun exposure to produce its disturbing consequences, the longer you live, the greater the chance you will experience those consequences.

If you have a family history of skin cancers or were excessively exposed to the sun, especially if you had severe sun burns during childhood, be aware that you are at greater risk. Likewise, if you have moles or a family history of moles, you need to be especially attentive in monitoring your skin for signs of a possible problem. Look for changes in the color, size, or shape of moles. If you note any changes, see your doctor immediately. A mole that looks irregular, has variable colors, or is larger than a quarter of an inch in diameter should be examined by your doctor. Examine yourself regularly, and have someone else check hard-to-see areas for any suspicious moles or changes in moles.

Always use a sunscreen with an SPF (sun protection factor) of at least 30 when you plan to be in the sun for thirty minutes or longer. The "30" means that you get thirty times the level of protection you would get if you wore no sunscreen at all. Everyone under the age of forty-five should use at least that level of protection, no matter how long he or she is in the sun. However, the SPF is only the beginning. More important, you need broad-spectrum protection.

Ultraviolet (UV) rays are what damages the skin, and the sun emits three basic types. Ultraviolet A (UVA) rays have the longest wavelength and produce a tan. These are the safest of the ultraviolet rays but can cause cancers and definitely promote wrinkles. Ultraviolet B (UVB) rays are somewhat more dangerous and are the most common cause of sunburn and skin cancers. Ultraviolet C (UVC) rays—those with the shortest wavelength—are the most dangerous, causing high rates of cancers. Luckily, the ozone layer blocks out most of these rays, although in such Southern Hemisphere countries as Australia and New Zealand, where the ozone layer is damaged, you need to be particularly careful and use a sunscreen that protects against UVC exposure.

Different sunscreens use different chemicals for blocking out the three types of UV rays. Some sunscreens use paraminobenzoic acid (PABA) and others use benzophenones or Parasol 1789. Each composition is better than the others at blocking out a particular type of UV ray. Studies on albino rats show that mixing all three provides the best overall protection. Consider using two or three different sunscreens at once, a PABA-based one, a benzophenone-based one, and a Parasol 1789-based one. If you are going to be out a long time, you should also use zinc oxide on areas particularly vulnerable to skin cancers, like the lips and nose. If you are planning on exercising or being in the water, make sure to apply water-resistant or, better yet, waterproof products. Finally, apply products liberally and often. The consistent use of sunscreen helps preserve your skin, preventing skin cancers and wrinkling. If you are out in the sun for more than an hour, or go in the water, consider reapplying your sunscreen, even if the manufacturer calls it "water-resistant."

Don't make the common mistake of protecting your face but neglecting other parts of your body. Skin cancer can affect any area of the body, even if it has not been exposed excessively to the sun. Although cancers are more likely to occur in areas exposed to the sun, too much sun can cause cancers anywhere on the body. For example, construction workers who only tan on their necks and arms can still get skin cancers on parts of their bodies that have never been exposed to the sun.

Finally, avoid tanning beds, which emit a lot of UVA rays. Remember that UVA rays cause wrinkling. If you decide to use a tanning bed, do not expose yourself for more than ten minutes a day and wear a physical-block sunscreen such as titanium dioxide or zinc oxide on vulnerable areas (lips, nose, ears, and shoulders). If you still want a tan, consider using the no-sun tanning cream dihydroxyacetone (DHA). It poses no known risks, so most experts believe it is safer than baking in the sun.

Table 5.2 shows the effect of sun and vitamin D on your RealAge.

Table 5.2	The RealAge Effect of Sun and Vitamin D

FOR MEN:

Daily Sun Exposure and Vitamin D*

CALENDAR AGE	No sunburn blisters; 10 min of sun a day or 400 IU vitamin D a day†	No sunburn blisters, no regular sun, and no vitamin D	Blisters after age 30, regular sun‡	Blisters before age 30, regular sun‡
		REALAGE		
35	34.6	35.9	35.5	36.0
55	54.6	56.8	55.7	56.5
70	69.8	71.9	70.8	71.7

FOR WOMEN:

Daily Sun Exposure and Vitamin D*

CALENDAR AGE	No sunburn blisters; 10 min of sun a day or 400 IU vitamin D a day†	No sunburn blisters, no regular sun, and no vitamin D	Blisters after age 30, regular sun‡	Blisters before age 30, regular sun‡
		REALAGE		
35	34.6	36.0	35.5	36.0
55	54.6	56.9	55.7	56.4
70	69.7	72.1	70.8	71.5

*See Table 10.6 in Chapter 10 for the benefits of different amounts of vitamin D.
†Increase vitamin D to 600 IU if over age 60.
‡"Regular sun" means 10 minutes or more a day in an area where the sun has enough energy to convert precursor vitamin D to vitamin D.

Get a little sun every day, in moderation. Getting a little sun promotes production of vitamin D and helps prevent certain kinds of depression. But don't overdo it, and protect yourself if you're going to be outside for a long period of time. Overexposure can make your RealAge more than 1.4 years older.

Table 5.3   The RealAge Effect of Dental Disease

FOR MEN:

Gum Disease and Tooth Loss

CALENDAR AGE	No Disease	Gingivitis	Periodontitis	Periodontitis and Tooth Loss
			REALAGE	
35	32.9	34.7	36.3	37.1
55	51.3	54.5	56.7	57.7
70	63.5	69.6	73.5	73.7

FOR WOMEN:

Gum Disease and Tooth Loss

CALENDAR AGE	No Disease	Gingivitis	Periodontitis	Periodontitis and Tooth Loss
			REALAGE	
35	33.6	34.7	36.2	37.0
55	51.6	54.8	56.5	56.6
70	64.4	69.8	73.3	73.4

Keep Smiling: Keeping Your Teeth—and Heart—Young

Did you know that flossing your teeth is one of the best and easiest ways to keep your immune system young? Many people make the mistake of thinking that tooth and gum care are just a matter of vanity. But that's not true at all. Of course, none of us wants to lose teeth because of cavity or disease, and nothing says "old age" more clearly than a pair of dentures. But dental disease and tooth loss don't just make us look and feel older, they actually do make us older. In fact, periodontal disease can make our RealAge more than 3.7 years older.

Cavities are no fun, and can lead to the need for dentures at an earlier age, but they don't seem to make a difference in your overall health or longevity. What really affects our rate of aging is the presence of gum disease (gingivitis) or diseases that destroy the underlying jaw bone (periodontal diseases). Studies show that the presence of periodontal disease, a disease most common in people with tooth loss, actually affects longevity. The best of these studies, done at Emory University in conjunction with the Centers for Disease Control, showed that people who have gingivitis and periodontitis have a mortality rate 23 to 46 percent higher than those who don't. In terms of RealAge, these dental diseases make you as much as 3.7 years older. Why? They are linked to increased rates of cardiovascular disease and strokes, as well as to an increase in mortality from other causes, such as infections. Conversely, the absence of periodontal disease makes you 3.4 years younger than the average person. Table 5.3 shows the effect of dental disease on your RealAge.

I myself had once regarded dental health as a primarily cosmetic issue. So when I first read these studies, I was shocked. It had never occurred to me that dental health might affect immune and arterial health. At first I assumed that the correlation between dental disease and higher death rates was due to "confounding factors" (the presence of other factors that might also be producing an effect). I assumed that people with other bad health habits—smoking, overeating, excess alcohol consumption—would also be more likely to develop dental disease. But I was wrong—very wrong. The surprising truth is that simply flossing your teeth every day can actually make your arteries younger. The probable reason is that flossing helps keep your immune system young by preventing gum and periodontal infections. For example, men under fifty who have advanced periodontal disease are 2.6 times more likely to die prematurely and three times more likely to die from heart disease than those who have healthy teeth and gums. Why would this be?

We don't know the answer for certain, but one theory is that the same bacteria that cause periodontal disease also trigger an immune response that causes inflammation of the arteries. In fact, a strain of bacteria commonly found in tooth plaque has also been found in the fatty deposits that can clog the arteries. Studies have shown that periodontal disease leads to a higher white blood cell count and an increase in C-reactive protein (hs-CRP; see Chapter 4), both indicators that the immune system is under increased stress.

Why is inflammation harmful? Inflammation of the arteries causes swelling of the artery walls. This constricts the arteries and reduces blood flow. Swelling also causes the blood flow to become turbulent—that is, not smooth as it should be, but swirling. Turbulent blood flow makes potholes more likely to form in the walls of the arteries, and these potholes provide places where lipids and white blood cells can seep into the wall of the artery. The resulting buildup of lipid deposits along the artery walls (plaque) reduces the diameter of the blood vessel and blood flow even more. All of these events promote inflammation at the tip of the plaque, and clotting at that inflammatory focus, and subsequent cardiovascular disease.

In addition, inflammation destabilizes already existing plaques. A clot in a pothole can break off and travel to a smaller vessel in the heart, brain, other organs, where it can cause major damage. One of the ways to detect such inflammation is measurement of high-sensitivity C-reactive protein (hs-CRP), as described in Chapter 4. A high level reflects a greater risk of arterial aging. Each risk of arterial aging magnifies other risks. So gum disease increases arterial aging even more if you have an elevated LDL cholesterol level or if you have high blood pressure.

Periodontal disease has also been associated with miscarriage. If you have periodontal disease, the risk of miscarriage is more then three times higher than if your gums and jaw are healthy. It's not a mystery as to why. If arteries become inflamed, they deliver less blood, and you are thus more likely to have heart disease. Inflammation in the arteries to your uterus results in inadequate blood supply to your baby, and miscarriage.

I believe that the same plaque that causes tooth decay—that sticky coating of bacteria, saliva, and food deposits—also needlessly ages both your immune system and then your arteries. Regardless of whether or not the arterial-pothole theory is true, my "confounding factors" theory was definitively shown to be incorrect. What I didn't realize when I first read the data was that all the major studies done on dental disease and longevity had adjusted for the very confounding factors I suspected were actually responsible for the aging. Even after making allowances for these unhealthy choices, researchers still found a distinct relationship between the incidence of periodontal disease and shortened life span and reduced quality of life. Therefore, be aware that good oral hygiene is an important element in your RealAge Makeover.

We now think that strengthening immune or other mechanisms to prevent inflammation of arteries is key in preventing arterial aging. If you use statistical techniques that factor out low socioeconomics status as a cause of increased aging, then periodontal disease does not seem to increase arterial aging. I look at it the other way: people of lower socioeconomic status may not care for their teeth and gums as much or as well as people of higher status. As a result, they have chronic gum infections, greater immune dysfunction, subsequent inflammation, and a higher risk of arterial aging, heart disease, stroke, memory loss, impotence, miscarriage, and even wrinkling of the skin. Thus, one of the ways to mediate the adverse effects of lower socioeconomic status may be to take care of teeth and gums. At first I thought this goal could be accomplished simply by brushing and flossing. However, routine professional dental care, customized to the person's individual rate of plaque formation along the gums, is also an essential part of the protective process to can prevent plaque from making your RealAge older. Even with optimal brushing and flossing techniques, each of us develops the plaque around our teeth at different rates.

This new understanding of the importance of great dental care—both at home, and at the dentist's office—means we have another weapon in our RealAge arsenal. Chances are, the lifestyle choices regarding your teeth and gums that you should add to your RealAge Makeover plan are things you already know you should do. Brush your teeth with a fluoride toothpaste several times a day, especially after eating. If you cannot brush after a meal, chew sugarless gum. When you brush, make sure to brush your tongue to get rid of bacteria there. The best way to brush your teeth is to brush at an angle into your gums. Brush about two minutes each time. Some of the at-home ultrasonic cleaners prevent gum disease as well and clean your teeth faster. Two minutes of brushing into your gums, flossing every day, and seeing a dental professional periodically seem to be the best and most important actions you can take to prevent periodontal disease. Flossing may be the element of our daily routine that we are most likely to skip. Of all the men who've taken the RealAge program, only 16 percent say they floss regularly (at least four times a week).

In addition to this good self-care, there are other things you can do for the sake of your teeth and gums. One is to quit smoking—so there's yet another incentive for quitting smoking (see Chapter 6). Another is to learn to manage stress (see Chapter 7). And keep smiling, because every time you floss, you're making yourself younger.

What If You Get Cancer? How Does It Affect Your RealAge?

With rates of cancer so high in this country, you probably know at least one person who has had cancer, and you might know several. Or you yourself might be a cancer survivor. If so, you're probably wondering what effect your brush with cancer has had on your RealAge. The answer to that question will vary greatly, depending on what kind of cancer was involved. Some cancers attack the body quickly and aggressively. In contrast, some cancers grow slowly and result in little damage. There are numerous therapies including tumor removal, chemotherapy, immune therapy, and radiation which can often stop the spread of cancer throughout the body. Clearly, a diagnosis of cancer is not a death sentence. A person in his or her thirties might have a tumor removed and then live for another fifty years. The affect of the disease on your aging depends on your attitude and choices, the type of cancer you have, how it is treated, and how long you are free from cancer after treatment.

As a concrete example, let's consider a fifty-eight-year-old woman who has had a malignant lump successfully removed from her breast. There is no indication of significant spreading in the lymph nodes. At the time of the surgery, she has a RealAge of sixty-five. If that same woman undergoes chemotherapy and still shows no signs of tumor growth during the following five years, her RealAge would change as a result of having had cancer from being seven years older to being only two years older than her calendar age. The general rule is that the longer a person remains cancer-free after treatment, the less effect the disease has on his or her RealAge. Of course, if after consultation with her physician she chooses to do other healthy behaviors, such as eating 10 tablespoons of tomato sauce a week, taking an aspirin a day, and doing all three forms of physical activity, she can make her RealAge substantially younger than her calendar age.

Scientists have been working hard for decades to find a cure for cancer, but we have yet to find the magic bullet. That we haven't made huge progress is reflected in the rate of cancer deaths in our population, which has not changed significantly since 1970. One of the reasons scientists haven't yet found a cure is that the causes of the disease are often extremely complex. In fact, the term cancer describes a phenomenon—the growth of tumors—and defines a general category that contains a broad range of diseases.

However, even though we haven't managed to find a cure for cancer, we certainly do have treatment options. If a tumor is found early and can be removed surgically, in approximately half of the cases it will not reappear. And much of the time, treatment delays spread of a cancer. Once a cancer has metastasized, the likelihood that radiation or chemotherapy would actually stop the disease is only about 10 percent—not especially promising. Several new gene-targeting drugs, and drugs targeted to stop the blood vessel growth that is necessary for tumor growth, appear very promising. However, these drugs are still in development and are several years away from being standard treatment procedures.

Dr. Judah Folkman's wonderful theory that we may be able to prevent a cancer from growing by depriving it of new blood vessels has generated much study. A cancer can't grow if it doesn't have nutrients, so this stopping of the blood vessel growth is important wherever and whatever the cancer is. Although the theory is valid when tested in animal models of cancer, scientists have had two major problems in applying this theory successfully in human beings. The first is that we have trouble giving the drug in a way that actually stops the growth of blood vessels to cancer tissue. Only recently have scientists been able to target such blood vessels or the growth factors, signaling chemicals, and immune inhibitors that stimulate or allow such vessels to grow. The second problem is that all of us need new blood vessels from time to time. When we get a cut or break a bone, we need new vessels to grow to that area so we can regrow that skin, bone, or other tissue. Selecting only the vessels that feed a tumor and not those we need for other reasons is not an easy task.

Recently, a few biotechnology companies have had very strong success in employing this blood vessel treatment in phase II of Food and Drug Administration trials. At least two companies seem to have found a solution to the administration and selectivity problems. This is an exciting development that means we may be only a few years away from this dramatic and wonderful technology. In the meantime, we have to wait.

The best behavior, of course, is to avoid cancer altogether, and that means avoiding cancer-causing substances, avoiding nutrient deficiencies that lead to defects in repair processes, avoiding nutrients that increase propagation of cancer cells, and strengthening the immune system so that it can effectively scavenge early cancers. When you are as young as you can be, your immune system will be better able to wipe out any possible cancer cells in your body.

Food choices, vitamins, exercise, and prevention or management of stress are all key ways of slowing aging of the immune system. Let's consider one example of immune system aging—prostate cancer—and see what you can do if you do get it. Here is how one person is living with cancer.

The intriguing story of Michael M. illustrates the power of your choices. He found he had prostate cancer that had spread beyond the prostate. His prostate-specific antigen (PSA) levels were extremely high, even after his prostate was removed. If your prostate is gone and your PSA levels are still sky high, it means your prostate cancer has spread elsewhere. In Michael's case, at least to bone. But he didn't give up. He started researching and learned that saturated and trans fat may increase the growth of prostate cancer, and that lycopene, selenium, and vitamin E may decrease propagation of those cells.

Michael M. is still alive more than ten years after the discovery of his tumor, when most urologists wouldn't have given him two more years to live. His PSA levels have decreased steadily as he's changed his diet and habits, and done many of the things this book advocates to retard or reverse aging of the immune system. He avoids saturated and trans fats, and gets adequate amounts of folate; vitamins B_6, B_{12}, D, and E; selenium; lycopene; and sleep. He decreases stress and does all three forms of physical activity. He strengthens his immune system with uncommon passion and devotion and has not succumbed to his cancer. Instead, he has opposed it and has lived longer than anyone would have thought possible because his immune system has kept the cancer at bay.

The Immune System: The Final Word, or Just the Beginning?

The great news about the immune system is that there is so much we can do to keep it young and healthy so that it can efficiently perform its most valuable function—keeping serious disease at bay. Start looking at your lifestyle choices recommended to you by the computer or chart that pertain to immune system health, and consider incorporating a few into your RealAge Makeover plan. *All of us can do things to keep our immune systems strong and young, and there's no better way to prevent cancer and the myriad other autoimmune diseases that age us.*

Live Smart in the Aging Environment Around You

Choices That Can Give You a Daily RealAge Makeover

A RealAge Makeover Success Story: Donna S.

Donna S. was a thirty-nine-year-old woman who dreaded turning forty. She smoked and didn't exercise. Then she took the RealAge test and found her Real-Age was 44.4. She knew she needed help and gave me a call. She decided she wanted to be thirty-five. At first, she simply started walking every day. Then she started lifting weights. After three months she decided to try something really difficult, to quit smoking. With the help of walking, supportive phone calls, a medication and the patch (described later in this chapter), she was able to quit. She continued to get younger, and after thirteen months, she was more than nine years younger than she had been.

At Christmastime, Donna decided to visit a friend, Michelle, whom she hadn't seen for a year. To Donna's amazement, Michelle didn't know who she was. After Donna identified herself, Michelle said, "Oh, my God! You look twenty years younger," and then asked if she had had plastic surgery. "No, I just decided to give myself a RealAge Makeover. I lost all the wrinkles soon after I stopped smoking." Donna had transformed herself from a RealAge of forty-four to just under thirty-five in less than a year and a half. She not only felt younger but also looked much younger, too.

The world is full of hazards: some you can see, like an open manhole in the street, and some you can't, like radon seeping into your home. But giving yourself a RealAge Makeover helps you to live young, even in a world that isn't designed to keep you young—all it takes is a little thought and planning. Simple actions like buckling your seat belt and asking guests to step outside to smoke help you to stay young. So will avoiding accidents which, along with unintentional poisonings, are the third leading killer in the United States. Even though we don't equate accidents with aging, they can instantly decrease your quality of life. Other factors such as cigarette smoke, pesticides, or air pollution can also age you—not instantly, but over the long term. Whether by not smoking, avoiding illicit drugs, or having safe sex, you can help keep yourself young. Learning how to live safely in the world around you will make your RealAge as much as twelve years younger.

- I doubt you'll be surprised to hear that smoking makes you older fast. In fact, smoking can make your RealAge eight years older. It ages your arteries, increasing your risk of heart disease, stroke, memory loss, impotence, decay in the quality of orgasm, and even wrinkling of the skin, and weakens your immune system, promoting cancer, stroke, and lung disease. And just because you get your nicotine from a different source doesn't mean it's safer; smokeless tobacco (chewing tobacco and snuff) and cigar smoking can cause just as much damage as cigarettes, if not more. If you yourself don't smoke, but live or work in a smoke-filled environment, that will age you too; spending just one hour in the presence of secondhand smoke is the equivalent of your smoking four cigarettes.

  If you're a smoker, the best thing you can do for your RealAge Makeover is to quit once and for all. It's not impossible, and celebrating your "years-younger" parties, taking walks at lunchtime, and making bets with other quitters can all help you accomplish this goal. With a little preparation, you'll be able to ride out the roller coaster of stopping and starting while on your way to becoming smoke-free. The RealAge benefit of quitting smoking is that you get back seven of the eight years that smoking has taken from you. How's that for giving your RealAge Makeover a boost?
  Difficulty rating: Most difficult

- The vast majority—eighty percent—of all accidents are avoidable. So why age unnecessarily? Make a habit of taking proper safety precautions in everything you do, at home and on the job. It can help make your RealAge one to six years younger.
  Difficulty rating: Moderately easy

- Most people would never think that making sure to buckle up before driving off is a part of a RealAge Makeover, but it is. By taking routine safety precautions in everything you do that involves movement, such as wearing a helmet when biking, you can make your RealAge 0.6 to 3.4 years younger. You can't keep all accidents from occurring, but by taking such steps as wearing protective gear and buckling up, you can reduce their impact.

Difficulty rating: Quick fix

■ Air pollution, exposure to mold toxins or toxic chemicals, and living with high levels of radon or asbestos can dramatically increase your risk of cancer to that of someone five to ten years older. Learning how to recognize potential environmental hazards and avoiding exposure to toxins can make your RealAge 2.8 years younger.

Difficulty rating: Moderately difficult

■ Sex and drugs are the symbols of wild youth; the truth is that they can make us old, fast. But sex can also make us young, too. Having great sex within the confines of a mutually monogamous relationship is a great part of a RealAge Makeover. For those who are not in a monogamous relationship, practicing safe sex during casual sexual encounters, avoiding high-risk partners and knowing their sexual histories, and always using a condom correctly are all ways to stay young. In fact, having a lot (men) of high-quality (women) sex more than the national average of once a week makes your RealAge younger, a lot younger. Although these data are preliminary, several studies have indicated that having high-quality sex more frequently could make your RealAge two to eight years younger. We do not have enough data on masturbation to know if that practice provides a RealAge benefit. By not using drugs and seeking counseling if drug use is a problem, you can make your RealAge more than eight years younger.

Difficulty rating: Moderately easy to most difficult

It is easy to understand how damaging your arteries or weakening your immune system might make you older. But how do preventing accidents, avoiding environmental hazards, and reducing the risk of injuries help keep you young?

We are constantly interacting with the environment around us, and whether or not that interaction ages us is at least partly under our control. Your environment consists of everything that is not the body itself: the air you breathe, the city you live in, the food you eat, and the people you know. Learning to navigate through the world around you so that it doesn't harm you is one of the keys to staying young and avoiding disability. That means using some common sense.

Although we don't tend to think of wearing seat belts or bicycle helmets as related to aging, they very much are. Of course, if you're a parent, you need to protect not only yourself but also your children. When our kids were growing up, Nancy and I always insisted that they wear safety gear, and periodically checked that it was in working order. Even when they became teenagers and didn't think it was cool, we still insisted. One day, my son Jeff's friend CK came over to go rollerblading. He didn't have a helmet. They grumbled, but I wouldn't let them leave until he put one on. I felt like an ogre but later I was awfully glad. The boys went rollerblading near the deliveries ramp of the University of Chicago Library. It was well after hours, and they thought they would have the place to themselves. However, someone had parked at the bottom of the ramp and was now pulling out. Jeff and CK didn't see the car until it was almost upon them. My son escaped serious injury, landing on his wrist and knee protectors, but CK could not avoid the car and ended up on the front windshield.

Thank goodness he had the helmet on! It saved him from serious brain damage. His leg was broken in several places, but rehabilitating from even a multiple fracture is a lot easier than from a brain injury. Today he's a successful professional instead of a person living with neurologic disabilities, simply because he wore a helmet that day.

The harm caused by accidents isn't cumulative but sudden, the kind of "instant aging" all of us hope to avoid. As in CK's case, much of that aging can be prevented. Many accidents, particularly auto accidents, are fatal, and these fatalities can often be avoided. An injury from an accident can trigger a chain reaction that makes you give up other Age-Reduction strategies as well. For example, if you get into a car accident and aren't wearing your seat belt you might very well injure your back. That prevents you from staying active and exercising. When you quit exercising, you gain weight, so your LDL cholesterol, blood pressure, and stress levels all increase, and your arteries begin to show signs of age. Or you rupture your bladder in a car accident and need treatment for life. All of a sudden, you are living the life of someone much older. Just because you forgot to buckle your seat belt.

The same is true for toxins in the environment. Whether it's cigarette smoke in a restaurant or radon in your home, these toxins can lead to increased aging. When Nancy and I were buying our home, I was not really concerned about radon, but had learned to stipulate for its removal in the purchasing contract. (Radon, a naturally occurring gas, is a known carcinogen. It is the product of decaying radium and uranium in the soil, and can seep into a house from the ground below.) The real estate agent thought I was crazy, but I insisted on writing into the contract that radon testing be done in three places, and that if radon were detected, it would be reduced to an undetectable level as a condition of our purchase of the house. The sellers thought nothing of accepting these conditions, because they had lived in the house for eight years without a problem. They were very surprised to learn that the radon level in their home was very high. The irony is that a simple remedy could have brought the radon level down to what the Environmental Protection Agency considers safe. However, our contract required that radon levels be undetectable, and achieving that goal required more work. The extra cost was only around four hundred dollars, a small price for keeping yourself from getting older needlessly.

Take a little extra precaution when you're buying a home to make sure there is no asbestos, no radon or other pollutants, and no molds. It takes a little more effort, but most sellers will agree to your proposals. Avoiding exposure to known carcinogens, whether they are pesticides or asbestos, can help keep you young longer.

Tobacco: Where There's Smoke, There's Fire

Even the tobacco companies now admit that smoking is deadly. Smoking can be blamed for nearly half of all premature deaths each year, more than four hundred thousand. Smoking remains the greatest public health hazard we face. We all know that smoking can cause lung cancer, but we can't predict which smokers will get it and which will not. However, what is predictable from cigarettes is aging of the arteries, the most important aging effect of cigarettes. Every smoker will get it. Aging of the arteries inevitably causes wrinkling of the skin, impotence, and decay in the quality of orgasm, as well as heart disease, stroke, and memory loss. Whether they travel to your reproductive organs, skin, or heart, bad arteries cause the same problems throughout the body.

And the effects don't show up thirty years down the line but right now, today. You'll see new wrinkles in your face. Donna's story at the beginning of this chapter illustrates this point.

Smoking cigarettes ages the skin prematurely by two mechanisms; first it ages your arteries; and second, it decreases the ability of your lungs to provide oxygen to your blood. By these two mechanisms, smoking decreases the amount of oxygen that gets to your skin cells, causing them to age faster than they should. It also causes shortness of breath that results from emphysema. The lack of oxygen further ages your lungs by diminishing the ability of your immune system and lung protective systems to work normally, leading to a high incidence of respiratory illnesses, plus a loss of stamina and energy. Smoking clogs your arteries with inflammation that can lead to high blood pressure that further ages your arteries; it is a nasty positive feedback loop to make you older by making you more vulnerable to infections and raising your blood pressure.

For the American population as a whole, smoking makes us more than 250 million years older than we need to be. At $350 billion in settlements, the tobacco industry is getting off cheap. If we valued each year of life lost to cigarettes at fifty thousand dollars, the tobacco companies would owe us thirty-six times that settlement. If you're a smoker and have a pack-a-day habit, consider yourself eight years older. Think you're forty? Try forty-eight on for size. Think you're fifty? More like fifty-eight. Even if you smoke just four cigarettes a day, which is barely any at all, your RealAge is 2.6 years older. Even if you don't smoke but live with a smoker or work in a smoke-filled environment for just four hours a day, your RealAge is almost seven years older.

Recently laws have been passed that prohibit smoking in bars and restaurants in some localities, and the biggest winners are the employees. Senate leader Joe Bruno and the state legislators who pushed through the antismoking law in New York probably saved restaurant and bar owners and workers more than 4 million years of aging and hundreds of millions in lawsuits. And it's not only New York. As of the summer of 2003, California, Delaware, Florida, and Connecticut had statewide laws in effect to prohibit smoking in workplaces.

Beyond the Smoke Screen: How Smoking Ages You

If you're a smoker, you're probably tired of your family and friends nagging you to quit. You're probably sick of the self-righteous attitude nonsmokers can have and how hard-hitting they can get. And maybe some of your annoyance is a defensive reaction, masking a deep down fear that you can't quit. I don't blame you for having these feelings. And I know that lecturing never solves anything. So instead I will just give you the facts, explain how it truly is within your power to quit, and let you decide what to do. That's how I've helped 309 of 315 smokers to kick the habit. I'll simply present the studies and explain scientifically how smoking ages you. And I won't lie about it or candy-coat it. But my patients—even the ones who really struggled to succeed—tell me it's the best thing they ever did for themselves. And I can almost guarantee that you'll feel that way, too.

The process by which smoking ages the body is multifactored and affects the whole body. It causes inflammation in all the major systems and organs. Most of us now know about LDL cholesterol contributing to arterial aging (see Chapter 8 for the latest information), but most heart attacks, strokes, impotence, and memory loss occur in people with relatively or absolutely normal LDL cholesterol levels. Just like Michael Bishop in Chapter 5, I now also believe inflammation is one of the culprits—if not *the* leading culprit—of aging of our arteries, and smoking fosters inflammation of the arteries and immune systems. Scientists believe this inflammation allows LDL cholesterol to accumulate in the wall of the artery as plaque, even when you have normal levels (and to a greater degree if you have increased levels). In this fashion, smoking causes arterial and heart disease and is responsible for more than 80 percent of all heart-disease deaths in those under fifty. And, of course, smoking causes cancer, lung disease, and emphysema. In addition, smokers have more colds, pneumonias, and other infections than nonsmokers.

Smoking and Cardiovascular Disease

Cardiovascular disease is just one example of the many health problems caused by smoking. Doctors have known for decades that smokers suffer considerably more heart attacks than nonsmokers. Heavy smokers are ten times more likely to have heart attacks than nonsmokers. Studies have reported that as many as 40 percent of all stroke victims are smokers. Smoking is one of the top three causes of impotence and decline in the quality of orgasm in both men and women. Also, smokers have the same amount of wrinkled skin at age forty as someone twenty years older. All of these are signs of inflammation in the arterial system or aging of the arteries. How exactly does smoking cause aging of the cardiovascular system?

The inflammation of the arteries caused by smoking has three effects.

1. It causes swelling like the redness and swelling in your skin when you get an infection. The swelling of that artery in turn decreases the space inside the blood vessel for blood to flow through.
2. Inflammation thickens the artery with that swelling, increasing the swirling of blood.
3. Inflammation also causes potholes in the artery walls. These potholes are places where cholesterol and other precursors of fibriotic material can get beneath the lining and accumulate into plaques. Inflammation of the arteries thus inhibits the ability of arteries to expand properly, prohibiting the proper delivery of nutrients to all cells and sapping energy.

Why does it sap energy? When you use your muscles, you need nutrients. One of the ways the muscles get more energy is for the arteries to dilate. When the arteries to your muscles can't dilate, the muscles feel acutely tired and sore. Thus, you can't do as much, you feel older and *are* older. Even if you smoke only five cigarettes a day, the ability of your arteries to dilate is only 50 percent of

Table 6.1	The RealAge Effect of Smoking

FOR MEN:

History of Smoking*

CALENDAR AGE	Never Smoked	Ex-Smoker	1 to 19 Pack-Yrs	20 to 39 Pack-Yrs	40 or More Pack-Yrs
			REALAGE		
35	34.2	34.9	39.0	39.7	40.3
55	53.6	54.8	58.8	61.5	62.0
70	68.2	69.7	77.2	77.9	80.1

FOR WOMEN:

History of Smoking*

CALENDAR AGE	Never Smoked	Ex-Smoker	1 to 19 Pack-Yrs	20 to 39 Pack-Yrs	40 or More Pack-Yrs
			REALAGE		
35	34.1	35.1	38.9	40.0	40.6
55	53.9	54.9	59.9	61.6	62.2
70	68.2	69.9	76.0	80.2	80.7

*"Pack-years" quantifies a person's history of smoking in a standardized way. It is calculated as the fraction of a pack smoked per day times the number of years smoking occurred at that rate. For example, if you smoked an average of one-half pack of cigarettes a day for six years and then one pack a day for twelve years, your history of smoking would be $(0.5 \times 6) + (1 \times 12)$, or 15 pack-years.

those never exposed to tobacco smoke. This sapping of energy occurs even in passive smokers, people who are exposed to secondhand smoke.

Smoking also makes it more likely that bad (LDL) cholesterol will accumulate in the walls of the arteries. For reasons that are not yet clear, smoking reduces the level of good (HDL) cholesterol—the type that removes the LDL cholesterol—in your bloodstream.

One study found that women who smoked a pack and a half a day had five to seven times the risk of heart attack as women who had never smoked. However, no level of smoking is safe. Even women who smoked only one to four cigarettes a day were two and a half times more likely to have a heart attack than nonsmokers.

Smoking and Cancer

Lung cancer is the health problem most closely associated in people's minds with smoking. And more than 90 percent of lung cancers in the United States occur in the approximately 30 percent of the population who smoke. Smoking is responsible for more than 157,000 deaths from lung cancer annually. And, the impact of cigarette smoking is not gender-specific: both men and women suffer from the ill health caused by smoking. It is the most common cause of death from cancers, accounting for 31 percent of fatal cancers in men and 25 percent of fatal cancers in women. For women, the number of deaths from lung cancer is growing rapidly. Just five years ago, lung cancer was responsible for just 18 percent of the fatal cancers in women. Since the total number of cancer deaths was approximately the same, the increase in the percentage means that each year, every year, women are experiencing approximately 20,000 additional deaths from lung cancer. The increase in breast and lung cancer in women is directly related to the fact that women started smoking a great deal more about twenty years ago. Because of this increased smoking, women are fast becoming almost equal to men in aging and cancer deaths. So it's horrible but true, "You've come a long way, baby," as the ads so ironically says. For men, the percentage of cancer deaths caused by smoking seems to have peaked and has started to recede in parallel with the decline in smoking in men from its peak twenty-five years ago. Unfortunately, for women in the United States, the peak from smoking, and therefore suffering and dying from lung cancer, still lies ahead.

Among the 4,000 chemical compounds commonly found in cigarettes, more than 40 percent are known to directly interact with DNA to cause genetic changes that lead to cancer. Many of the components of tobacco smoke are oxidants—agents that promote chemical reactions with oxygen. Therefore, they also increase free radicals, the by-products of such reactions. Free radicals are temporarily unstable atoms or molecules with extra or unpaired electrons, which react with other atoms or molecules to produce yet another unstable molecule. Free radicals can cause inflammation and can damage our organs and DNA; they cause premature aging of the cells and promote cancers. Our body can get rid of them when antioxidants and some other molecules bind with unstable free radicals to make them neutral or stable. Then they can be washed harmlessly out of the body in urine.

Damage by free radicals to your DNA occurs with exposure to even a very small amount of cigarette smoke. In studies, dogs exposed to the smoke of just one cigarette—not even enough to increase heart rate, blood pressure, or other physiologic measures—had twice as much free-radical damage as dogs not exposed to cigarette smoke. This free radical damage is one reason that secondhand smoke is so harmful.

The effect of tobacco on the immune system is twofold. First, it contains toxins that damage DNA, causing cancers. In addition, smoking knocks out the body's two protective systems that fight aging of the immune system in general and cancer in particular (see Chapter 5). Smoking makes the immune system less vigilant about catching cancer.

Nitrosamines, by-products of cigarette smoking, interact with the body's enzymes to create a new chemical that is highly inflammatory and highly carcinogenic, or damaging to DNA. Some people have much more or much less of the human acetylator enzyme that helps the body remove certain carcinogens from the body. The "slow acetylators" who produce less of this enzyme than others are predisposed to breast cancer, as well as other kinds of cancer. There are always a few die-hards who smoke a pack a day from age eighteen and live to be ninety: a very few people are physiologically less susceptible to the arterial aging and carcinogenic effects of cigarette smoke than the rest of us. These people have higher levels of specific enzymes that deactivate the carcinogens contained in smoke. Don't assume you're one of those rare people who have better mechanisms for preventing inflammation and for fighting cancer. The ingestion of any tobacco product, whether through smoking, chewing, or inhaling secondhand smoke, increases aging of the immune system and of the arteries. The single best way to safeguard yourself against the carcinogenic effects of tobacco is not to use it at all.

Smoking, Lung Infections, and Emphysema

Smoking is a primary cause of emphysema and premature aging of the lungs. More than 2 million people in the United States (and possibly many more) suffer from emphysema, the fourth leading cause of death in the United States. Emphysema occurs when the air sacs in the lungs die. Scientists have long suspected that emphysema is caused by an autoimmune response, a chemical reaction in the smoker's body that causes the body to kill its own lung cells and air sacs. Normally, the immune response is well-gauged to react to the low-level assaults of everyday living. The immune system habitually kills off single cells that show signs of distress. When lungs are exposed to the constant irritation of cigarette smoke, this normally protective system overreacts. When many, many cells show signs of distress, the body begins to kill off its air sacs en masse, and this leads to emphysema. Cigarette smoke also inhibits the ability of the breathing tubes to clear secretions. Since smoker have decreased immunity because of the aging of their immune system caused by inflammation, they are more prone to respiratory infections. Because of the decreased immunity and decreased ability to clear secretions, smokers may get bronchitis, as well as many more respiratory infections, and may develop infections in those damaged air sacs. It's more difficult for such infections to clear up, because cigarette smoking increases carbon monoxide in the blood and decreases oxygen going to the heart, lung, and other tissues. Finally, when many of the cells needed for taking in oxygen and expelling carbon dioxide are gone, the smoker has a much more difficult time breathing.

Smoking and Other Aging Effects

As if all the serious health problems covered were not enough, smoking has been tied to other kinds of aging effects, as well. Smokers are at a higher risk of macular degeneration, an eye disease commonly associated with old age, at a rate more than two and a half times that of nonsmokers. Smokers are also twice as likely to get diabetes, and diabetics age at one and a half times the normal rate if the disease is just managed only typically (as opposed to with tight control of blood pressure and blood glucose and some exercise—see Chapter 12). For the over 10 percent of Americans with mild thyroid disorders, heavy smoking can trigger thyroid failure, seriously raising cholesterol levels and further accelerating arterial aging.

The dangers posed by smoking interact with other potential health problems, causing your odds of an event occurring to increase exponentially. If you come from a family with a history of heart and arterial disease and you smoke, you have fifteen times the risk of heart attack as someone from the same family who does not smoke. Similarly, if you have high cholesterol and you smoke, you have a risk level of a heart attack thirty-five times someone with high cholesterol who does not smoke. Alcohol and cigarettes are another deadly combination: people who both drink alcohol and smoke are at much higher risk of mouth, throat, and liver cancers than people who do either one or the other. Alcohol causes the body to make enzymes that metabolize tobacco smoke into highly carcinogenic substances.

A health event such as a heart attack could have devastating effects on your longevity and well-being. Most smokers are at least partially aware of how much they are damaging their health. So why do they keep smoking? The answer lies in the extraordinary power of an addiction to nicotine, which at times can feel overwhelming. So how do you give your RealAge Makeover—as well as your self-esteem—a huge boost by beating that addiction?

How to Stop Smoking the RealAge Way:
Getting Younger and Thinner
A RealAge Makeover Success Story: Dan W.

Dan W. was the lawyer for the mayor of a major city. But he had a problem. He smoked five packs a day. He would always have a cigarette in his hand. Sometimes he had one in each hand. He would almost always use one cigarette to light the next. When people saw him a year after I worked with him, and then two and three years later, they couldn't believe their eyes. They said that anyone who could get Dan to stop smoking, not gain weight, look so much younger, and be so much more vigorous must have a magic potion.

I have no magic potion. It's just a systematic process that has helped many people to quit smoking and regain their lives, and it can help you, too. It's a difficult process; I won't pretend it's not. Nicotine addiction is very powerful.

About two years after he stopped smoking, Dan called me. "Mike, do you understand what it is to quit smoking? I had a dream last night. I dreamed I died. It was a pleasant dream because when I got to heaven I was able to smoke. That's why it was so pleasant."

I asked Dan if he had ever had "just one."

"No," he said. "It was so hard to quit that I will never start again. I know that if I had just one, I would be hooked all over again."

And he was probably right. There are people who are genetically addicted to smoking. With just one cigarette, they are hooked. (If you dream that you don't mind dying because you can smoke in heaven, you are probably genetically addicted.) This is the case for about one third of the smokers I have come across. The rest are physiologically and psychologically addicted but don't have the same huge genetic predisposition. They are just as hooked, but for them it is both a little easier to avoid getting hooked in the first place and a little easier to quit. Make no mistake, however: quitting is hard for everyone. That's why nearly one in three Americans over age fifteen who smoke—30 percent of all men and 27 percent of all women—continue to smoke despite the warnings, and despite repeated attempts to quit.

Quitting smoking is difficult because cigarettes are so highly addictive—but that's just a part of it. Another reason is that it's so easy to justify waiting to quit tomorrow instead of today because we believe the ill effects won't occur until the distant future, so there's no urgency. But that is flawed thinking. Smoking zaps your energy and makes you look, feel, and actually be older today.

Talk about a RealAge Makeover—if everyone stopped smoking today, the health of the planet would be transformed. Thirty percent of all deaths related to cancer, 30 percent of all deaths related to cardiovascular disease, and 24 percent of all deaths related to pneumonia and influenza would be eliminated. But it's not easy. Of the 50 million Americans who smoke, 70 percent want to quit, and more than a third of them try each year. Unfortunately, only about 3 percent actually succeed. Fortunately, there's good news. Those who use the RealAge program on-line have had greater success in their efforts to stop smoking.

You're giving yourself a RealAge Makeover, and have learned to become aware of daily lifestyle choices. Well, smoking is a choice. Every time you choose to smoke a cigarette, you are making a choice to get older. By the same token, every cigarette you don't smoke—every time you fight that urge and win—is a choice you make to get younger.

Many people fear that they'll gain weight when they quit, but the technique we describe actually causes the vast majority to lose weight.

As I mentioned in Chapter 1, I first developed the RealAge concept to help a friend quit smoking. Those eight extra years caused by smoking were enough to make him sit up and take notice, and he kicked the habit. In the past eighteen years, Simon has gone from a RealAge that was fourteen years older than his calendar age (when all factors were considered; eight years older just from smoking) to one that is more than eight years younger than his calendar age. Back then he was forty-nine with a RealAge of sixty-three (fifty-seven just from smoking); now he's sixty-seven with a RealAge of about fifty-nine. He lives younger now than he did eighteen years ago, with much more vigor and energy than he ever could have imagined. If you are a smoker and give up the habit, you will get younger, too.

When I talk about a RealAge Makeover I talk about getting younger and healthier on both the inside and the outside, and about turning back the clock. Nowhere is this more obvious than when it comes to quitting smoking. While the effects of smoking are terribly insidious, they are also largely reversible if you quit soon enough. And quitting really does make most smokers look younger, just as it did for Donna S. The wrinkling caused by smoking seems to be reversible in a noticeable way within a year or two of quitting. Although smoking a pack a day makes a person eight years older in RealAge, cessation of smoking can earn back seven of those years. Of course, the number of years you smoked before you quit determines somewhat how many years you get back. The sooner you quit, the better. In fact, if you quit before you smoke twenty pack-years and before age thirty-five, you get back almost eight years that you aged. The net effect of being a former smoker is that a person who stopped a one-pack-a-day habit at age forty-five is only about one year older in RealAge by the time he or she reaches fifty. So, while his or her calendar age has become five years older, he or she is really two years younger (and maybe even more if that former smoker has adopted other RealAge Makeover strategies).

Although it often takes several weeks to feel better, the benefits of not smoking start almost immediately. Within just twelve hours of quitting, the body begins to get younger. Carbon monoxide levels decrease, and the blood can carry more oxygen to the cells. In only a few weeks, damaged nerve endings in the mouth and throat begin to regenerate, and the bronchial tubes begin to open. When the bronchial tubes start to open, coughing and clearing of secretions increases. You may feel as though you have a cold for as long as eight months after you stop, but that is really a sign that you are cleaning junk from your lungs.

Once you've gone two months without smoking, you can throw yourself a one-year-younger party. Go ahead, have a real chocolate cake—you'll see it's already easier to blow out the candles. After five months, you reach the point where the nicotine cravings subside, and you start feeling substantially better overall. (You no longer wonder if you are trying to fool yourself that you feel better; by five months, you are sure that you do feel—and look—younger.) The evidence that your immune system is getting younger and more efficient will be that you'll probably get fewer colds and other respiratory tract infections. The RealAge gain: two years younger. Within eight months, your lungs will be clearer and your stamina greater. After one year of not smoking, you will be three years younger. How's that for a wonderful gift to give yourself? A three-years-younger RealAge Makeover in just twelve months.

Some people recommend that after one year of not smoking, you get a fast spiral CT (computed tomography) scan of your lungs, a specialized procedure that uses x-rays to produce cross-sectional pictures of the body. This diagnostic test can show whether you have small tumors. About 2.5 percent of smokers harbor a tumor under 1 centimeter in diameter, and removing them can save your life. However, the benefit of getting CT scans after quitting smoking is still controversial, as 10 to 25 percent of people will get a false positive result. This could mean that they will get many follow-up x-rays their whole life, possibly without benefit. Because there is a risk as well as a benefit, and at present no clear preponderance of benefit over risk, each ex-smoker should discuss this matter with his or her physician.

In two years after you quit, your risk of having a heart attack or stroke will decrease considerably, and after five smoke-free years, your levels of arterial aging will return almost to the level of people who have never smoked. Your risk of developing cancer and other forms of immune system aging will equal the average risk of nonsmokers. Another way of saying it is this: if you give up a pack-a-day habit, you will become a year younger (and can celebrate year-younger parties) at two, five, eight, thirteen, twenty-two, thirty-two, and sixty months from the time you quit.

If you think you're too addicted to quit, you should know that I have seen patient after patient who felt exactly the same way, and then went ahead and successfully quit. One such person was Mary Jane.

A RealAge Makeover Success Story: Mary Jane

Mary Jane had been a smoker for thirty-five years, and it was taking a terrible toll on her health. She was asthmatic, diabetic, and sixty pounds overweight. She routinely missed more than her allotted number of sick days, suffering recurrent bouts of upper respiratory tract infections.

It wasn't that she didn't want to quit—in fact, she'd tried numerous times. But for every morning that she said, "I'm never going to smoke again," by the end of the day she'd be lighting up. Then one day, everything changed for Mary Jane. She found she needed a major operation. Her diabetes and asthma were both out of control, and it was clear to her that her health was in a crisis. The prospect of dying put it all in perspective. "In life, you have to make choices. I had to make the choice: Was I going to live or die? When you realize that the alternative is dying, quitting is not that hard."

Mary Jane started walking thirty minutes a day. About a month later she and her doctor agreed on nicotine patches and pills to helped ease her cravings. She stayed physically active and avoided situations in which she might encounter smokers.

This is not to imply that the process was easy. In fact, giving up smoking was one of the hardest things Mary Jane ever did. Those first few months were especially difficult. But finally being able to quit is not even the best part. She's also managed to get her diabetes and asthma under control, and she has lost sixty-five pounds. "I feel 100 percent better," she told me proudly. "I can't imagine going back to smoking again."

We celebrated Mary Jane's first year-younger party just two months after she smoked her last cigarette. A year later, at her third year-younger party, the company where she worked gave Mary Jane some of those days she used to take as sick days as vacation days—her reward for all the new energy she was putting into her job, and for sticking to her commitment to kick the habit once and for all.

Unfortunately, addiction is very powerful, and Mary Jane is only human. One day she decided to have "just one" and was immediately hooked again. However, within three weeks, she managed to quit a second time. She continues to fight the smoking urge daily, she says, but she is active, takes good care of herself, and gets a little bit younger every day.

No More Cigarette "Buts": Kicking the Habit

For most smokers, quitting is not a one-time event; it's an on-again, off-again routine. They stop. They struggle with it for a few days, weeks, or months. Then the craving gets to them and they decide, "What's one cigarette?" They light up, and then they're hooked again and back to square one.

Cigarettes are psychologically and physiologically addictive; we know that beyond the shadow of a doubt. In studies on smoking, laboratory mice learn what times of day they will be given their smoke exposure and at the appointed time race expectantly to the side of the cage where the smoke comes out. They need their smoke! Of course, having never been a smoker, I have never personally struggled with that addiction. But at this point I have helped and witnessed so many people struggle with (and overcome!) the nicotine habit, I do know that it's a major battle. At the same time, there's no better fight to win. People who successfully quit and stay away from cigarettes deserve a lot of credit.

It's taken years of research to start to understand exactly how and why the body becomes addicted to nicotine. Dopamine is a naturally occurring chemical that dulls the body's response to pain and produces a pleasurable feeling. Many addictive drugs, including cocaine and even caffeine, trigger a dopamine reaction. Studies using brain scans show that smoking triggers a release of dopamine in the brain. Unfortunately, the more you smoke, the more your body adjusts to a higher level of dopamine release. What used to be an elevated dopamine state is now normal, and so when you don't smoke, the body goes into withdrawal. The good news is that in time, your dopamine state goes back to normal, and you don't require those levels. The challenge is how to stay smoke-free long enough to let your body and brain readjust.

One of the problems with quitting is that at first you feel worse. For the first several weeks, you feel intense cravings and, since nicotine is a stimulant, rather sluggish. After a few weeks, those feelings will subside. Just stick to your guns.

There are many, many services and information sources that help smokers quit—from high-priced inpatient clinics to free support groups at community centers. If you are serious about quitting, talk to your physician, search out smoking-cessation programs and support groups in your area, buy a few books about kicking the habit, and consider pills and nicotine patches or chewing gum to help ease your cravings. Different methods work better for different people. Thinking about quitting in terms of aging may be just the ticket for you: eight years is a lot of time to lose for just one habit.

Only 2 percent of smokers who try to quit "cold turkey" can successfully stop the first time. Using nicotine patches doubles the success rate to 4 percent. One study found that combining the patch with anti-craving pills boosted the effectiveness to almost 60 percent. In my own practice, the success rate has been much higher: Three hundred nine of the last 315 patients who have tried to quit have been able to do so. Many have been pack-a-day smokers for at least a decade.

Since this book is about the effects of aging rather than the techniques for beating an addiction, I am not going to go into all the details here, but I will describe the program.

The first step is to start walking thirty minutes a day, every day—no excuses. Not bad weather, not fatigue, not lack of time, and not back pain—no excuses. Then, call someone to report that you did take your walk. The same person every day. At this point, you will still be smoking. That's all right; we don't want you to quit cold turkey. But we do want you to start walking. Walking for thirty minutes will not only help prevent weight gain when you stop but, more important, will also drive the message home that you have the discipline to quit. Of the 315 who have shown this discipline, 309 are former smokers, most for over three years now. Of the twenty smokers I tried to work with who wouldn't walk for thirty minutes a day, only six are now ex-smokers. Want to improve the odds? It seems to me you do when you walk thirty minutes and then call someone every day.

Then, after thirty days of walking every day, start taking Wellbutrin (bupropion). (There are contraindications to taking bupropion [such as high blood pressure and seizure disorder] so check with your doctor.) Take 100 milligrams (mg) of Wellbutrin once a day in the morning for the days 31 and 32. Keep walking every day, and keep phoning your support person to report that you're sticking to the plan.

Day 33 is your quit day. Throw away all your cigars, cigarettes, chew, lighters, ashtrays, and any other tobacco-related paraphernalia. On that day, put on a nicotine patch as prescribed by your doctor (these patches are available by prescription or over the counter). I recommend 7 to 10 mg if you smoke less than one-half pack a day, 14 mg if you smoke one-half to one pack a day, and 20 to 22 mg for a pack a day or more. For the few smokers I've helped who smoked more than three packs a day, I've prescribed two patches. At that time, day 33, I ask the (now) ex-smoker to start taking two Wellbutrin (100 mg each) pills a day—one in the morning and one in the evening. Keep walking every day, and phoning. Days 36 to 39 after you start walking—3 to 5 days after throwing away the cigarettes and quitting—will be the toughest. However, if you make it through day 39, you can look back and know you've survived the worst of it. The typical ex-smoker continues that regimen—walking thirty minutes, phoning your support person, two pills, and patch—with a few changes for six months: patch size decreases after two months and again after four months, and pills decrease to one a day, usually in month four after stopping, and to none after month six. The walking (with the addition of strength training after day 60; see Chapter 9) continues forever.

By combining exercise, supportive phone calls, the patch, and the pills with RealAge planning, my patients have stopped smoking and started getting younger. And you can, too. Consider joining a program provided by a smoking-cessation clinic or community support group. Ease the physiologic cravings by getting patches and pills, and ease the psychological urge to smoke by walking and developing a support system that will keep you away from cigarettes. Don't forget to include "year-younger" parties in your plan: you need to celebrate your successes.

Much of what keeps people smoking is addiction, but part of it is habit, too. So while you're kicking your addiction, you might find it also helps to change your day-to-day habits. Increasing the amount of physical activity you get helps reduce the craving for cigarettes, and an increase in breathing and heart rate helps some people visualize that they are getting the nicotine out of their systems faster. Changing the environment where you choose to spend free time can help, especially going to places such as museums, libraries, theaters—and, increasingly, bars and restaurants—where smoking is prohibited. Small changes in daily habits can send you and your brain a powerful message that things are going to be different this time.

As I've said, quitting is tough, but it can be done, and nothing will give a bigger boost to your RealAge Makeover. Consider the story of Eddie E.

A RealAge Makeover Success Story: Eddie E.

Eddie's wife had been diagnosed with esophageal cancer and died only a month and a half later. He was left with a teenage daughter to counsel and care for all by himself. He was despondent and desperate, increased his smoking to four or five packs a day, and started drinking heavily. Three weeks later, I received a call from a mutual friend who was concerned about him. I immediately gave Eddie a call.

Three months later, Eddie had not only been smoke-free for a month and a half, but he had started weight-lifting, continued walking thirty minutes a day, called me every day, and was now nine pounds lighter. One day, he commented, "You know, I took my blood pressure this morning. I can't believe it's down thirty points on the upper number and nine points on the lower number. But that's what you told me would happen; I just didn't believe you." That is exactly what happens: the system heals itself if you get active and don't smoke.

Eddie E. lost weight when he quit smoking; so did Donna S., and Mary Jane, and most of the 309, and so can you. Let's talk about how.

Stop Smoking and Lose Weight

One of the biggest fears people have about quitting smoking is weight gain. On average, men gain about ten pounds within six months of quitting, and women, about eight. (This applies to all successful quitters except those who take the RealAge Makeover program.) However, weight gain should be the very least of your worries. The dangers of smoking are far greater than the dangers of gaining six to ten pounds. Besides, the weight gain is often temporary. Women may gain eight extra pounds within six months of quitting, but they commonly lose six within the next eighteen months. With careful planning, you can prevent weight gain altogether. Here are some tips:

- Make walking a part of your daily routine. It helps fight cravings and keeps weight off. After sixty days (twenty-seven off cigarettes), begin doing strengthening exercises (see Chapter 9) for ten minutes every day.
- Chew sugarless gum to help ease oral cravings.
- Have lots of chopped vegetables and low-fat snacks on hand. Popcorn without butter is a good thing to munch on (see the recipe for "Simon's Popcorn" on page 309 in *Cooking the RealAge® Way*). Fruits, especially small ones such as grapes and berries, are also great snacks.
- Start a "celebration of year-younger birthdays" fund. If you were a pack-a-day smoker, you're now saving five dollars or more a day, and this becomes celebration money. You might want to spend it on daily treats you didn't permit yourself before, like fine bottled water, a fancy tin of breath mints, or a gourmet low-fat cappuccino at your fa-

vorite coffee shop. Even better, save it for the two-month, eight-month and so on year-younger anniversaries, and celebrate with a gift to yourself or a celebratory year-younger birthday party with friends. Or you might want to save up toward a bigger treat, like a cruise, a piece of jewelry, or a vacation at a bed and breakfast. As you watch the fund grow a little every day, you'll know that you're getting younger.

- If possible, try to stop smoking some time other than the holidays. All that rich food increases the temptation to overeat. On the other hand, ex-smokers tell me that any time you're motivated to quit, that's the best time to do it.

- Find something to do with your hands. Many smokers find comfort in having something to hold. Buy yourself a bunch of desk gadgets or other objects to fiddle with and divert all that nervous energy.

- When you feel the temptation to smoke, close your eyes and take a deep breath. Remember all the reasons you quit smoking in the first place. Keep a list of those reasons and add to the list as you discover new benefits of being a reformed smoker: "more energy," "fewer colds," "years younger." Call your support person and talk about the craving; start walking or lifting weights in a smoke-free area.

- After you've discontinued routinely taking the Wellbutrin pills for about six months, still carry a small pillbox that contains some of them. If you feel the urge to smoke, take a Wellbutrin, even if it's been months since you quit. Take it with a gulp of water and walk around for thirty minutes. If you still feel the urge, call your support person before you light up. Even if you fall off the wagon for a drag, get back on immediately. Do not have the second cigarette, ever.

- Don't downplay your accomplishment. Reward yourself for quitting. Being smoke-free is something to celebrate.

It helps to avoid not just the cigarettes, but anything you associate with smoking. For some people this may be coffee or alcohol. Others do not need to avoid these things and, in fact, find coffee or iced tea helpful. Others drink lots of water, fruit juice, and herbal teas. Eating several small meals instead of one big one keeps blood sugar levels constant, which helps quell the nicotine craving. Avoid behaviors and situations you associate with smoking. If you used to smoke right after meals, try doing something else at that time, such as taking a walk or doing the dishes. In addition, do positive things that boost your self-image. Go to the dentist and have your teeth cleaned. You might also have the dentist whiten them, or try some whitening strips yourself: remember, you're no longer a smoker. Have your smoky-smelling clothes cleaned at the dry cleaners. *Reward yourself.*

If you fall off the wagon and have a cigarette, it's not the end of the world. Don't use it as an excuse to go back to your old lifestyle. Instead, get right back on board. The fact is that each time you quit, your odds of being successful increase. Each time, you'll get closer to your goal.

And don't think you're too old to benefit from kicking the habit. Don't tell yourself, "I've smoked this long, why quit now?" Almost everyone, at every age, can benefit from beating a nicotine addiction. Smoking is to aging what putting the gas pedal to the floor is to driving. Even if you've smoked for ten, fifteen, or twenty years, you have a lot to gain by quitting.

Cigar Smoking

In the last decade, cigars became newly chic. Since 1985, cigar use in the United States has quadrupled. More than five billion cigars were sold in 2001 alone. That trend of rapid increase is finally starting to fade. Since cigar smokers smoke less frequently and do not inhale as much smoke, they often believe they are at a lower risk than cigarette smokers. They are wrong.

Cigars are a particularly dangerous way to smoke tobacco. Just like cigarettes, they produce benzopyrene, hydrogen cyanide, and ammonia. They produce more carbon monoxide and more particulate matter than cigarettes. The greater amount of particulate matter that cigars produce makes them more dangerous not just for the smoker but for those around him or her as well.

Cigars produce a more toxic form of secondhand smoke than cigarettes, so don't think that sitting in a cigar bar and not smoking isn't doing you any harm. And although cigar smokers claim not to inhale, this is often not true. Most former cigarette smokers continue to inhale when they take up the cigar habit.

Cigar smokers are more likely to get cancers of the lip, mouth, pharynx, and esophagus than cigarette smokers, and are about six times more likely than nonsmokers. Such cancers can often be fatal; and even when they're not fatal, they can age and disfigure you.

No comments, please, about Winston Churchill and George Burns. Although we don't know why these cigar smokers were fortunate enough to live so long (perhaps good genes or good habits), we do know that other well-known cigar smokers such as Babe Ruth and Ulysses S. Grant died young from throat cancers caused by cigars. Smoking one cigar a day makes your RealAge 2.6 years older. Smoking five cigars a day makes your RealAge eight years older.

Passive Smoking

No longer exposing your lungs to cigarette smoke—whether your own or others'—will give a big boost to your RealAge Makeover. If you are a smoker who has to kick a nicotine habit, you are facing a difficult but entirely doable task. If you are a nonsmoker who is exposed to secondhand smoke, you have a far less difficult challenge, with many of the same RealAge benefits. All it takes is some tact, perseverance, and a willingness to take a stand for the sake of your own health.

Start by making your house a smoke-free environment. Smokers—whether guests or family members—will have to step outside for a puff. While you may feel uncomfortable when you first implement this policy, the message you'll be sending is that you can no longer tacitly condone a practice that does so much damage to the people you care about. If you meet with resistance, you might talk about your RealAge Makeover plan, and how their secondhand smoke affects it. Once you explain that spending more than four hours a day in a smoke-filled environment can make your RealAge as much as 6.9 years older, they will better understand why you're insisting they step outside.

If it's your work environment where you are affected by secondhand smoke, it will probably be much easier to implement a no-smoking policy, because such policies have become so prevalent in the workplace. If your office doesn't yet have a no-smoking policy, talk to your boss or office manager about implementing one. If nothing is resolved, talk to your local board of public health or Better Business Bureau to find out if a local or state no-smoking ordinance exists. The federal Americans with Disabilities Act requires employers to provide a work environment that accommodates employees with disabilities. Therefore, employers must provide a smoke-free environment for employees who have asthma or are allergic to smoke.

Smokeless Tobacco

More than 10 million Americans use smokeless tobacco, and its use is on the rise. Over the past thirty years, its use has increased sixfold, making it the fastest growing segment of the tobacco market. Because they do not inhale smoke, many people think they are reducing their risk. Unfortunately, this is not the case. Although the risk of lung cancer is lower among people who use chew or snuff, the risk of other cancers is considerably higher.

Smokeless tobacco causes mouth and throat cancers, dental problems, cardiovascular disease, and nicotine addiction, just as cigarettes do. And since it causes nicotine addiction, it's just as hard to kick the habit. In fact, the amount of nicotine and other chemicals found in the blood of people who chew is even higher than that found in the blood of smokers.

Accident Prevention: Protect Your Youth

A RealAge Makeover Success Story: David Q.

Dear Dr. Roizen,
I have to thank you—you probably saved my life. I read your chapter about accident prevention about a year ago. I had a helmet that had a crack in it, so I didn't wear it very often, especially when biking around home. But after reading your chapter, I learned I could send the helmet back to the manufacturer and they would give me a new one, so I did.

Less than a month later, a car swerved to avoid a dog and hit me. I was thrown about twenty feet and landed on my head and shoulder. That new helmet saved my life. My collarbone and my arm were broken, but I'm rehabilitating and I'll be fine. Thank you for your warning.
David Q.

P.S. I have recently taken the helmet back to the manufacturer again because it got destroyed when I landed on it, and again they replaced it for free.

Although you might not have thought that avoiding injury from accidents is something you add to your RealAge Makeover plan, it certainly is. I hope that you will make yourself younger in this way as much as David Q. did by reading this part of the chapter. In 2001, approximately 150,000 Americans died from injuries; 61 percent of these were considered accidental deaths. Eighty percent of those accidental deaths were preventable. For American adults thirty-five to forty-five years of age, accidental poisoning (primarily drug overdoses), motor vehicle accidents, and firearm accidents are the first, second, and third major causes of death according to the National Center for Health Statistics. Motor vehicle accidents are the third leading cause of death among Americans under the age of sixty-five, producing more than 43,500 deaths and 500,000 serious injuries each year.

Not only do you risk aging and death in traffic accidents and in accidents such as falls (the second leading cause of accidental deaths) but also the injuries you sustain are likely to cause aging because they can make you less mobile and more prone to chronic pain. In addition, accidents tend to have a snowball effect. After being injured in an accident, a person may become chair- or bedridden, further aging him or her.

As a doctor, what I find maddening about the accident statistics in the United States is that so many accidents are preventable. For example, drunk driving is a leading cause of car accidents, accounting for about 40 percent of all traffic deaths and 9 percent of injuries (see Chapter 11 on alcohol use and abuse). Although we all know better than to drink and drive, too many of us still do it. The cost of a cab is nothing compared with the cost of your life. But we persist. Why tempt fate?

I ask that question every time I see a patient who gets hurt because he didn't bother to wear proper protective gear before trying to chop down a tree in his front yard. Or because he thought he'd impress his friends by popping a wheelie on his motorcycle. Or because she didn't think she needed a lesson before waterskiing for the first time. While many accidents are one-of-a-kind in their particulars, they often have one thing in common: lack of common sense. We all have a built-in alarm system—a feeling of nervousness or trepidation before an event when we know we're putting ourselves at risk—but we sometimes don't listen to that warning signal. If the little voice in your head says, "Don't do it," don't do it.

As well as protecting yourself, insist that your children use safety measures every time. I can tell you from personal experience that it's easier to live with yourself as an ogre than as someone who did not prevent a bad event. Don't let the accident-waiting-to-happen become the accident-that-happened. It's one of the best ways to keep yourself young.

Don't forget that you have to protect yourself at work, too, to keep yourself young for the time after work. Most Americans between age twenty-two and sixty-five (more than 120 million of us) spend 40 percent of our waking hours at work. Most jobs carry a certain amount of risk due to accidental injury—even the jobs we think of as very safe, such as desk jobs, where people sitting at a keyboard all day long are prone to carpal tunnel syndrome. And then there are the more obviously risky jobs, like being a painter on high scaffolding or window-washer (talk about aging events: my patient the window-washer was on a suspended platform outside the 38th floor at the Bank of America building when the 1989 earthquake hit San Francisco; he had to use his squeegee just to try to slow down the platform's rocking movement). Each year, 6,500 Americans die from work-related injuries, and 13.2 million suffer nonfatal injuries. Think about the risks you face on the job and the steps you can take to avoid them.

Make choices that help protect your youth. Is something that is possibly correctable at your job really worth getting older for? Why not try to correct it?

We've discussed safety as a general issue. Now let's look at specific areas of your life in which you can make good RealAge choices. Let's start with the biggest cause of accidents: transportation. Whether it's by car, bike, or motorcycle, you can make yourself younger while getting from here to there.

Seat Belts: Buckle Up, Youngster!

As we all know, a car crash can bring about devastating injuries in a matter of seconds. Every month, I see the victims of auto accidents as they are rushed into the operating room for emergency surgery, clinging to the last thread of life. Perhaps nothing brings it into focus like seeing one of your own there. A colleague of mine almost died; her child did die. A summer vacation in the mountains should have been perfect but wasn't. It was raining and the road was slick. Their rented van was winding up a curvy mountain road when a flash flood hit. The van hydroplaned and plummeted over a precipice. Everyone in the van was wearing a seat belt except my colleague and her child, who were thrown from the van. The child was killed, and my colleague suffered serious internal injuries and broken bones. The fact that she survived at all was a miracle. No one wearing a seat belt was hurt at all. This tragic story drives home a very clear message: buckle your seat belt, because it can save your life.

A recent study estimated that seat belts and air bags reduce the risk of severe injury by 61 percent. Simply using a three-point seat belt—one that crosses over both the lap and the shoulder—reduces risk by as much as 45 percent.

Because seat belts have a proven safety record, most states now require that you wear one whenever you are riding in a car. Strap on a seat belt every time you get in a moving vehicle, whether it's your car, a cab, or anything else with wheels. Don't think you need to use a seat belt in a cab or limousine? Just remember what happened to Princess Diana. I'm awfully glad it's mandatory in New York for cabs to have seat belts in working order. Although it's sometimes difficult to get them on, I routinely do it because it makes me younger and keeps me safe. Wear a seat belt even if you are sitting in the back seat, and make sure that all belts have both a lap and shoulder harness. Keep all seat belts in good working condition. If you have an older car, make sure the belts are up to standard, even if it means replacing the old ones. If you are under 5 feet, 2 inches tall, have a small frame, or have children who regularly ride in the car, check to make sure the shoulder harnesses fit properly. If they don't, have them adjusted. Don't deliberately slip out of the shoulder strap, either. The shoulder strap significantly reduces the amount of internal organ damage that would occur in an accident. Almost all of the deaths among adults have involved people who were not wearing seat belts.

A trip to your local mechanic should be part of your safety plan, too. Have your car inspected annually or every 5,000 miles. Have the oil, tires, and engine checked. If you are about to go on a long trip, a professional should inspect the car to make sure it's in good working order. Finally, by making safety a priority when shopping for a car, you are choosing to get younger. Look for cars with a strong safety record. It's worth a little more money for the added youth protection it provides.

Air bags are required in new cars. If you own an older car that doesn't have them, consider trading it in for a car that does. Air bags reduce the risk of death by 9 to 16 percent among drivers already using a seat belt, and by as much as 20 percent among drivers not wearing seat belts. Experts estimate that air bags have prevented approximately 56,000 fatalities and a lot more disability from head-on collisions over the last ten years.

In recent years there has been concern about air bags because in rare instances they have hurt or even killed the passengers they were supposed to protect. Despite these rare tragedies, car by car and accident by accident, air bags still prevent disability and save lives. They have been shown to pose a risk for only two groups: small children, and adults shorter than 5 feet, 2 inches tall. Another new safety invention is side air bags; if you're buying a new car, make sure it's equipped with them. They make the average driver 0.15 years younger, and the under-twenty-five male driver, almost a year younger.

Pregnant women can make themselves much older by "rushing" ahead in a car. This problem occurs especially during the third trimester when seat belt usage, steering wheel position, and even quick stops increase pressure on the uterus and fetal living environment. More than 4 percent of pregnancies are lost to auto accidents, most due to trauma in the last trimester. And most due to minor accidents (because of the increased pressure on the uterus caused by the sudden deceleration when braking suddenly). So it is especially important for pregnant women to drive or be driven slowly with real caution.

Another way to make yourself younger while driving your car is to stay within five miles an hour of the speed limit. It can make your RealAge three years younger. Apparently, this one is far easier said than done. More than 5 million people have filled out the full computer questionnaire that calculates their RealAge on our website. A vast majority admit to speeding on a regular basis. When asked if they would be willing to modify their behavior, most of them say, "No." Indeed, more people say that they would rather give up smoking than speeding! It is amazing that so many people refuse to budge on this one, because slowing down and staying close to the speed limit is a reliable way to keep your RealAge younger.

Try to drive for a while within four miles of the speed limit. It's not that difficult. As with many of the RealAge choices, sometimes it's just a matter of replacing one habit (speeding) with another (keeping closer to the limit). You'll get used to it before you know it. And if nothing else, you must always stay within fourteen miles of the speed limit. Accident rates and aging go up dramatically when you go fifteen or more miles over the speed limit. (And the answer is not increasing the posted "speed limit".) Indeed, for drivers under age thirty-five, the most frequent cause of auto accidents is speeding (see Table 6.2). For drivers over the age of seventy-five, the most frequent cause of accidents is unsafe or ill-timed left turns against traffic. Finally, if you can do so, use a cell phone only when you are not driving; using a cell phone when driving focuses your attention on the conversation. This diversion of attention increases the accident rate.

Motorcycles: Don't Forget the Helmet

We sometimes associate motorcycles with wild youth. The truth is, few things can age you so quickly. Five seconds is all it takes to go from "young" to "dead." A motorcyclist is thirty-five times more likely to be killed on the road than the typical car owner. Not surprisingly, most motorcycle deaths and serious trauma come from head injuries. Sometimes emergency room doctors crudely refer to motorcyclists as "organ donors," because so many victims arrive at the emergency room brain-dead but with the rest of their vital organs intact. It sounds harsh, but it should stimulate thought. The motorcyclists who do survive accidents often endure injuries that are disabling or crippling, including severe and multiple fractures, and loss of limbs, paralysis from spinal cord injury.

If you think such shocking and horrible injuries are rare, think again. In Syracuse, New York, we have two hospitals that have rehabilitation units busy just caring for patients who have been paralyzed from spinal cord injuries.

When it comes to your RealAge Makeover, riding a motorcycle may send you off in the wrong direction; it may make you older. If you can't resist the urge to use a motorcycle, try to avoid roads with lots of traffic, go at moderate speeds, wear protective clothing, and make the most important choice for youth—wear a helmet. Helmeted riders have 27 percent fewer fatal accidents, and 50 to 75 percent fewer head injuries, than nonhelmeted riders. Helmets don't make motorcycle riding safe, just safer. After California passed a mandatory helmet law, serious head injuries in motorcycle accidents decreased by 34 percent. In the

Table 6.2 — The RealAge Effect of Speeding

FOR MEN:

Driving Over the Speed Limit:

CALENDAR AGE	Less than 5 mph	5 to 9 mph	10 to 14 mph	15 mph or more
			REALAGE	
35	34.6	35.8	36.8	43.4
55	54.8	55.2	55.5	59.4
70	69.9	70.1	70.4	72.8

FOR WOMEN:

Driving Over the Speed Limit:

CALENDAR AGE	Less than 5 mph	5 to 9 mph	10 to 14 mph	15 mph or more
			REALAGE	
35	34.8	35.4	35.6	42.4
55	54.8	55.2	55.4	57.5
70	69.9	70.0	70.2	71.2

year after passage of a helmet law in Texas, the number of motorcycle fatalities due to head injuries decreased by 57 percent, and the number of severe head injuries in motorcycle accidents declined by 54 percent. In Italy, the law was revised to mandate helmet use for those over age 18 on motorcycles and mopeds (it had been required for those under age 18 since 1986). In the year following introduction of the revised law, in the Romagna region helmet usage rose from 19.5 percent to over 97.5 percent with strong police enforcement. And 66 percent fewer brain injuries requiring admission to hospital occurred. Do not wait for a law to make your RealAge younger. If you drive a moped or a bike or a motorcycle, take charge of your brain's age now.

Here are some other safety tips for motorcyclists: keep your headlights on at all times. The risk of fatal daytime crashes decreases by 13 percent simply by keeping the lights on. Always wear motorcycling gloves, which have special protection across the palms, because it's an instinct to put out your hands when you go down. If you do this with bare hands while going forty miles an hour, your hands will suffer terrible injuries. You should also wear heavy leather boots and thick clothing (heavy jeans and a leather jacket) when riding, keeping your arms and legs covered. This helps prevent injury to the feet, legs, and arms. I was shocked to learn from a television sports producer who had covered motorcycle races that professional motorcycle racers rarely finish their careers without losing at least part of a foot. That's not something to look forward to as you age.

It should go without saying that you should never drive or ride on a motorcycle when under the influence of drugs and alcohol, but unfortunately it apparently does not. True to the rebel image we associate with motorcycle riders, the rates of driving under the influence are much higher for motorcyclists than for those who drive cars and other types of motor vehicles. Of course, either statistic could be wrong, but driving any vehicle and alcohol do not mix. If you read the statistics from many states, you would think that alcohol-related driving accidents are decreasing. One reason for these statistics may not be due to a decrease in actual alcohol-related accidents; it may be that the rules about hospital reimbursement create a false impression. For example, hospitals in New York State are not reimbursed by insurance companies for auto accident victims if the accident was caused by alcohol. Therefore, if hospitals and emergency room doctors were to test all drivers involved in all accidents with injuries for alcohol and report all accidents in which alcohol played a factor, revenue for the hospital, emergency physicians, and their departments would decrease substantially.

So, of course, the natural response of the emergency room doctors is not to do as many alcohol tests, because they don't want either the hospital or their own payments disadvantaged. What's the result? The statistics show a 70 percent decrease in alcohol-related traffic injuries that probably doesn't really exist. Although new laws may be playing a part in the decreasing numbers, we have no way of knowing exactly how much of a decrease there is, as long as all the accidents in which alcohol played a factor aren't reported as such. But even now, more than half of those injured in motorcycle accidents have elevated blood alcohol levels, and more than 40 percent test positive for marijuana use.

Bicycling: A Hardhead for Youth

Exercise is a vital part of your RealAge Makeover, and perhaps you've added bicycling to your physical activity plan. Great. You'll burn more than 450 calories an hour just bicycling at a moderate pace, as well as making your RealAge as much as 6.4 years younger (see Chapter 9). On that very same bike ride, you can do something else that will help make you even younger still: wear a helmet. Wearing a helmet can help make your RealAge 0.4 years younger than nonhelmeted riders, when calculated at a rate of fifty days per year of bike riding.

Each year, more than half a million Americans will end up in emergency rooms because of bicycle accidents. Head injuries account for one-third of the emergency room visits, two-thirds of the hospitalizations, and three-fourths of all deaths. Also, cyclists who have head injuries are twenty times more likely to die than those who have injured some other part of their body. A recent study found that use of helmets by bicyclists reduced the risk of head injury by 85 percent, and reduced the risk of brain injury by more than 88 percent.

Does wearing a helmet mean you won't get a head injury? No. But it does make it less likely. In the event you do hit your head, see a doctor—even if you were wearing a helmet. Surprisingly, many cyclists who fall and hit their heads but don't have any other injury requiring medical care often do not go to the doctor. Head injuries can be very serious and often don't produce symptoms right away, and sometimes not for months or even years. If you receive a hard knock on the head, it's always best to have a physician look you over.

And once you've recovered, replace your helmet. Even though it may not look damaged, it could be. Many manufacturers have a crash-protection guarantee and will replace a helmet for free if you are in a crash, as the helmet manufacturer did twice for David Q. Helmets should be treated carefully, and not be exposed to extremes of hot or cold, which can damage them. Consider replacing your helmet every five years, as helmets can begin to deteriorate internally with time and use. The quality of helmets has improved so much in the last ten years that you should replace any other helmet now. And the helmets manufactured five years from now will probably provide even better protection.

Like your car, your bike helps you stay youngest when it's in top working order. Have it tuned up regularly and make sure you have good tires, the brakes work, and, of course, that the bike fits you properly. Try to ride on bike paths and avoid roads with heavy traffic. While both having a dog and going for a bike ride keep you young, don't bike with Fido's leash tied to your bike; that can increase the risk of a crash, making you older. Wear reflective clothing when riding on roads with automobile traffic, especially at night, and have reflectors or lights on the bike itself. You might even get a light for the back of your bike. Since you're making such a committed effort to make yourself younger, you might as well do these few small, easy things, too.

Other Precautions: Making Safety an Issue

As you get younger and have more energy, chances are you'll keep adding to your RealAge Makeover with new activities, hobbies, and sports. That's terrific. Just make sure you do so with the proper equipment and training. No matter what the activity, if there's a chance of head injury, wear a helmet. If you play a racket sport or basketball, wear eye protection. All you have to do is look at professional basketball players with their wraparound glasses, or professional bikers with their helmets on, to know that the people at the top of the game take safety seriously. Even (especially!) sports like skateboarding require safety precautions. Enter any emergency room on a nice Saturday afternoon and you will see skateboarders and rollerbladers who forgot to put on their kneepads, wrist guards, or helmets. Boating accidents are another common source of injury, often because people forget that drinking-and-driving rules apply to the waterways, too.

The Air You Breathe: Aging Pollutants

According to a 1991 report by the Environmental Protection Agency (EPA), 164 million Americans, fully two-thirds of the population lived in areas where outdoor air quality did not meet federal air quality standards. Luckily, it appears that since then the situation has improved. The data released in 2004 by an independent organization indicate that in the time since, there has been a significant decrease in the percent of United States population living with outdoor air that does not meet the 1991 standards (more than 80 percent of the areas have improved). Still, most of us are affected by aging due to pollution. How much? That depends on where you live.

The effects of pollution are difficult to quantify, because air quality varies so much from day to day, area to area, and even block to block. If one were to generalize about the effects of pollution by comparing the deaths from all causes in areas with heavy pollution with the deaths from all causes in areas with little pollution, the RealAge difference would be 2.8 years. That statistic, though, can be misleading, as different pollutants have different effects on health. (In addition, in heavily polluted areas, other factors may affect the death rate as well, such as a higher population density or increased crime.) Nevertheless, pollution appears to have a measurable aging effect. The outdoor air pollutants of greatest concern to the EPA are ozone, carbon monoxide, nitrogen dioxide, sulfur dioxide, and lead. Other less-regulated pollutants of concern include volatile organic compounds, dioxins, asbestos, and particulate matter. While data exist to correlate increased amounts of each of these pollutants to increased mortality rates, particulate matter is now believed to be a major source of increased death and disability rates in the United States and around the world. While the United States spends hundreds of millions of dollars on ozone reduction, particulate matter—especially in the 2.5 micron range or smaller (referred to as "$PM_{2.5}$")—is quietly responsible for the death of a hundred times more people than ozone, and disability of even greater numbers. This is why the federal government is getting ready to issue new regulations regarding particulate matter that will greatly affect outdoor air quality. These particulates are produced by combustion of diesel, gasoline, and other carbon-based fuels, and by burning of tobacco.

Air pollution can aggravate arterial and respiratory problems. A report in the *British Medical Journal* found that changes in the level of air pollutants—specifically, ozone and black smoke, a major source of $PM_{2.5}$—led to an increase in the rates of deaths from all causes, primarily because of an increase of as much as 5 percent in cardiovascular and respiratory aging. Air quality may also have a significant effect on the development of asthma, a disease that affects as many as 20 million Americans.

Recent data show how air pollution produces asthma, and it's quite surprising. Small particles from the polluted air get deep into the lungs. Even though the immune system responds, the particles impair immune function. That impairment allows infections to occur, which results in damage to lung tissue, and subsequent asthma. So pollution doesn't directly produce asthma, but instead causes immune dysfunction that allows infections to succeed in damaging the lung, which in turn leads to asthma. Asthma rates are increasing in intensely urban areas such as the inner-city areas of New York and Chicago, suggesting that poor air quality's ability to trigger the onset of asthma is a concern that actually can and does affect and age large numbers of us. Air quality also affects the number of sinus infections and respiratory illnesses people suffer.

Particulate matter differs from ozone, carbon monoxide, and other pollutants in that the term does not refer to a specific chemical but rather a very complex mixture of numerous particles of varying sizes and chemical properties. In general, the higher the concentration of particulate matter of a certain size, the more likely you are to prematurely develop heart and lung disease. The smallest and midsize particles seem to be the most potentially injurious. Particles that are 10 microns or less in diameter (PM_{10}) are the most easily transported via air—larger particles fall to the ground quickly—and therefore are the most commonly measured particles when air pollution is analyzed. Of these, particles in the range of 0.1 to 10 microns are most readily breathed in and retained in the lungs. Particles smaller than 0.1 micron but greater than in the nanotechnology range are breathed in and out, and thus not retained in the lung. (Nano-

Table 6.3	The RealAge Effect of Air Pollution

FOR MEN:

Effect of Exposure to the Following Concentration of Air Pollution Particles (PM$_{2.5}$ to PM$_{10}$) per Cubic Meter of Air (μg/m^3)

CALENDAR AGE	Less 9	9 to 12.6	12.6 to 15.8	15.8 to 17.4	More than 17.4
			REALAGE		
35	34.2	34.7	35.0	35.2	35.4
55	52.8	54.4	55.0	55.2	55.6
70	68.8	69.2	70.0	70.2	70.7

FOR WOMEN:

Effect of Exposure to the Following Concentration of Air Pollution Particles per Cubic Meter of Air (μg/m^3)

CALENDAR AGE	Less 9	9 to 12.6	12.6 to 15.8	15.8 to 17.4	More than 17.4
			REALAGE		
35	34.5	34.7	35.0	35.1	35.3
55	53.0	54.6	55.0	55.1	55.5
70	68.9	69.3	70.0	70.2	70.7

You can obtain the numbers for your specific area by consulting the EPA's website *www.epa.gov/ ttn/airs/airsaqs/archived%20data/downloadaqsdata.htm* (look at the PM 2.5 pollution numbers for any of 594 metropolitan statistical areas—called MSAs—in the U.S. for the current up-to-the-day data).

technology, a hot trend at present, refers to the development and use of devices that have a size of only a few nanometers, a nanometer being one billionth of a meter.) These greater than nanotech but less than 0.1 micron particles do not seem to cause immune dysfunction in the lung, making them less of a problem. Particles greater than 10 microns rarely make it into the lungs—the cilia in your airways block their entrance and clear them out. The most recent research focuses upon particles in the 2.5 and smaller micron range (PM$_{2.5}$) as perhaps being the most important for human disease (see Tables 6.3 and 6.4).

While outdoor air pollution has historically received the most attention, I believe the data and rapidly growing concerns over indoor air quality will force a change in our focus and priorities. Research now indicates that indoor air quality could be five times more aging for us than outdoor air. The news media regularly report mysterious cases of "sick building syndrome" and the debate of indoor mold and mold toxins is front-page news. Unfortunately there is much still to be learned about the causes of indoor air pollution, but one thing is clear. Air pollution does not only occur outdoors. Particulates have a remarkable ability to go everywhere, especially those which are the smallest, very difficult to see, and most dangerous for human aging. Indoor air quality can be worse since in some systems, the indoor air is not be diluted with the outdoor fresh air. Watch out for toxic fumes that come from household cleaning fluids, laundry detergents, exterminator pesticides, garden sprays, dry cleaning and rug cleaning fluids, and other household products. Tobacco smoke can add particles in the 0.1 to 2.5 micron range. "Building sickness," essentially a malady caused by poor indoor air quality, is a real illness. Workers in poorly ventilated buildings have more respiratory infections, and complain of fatigue, headache, and nausea. If you work or live in a building that could be causing health problems for you, have the building checked.

A particularly notorious indoor pollutant is radon. Reports in the *Journal of the National Cancer Institute* and by the National Research Council (NRC) estimated that exposure to radon contributed to 10 to 12 percent of lung cancer deaths. Smokers are at particular risk, because smoke and radon interact. The NRC report estimated that 6 percent of American homes had excessively high levels of radon. How do you know if your home is one of them? Remember, Nancy and I had the requirement of testing and remediation written into our contract before buying our house; you can probably do so, too. If you already own your home, you can buy a radon testing kit at your local hardware store for about fifty dollars. Choose one that is certified by either the EPA or the state. The best variety are called "alpha-trak" or "electre." Alpha-trak versions, which are used for ninety days, give a better reading than short-term monitors. Short-term monitors do not track changes in gas levels that can vary over the year. If your house has high levels of radon (over 4 picocuries of radon per liter of air), call the local public health board or the EPA hot line (1-800-426-4791) to find out how to fix the problem. The usual remedies include having the basement foundation properly sealed, and having appropriate ventilation systems installed. For our house, three systems were required, but the radon levels are now below the lowest detection limits.

Asbestos is another indoor pollutant that has been associated with higher incidences of lung cancer and other cancers. Asbestos is found in many houses and apartment buildings, especially those built in the 1940s through the 1970s,

Table 6.4 The Ten Worst Metropolitan Areas in the United States (2002)

Highest Concentration of Air Pollution (PM 2.5s)

	AVERAGE ANNUAL PM 2.5 CONCENTRATION (Gm/M³)
Riverside–San Bernardino, California	27.4
Bakersfield, California	24.1
Los Angeles–Long Beach, California	24.0
Visalia–Tulare–Porterville, California	23.2
Fresno, California	21.6
Pittsburgh, Pennsylvania	20.3
Detroit, Michigan	19.8
Baltimore, Maryland	19.1
Modesto, California	18.7
Merced, California	18.7

Highest Annual Per Capita Death Rates Attributable to Air Pollution

	DEATHS PER 100,000
Visalia–Tulare–Porterville, California	123
Bakersfield, California	122
Fresno, California	115
Riverside–San Bernardino, California	95
Stockton, California	93
Los Angeles–Long Beach, California	79
Steubenville, Ohio/Weirton, West Virginia	78
Las Vegas, Nevada	76
St. Joseph, Missouri	76
Phoenix, Arizona	74

Other cities and areas among the top fifty for premature deaths attributable to particulate matter air pollution include: Spokane, WA (ranking, 14); Cleveland, OH (20); Reno, NV (20); Tampa–St. Petersburg, FL (22); Philadelphia, PA (25); Pittsburgh, PA (28); San Diego, CA (28); Providence, RI (32); Omaha, NE (34); St. Louis, MO (34); Chicago, IL (37); Detroit, MI (37); Nashville, TN (37); Atlanta, GA (44); and Mobile, AL (46).

Data on mortality pertain to 1990–1994 and are taken from the 1996 publication of the National Resources Defense Council, *Breathtaking: Premature Mortality Due to Particulate Air Pollution in 239 American Cities.*

when asbestos was a major component of many building materials. Asbestos is found in insulation used to wrap water pipes, in certain kinds of flooring, textured paints, old roofing materials, and elsewhere. Asbestos is not a risk as long as it is contained in a properly sealed wrapping. However, those protective wrappings can crack with age, causing asbestos fibers to leak into the air. As airborne fibers, asbestos particles are extremely carcinogenic. Because it is so expensive to have asbestos removed from your home, most experts recommend leaving it alone unless it is exposed. There are ways of sealing asbestos-containing material so that they present no health risk. For more information, call your local health board or the EPA at the number provided above.

Mold is another indoor pollutant that's gotten a lot of press lately, perhaps for good reason. While there is much research yet to be done, there is growing concern over mold endotoxins (mold, dust mites, or other small and inhalable "body parts") and mycotoxins (biochemical toxins produced by molds to weaken or kill the organisms they live on or compete with). While the indoor air quality community debates whether or not "toxic mold" is a real problem, the Food and Drug Administration (FDA) and veterinary doctors everywhere worry very much about the ingestion of mycotoxins by humans and animals. A large number of mycotoxins have proven carcinogenic when ingested in quantity, and a few of the most recent studies have shown that when inhaled, these toxins are at least ten times more potent. Perhaps the most sobering fact is that two mycotoxins—aflatoxin and the tricothecene T-2—are considered by the U.S. military to be among the most likely biochemical warfare agents to be used by terrorists. A large body of data exists proving that when exposed to large quantities of mycotoxin over a short amount of time, animals suffer greatly; however, little information exists concerning the low-dose, long-duration exposure to these particles. It took over seventeen years to find that one of these mycrotoxin molds—aflatoxin, that grows on peanut shells—could cause liver cancer. These are difficult causes to determine; for example, if the mold that breeds in Roquefort cheese causes cancer twenty years later in one of twenty people eating a certain amount of it, it would be difficult to attribute such specifically to that mold. The data are still too new and still too sparse for us to be able to say clearly how much aging mold and mold toxins cause. I believe we will find this to be a significant source of human disease (including autoimmune disease) and aging. Obviously, airborne indoor mold can cause disability and aging. So you want to ensure that places where you spend a lot of time are free of mold.

Smoke and carbon monoxide are other indoor pollutants can cause aging and even death. These are a particular risk at home. About 15 percent of all adult deaths from poisoning are due to the inhalation of carbon monoxide or gas. Buy a smoke detector and keep it in good working order, with fresh batteries installed. Smoke detectors have been shown to reduce the risk of death and injury from smoke inhalation by as much as 70 percent in home and apartment fires. Having a carbon monoxide monitor in the home is another quick and easy way to protect your youth. A recent study by the Centers for Disease Control found that having a functioning and well-maintained carbon monoxide monitor could cut the risk of inadvertent carbon monoxide poisoning in half. Because deaths from carbon monoxide poisoning and smoke inhalation are relatively rare, the RealAge benefit is just six to ten days. Nevertheless, why risk that kind of aging when having two silent monitors can protect you?

Motorboat engines produce huge amounts of carbon monoxide if they're in relatively closed spaces. So don't stand behind the motorboat when it is first started, and don't stay behind it even if you are planning to water-ski. Make sure you're out in a clear area and not so close to the exhaust of the motorboat that you could get a lungful of carbon monoxide.

One of the hazards we may be facing in the future comes from nanotechnologies. The particles spun off by nanotechnology production and research are extremely tiny. In studies, these particles were able to radically hinder immune function, because they can get deep into the lungs. There they cause inflammation and inhibit immune function. Nanotechnology processes produce particles that are undetectable by normal mechanisms. You can't see them like the smog of a bad day in the Los Angeles basin or in Hong Kong, but I fear that those particles may be able to cause major aging problems. This nanotechnology particle problem is only speculation on my part and not yet grounded in hard science. I just believe that this is a logical conclusion, because of the tiny sizes involved and ease of tiny particles to move deep into the lung and cause immune dysfunction.

We've considered what you can do to minimize aging from toxins, pollution, and accidents. Now let's look at two subjects that are often considered taboo, but are a part of everyday life for many people: sex and drugs. When it comes to your RealAge Makeover, illicit drugs are a no-no. They make you older. But sex is a different story. Safe sex, quality sex, makes you younger. We say "all things in moderation" but when it comes to sex, the more, the better!

Sex and Drugs: A Prescription for Youth?

Nineteen ninety-six marked the year the first "baby boomers" turned fifty. Those who grew up during or after the age of "sex, drugs, and rock 'n' roll" now outnumber those who came before. Which means that sex, drugs, and rock 'n' roll aren't just for kids anymore. Fifty percent of Americans between the age of fifteen and sixty admit to having tried an illegal drug at least once. Also, the person who spends a lifetime with just one sex partner is increasingly rare. Just how do sex and drugs affect our RealAge Makeover plan?

Safe sex is great for you, but unsafe sex can age you. By enjoying sex within the confines of a mutually monogamous relationship, by practicing safe sex during casual sexual encounters, by avoiding high-risk partners, by knowing your partner's sexual history, and by always—and correctly—using a condom, you can make your RealAge as much as 0.9 years younger. (It may be even more if we consider the benefits of avoiding the chronic inflammation of our arteries that sexually transmitted diseases (STDs) can cause.) Also, having lots of safe sex can make you even younger. Having sex at least twice a week can make your RealAge 1.6 years younger than if you had sex only once a week. Having sex more frequently than that might make your RealAge younger still. By avoiding drug use and seeking counseling if drug use is a problem, you can make your RealAge more than eight years younger.

Sex: The Most Fun You Can Have Getting Young

Giving yourself a RealAge Makeover means that you'll have more energy, feel better about yourself, and—with healthier arteries—have a better quality of orgasm. All of these things lead up to one thing: the potential for a better sex life. But is more sex a good thing? Absolutely. Sex is one of life's greatest pleasures, and not one that we want to give up because we're too old. It helps us be emotionally, physically, and mentally satisfied. Remaining sexually active will help make your RealAge younger no matter what your calendar age. Why? Sex decreases stress, relaxes us, enhances intimacy, and helps form the foundation of strong and supportive personal relationships.

No matter what your calendar age, nineteen or ninety, sex is a great age reducer. Nevertheless, there are risks associated with sexual behavior. With the increase in divorce rates, the relaxation of social roles, an increase in sexual freedom, and changes in gender expectations, more and more of us have chosen and may choose to have sex with more than one person over our lifetime. However, having multiple partners or not practicing safe sex puts us at increased risk of sexually transmitted diseases. Some STDs are life-threatening—acquired immunodeficiency syndrome (AIDS), for example. Others are less deadly or do not cause immediately identifiable symptoms, but nevertheless have long-term health consequences. Exposure to human papillomavirus, for example, while causing no problems in the short run, increases the risk of cervical cancer later in life. Learning how to have fun while keeping safe is the key to getting the most out of your sex life.

Sexually Active: Quality for Women and Quantity for Men Make the Difference

Ever wonder if you have sex more or less frequently than most other people? Surveys show that the average sexually active American has sex about once a week (fifty-eight times a year, to be precise), although there is clearly variation among individuals. Married people tend to have more sex than single people. The frequency of sex also varies with age and economic, social, and ethnic status. One of the first studies to track again longitudinally, done at Duke University beginning in the 1950s, found that the frequency of sexual intercourse (for men) and the enjoyment of intercourse (for women) correlated with longevity. In other words, people who had more sex of higher quality more often, lived longer.

Other studies found that sexual satisfaction became a predictor for the onset of cardiovascular disease: both men and women who were less satisfied with their sex lives were more likely to have premature aging of the arteries. Although the early studies provided thought-provoking insights, they unfortunately failed to provide accurate data. They did not control for confounding factors and failed to consider underlying physiologic factors. Some new studies are beginning to fill in the gaps, although the data are still not conclusive.

The Caerphilly, South Wales, study suggests that men who have sex considerably more than the average once a week—more than two orgasms a week—have lower death rates from all causes combined. In RealAge terms, they stay younger longer. The results suggested that there might be a relationship: the more sex a person has, the less aging he or she will undergo. This study is preliminary, identifying only a correlation between sex and longevity and not a cause-and-effect relationship. Unfortunately, the study takes into consideration only men, and not women. In addition, the study only asked about orgasms, so we do not know if a mutually monogamous partner was involved. We do not have data from other studies to know whether masturbation is a benefit for those who do not have partners. Nevertheless, the Caerphilly study is the largest and strongest proof we have that quantity of sex for men can actually help men get younger, and stay younger. If the numbers from this study prove to be correct, we can say that having sex twice a week (twice the national average) can make a man's RealAge 1.6 years younger. If we extrapolate linearly, as the early evidence suggests that we can, the person who has sex almost every day (350 times a year) and is happy with his or her sex life could have a RealAge as much as eight years younger.

It's always surprising to me when I look at these studies on sexual happiness and quantity of orgasms to find that an increase in quality for women and quantity for men reduces all three types of age-related disease. Why should more sex—or higher-quality sex—decrease accidents, and why should it decrease immune aging? It seems that great sex should relieve stress and decrease cardiovascular aging, but maybe companionship, or satisfaction with life, or the lack of stress decreases all three major categories of age-related disease. However it works, I believe so much in the therapeutic value of sex that I have even prescribed it for several of my patients, going so far as to write it out on a prescription pad! What these patients needed wasn't another exercise or another vitamin or supplement pill, but more sex to keep them young.

Joe J. came to see me for an intensive one-day health planning session. He had completed his RealAge survey in advance. I saw how healthy he was and how good he was at making choices that were beneficial to his RealAge, which was fourteen years younger than his calendar age of forty-eight. In fact, he was in such great shape I wondered why he had come to see me. It turned out that he wasn't satisfied with his sex life. His wife didn't want as much sex as he did, even though she was physically fit and had a RealAge that was much younger than her calendar age. He said, "Doc, I came to see you because I read in *RealAge* that you'll write a prescription for more sex. Would you do that for me? My wife takes doctors' orders very seriously. I know she'll want me to do whatever the prescription says."

I wrote the prescription and also arranged for them to see a sex therapist. I've seen him every year since, and he seems much happier than before. He says they are enjoying what the therapist and Joe and his wife all call "Magnificent Sex" now. Do you wish all RealAge Makeover plans were so much fun? They are. Just try them and see.

By the way, more than one woman has come to see me for that prescription as well. In fact, one uttered the most unanticipated line I have ever heard in that setting: she was separated from her husband and wanted a prescription for better quality sex. After a serious conversation about the need for her and her spouse to see a therapist together and the options for doing so, I wrote the prescription she wanted: "Higher Quality Sex whenever desired." She neatly folded that prescription with the other two I had written for her, and then calmly asked me what pharmacy she should go to fill that prescription. I had to be picked up off the floor I was laughing so hard.

Sex-ercise

Sex is an important part of your RealAge Makeover. So is exercise. And sometimes my patients hope to combine them. I'm often asked, "How much of a workout do you get from having sex?" The answer is that men and women get various workouts depending on position, vigor, and duration, but the calories spent per orgasm are about the same. During their sex studies in the 1950s, Masters and Johnson found that both men and women burn seven to twenty-five calories per orgasm.

Unfortunately, very few studies have been done since then, so more recent data are lacking. Some recent studies do show that sex is good for cardiovascular health. However, there is little information on sexual interactions that do not include orgasm, or on the differences between women and men.

Sexually Transmitted Diseases:
The Downside of Sex

You are probably barraged with sexual images in the media, some of it quite explicit. Unfortunately, when the media tackles actual facts about sex, it isn't explicit enough. While the tragedy of the AIDS epidemic has made us all aware of the concept of "safe sex," we still have a Puritan streak that often keeps us from talking frankly about the actual nuts and bolts of sex. This shyness helps no one, because your health, and even your life, can be at stake.

As we all know, the safest sex is with a disease-free partner in a mutually monogamous relationship. For some people, though, this is not a realistic option. The next best thing is to use condoms. Using a condom every time you have intercourse, and using it correctly, drastically reduces your risk of contracting an STD.

Making careful choices when it comes to sexual partners is a key element of safe sex. Intravenous drug users, men who have sex with men, and ex-convicts and their sex partners—no matter what their gender—are all at higher risk. Get to know your potential sex partner before you actually have sex. Talk to your partners about their sexual history, and about yours. Don't assume that younger partners are less risky. Quite the opposite. Two-thirds of STDs are diagnosed in people under thirty-five.

When it comes to sexual health issues, AIDS is clearly the biggest worry. However, we shouldn't forget about other diseases as well. The Centers for Disease Control states that more than 65 million people in this country are living with an incurable STD, and about 15 million a year will contract an STD, about half of which will be incurable.

How much does having an STD age you? Statistically, only 0.9 years. However, this statistic is misleading. Contracting HIV (human immunodeficiency virus infection) is a way of becoming old overnight. A thirty-five-year-old man who contracts HIV experiences twelve years of aging from the disease in a short period of time, and more aging as the disease progresses. In light of current improvements in treatment, the aging effect correlates directly with the quality of care. His risk profile changes to that of a much older man as soon as he is diagnosed. Other diseases are more uncomfortable than life-threatening, but they can lead to long-term aging of the immune or cardiovascular system.

STDs are so varied, which is partly why data on the relationship between safe sex and aging is hard to correlate. One of the biggest problems with getting statistics on STDs is that it is virtually impossible to perform controlled studies on sexual behavior. We can't create the ideal study conditions that produce the most accurate results as we can, for example, in prescription drug studies. We can't tell a group of people that half of them should have lots of casual sex and the other half should be monogamous. We can't even divide the monogamous group into two subgroups and tell one to have sex only once a week, and the other, to have sex every day.

More important, statistics are only general trends. For example, although the group having the highest incidence of STD infection consists of unmarried people under the age of thirty-five, STDs can affect anyone. Don't fool yourself that because you're from an older generation, you don't have to worry about these things. Either through divorce or widowhood, a lot of people find themselves back in the "dating scene" when they hit their forties and fifties. And stories from the retirement community Sun City, Arizona, indicate that even people in their eighties need to protect themselves from STDs transmitted by their new partners.

While researchers have spent more than two decades trying to find a cure for AIDS, sadly we are not there yet. Although the new, better drugs have made it possible for many HIV-positive patients to live symptom-free for years after infection, the onset of full-blown AIDS, a fatal disease, may not be completely prevented, just delayed. Also, this delay is achieved only when HIV-positive patients initiate and maintain a sometimes complicated and expensive schedule of medications. If you believe that you may have been exposed to the disease, or are changing sex partners, it's a good idea to get an HIV test. If you think you've been exposed, early treatment (within one to four hours) can prevent permanent infection.

Although HIV is a fairly difficult disease to contract, exposure to other

STDs reduces the immune system's defenses and increases the likelihood that HIV will actually infect a person who has been exposed. Estimates are that a person with genital lesions (from syphilis or herpes, for example) is one hundred times more likely to contract HIV during a single sex act than someone who has never had an STD.

When it comes to safe sex, remember three rules:

1. *Look out for yourself. Always.* Don't depend on your partner for protection. No matter who your partner is or what your partner says, make sure you use a condom. No matter how it feels at the moment, don't take needless risks.

2. *Talk before you act.* Talk honestly and forthrightly with your partner about sexual history and safe sex before you ever get to the bedroom. Trust is an important part of sexual intimacy.

3. *Don't believe your partner.* Honest talks and full disclosure of past behaviors are essential for practicing safe sex. However, that isn't enough. Your partner may tell you in good faith that he or she has no STDs but may be wrong. Since many STDs are "silent" (not apparent), a person may be unaware of the infection but still be capable of transmitting the disease. Many people have problems talking about STDs, a potentially embarrassing topic. Surveys show that a large percentage of people say that they would lie if asked about past sexual behavior. A study of sexually active HIV-positive patients showed that four of ten had not told their partners about their disease status. Always use a condom.

A question I'm frequently asked is, "When is it okay to stop playing it safe?" After all, the tough truth is that there is a small loss of sensation with condom use. For the "Magnificent Sex" we aspire to as a result of our RealAge Makeovers, many people would like to give up condom use for maximum pleasure while still keeping themselves disease free. The answer of when it's okay to do so is complicated. When does the "new" partner become the "one-and-only" partner? When can we give up on the condoms?

To consider this you must be in, or be ready to be in, a mutually monogamous relationship. First, talk to your partner about it. Determine that his or her commitment to sexual fidelity is just as solid as yours. Then, both of you should go to a doctor for a full set of tests. That way each of you will know the facts. If one of you tests positive for an STD, then you can make an informed decision about the best way to proceed.

Women who are pregnant or considering getting pregnant should get checked

| Table 6.5 | The RealAge Effect of Sex Practices | | | |

FOR MEN:

Casual Sex Practices

CALENDAR AGE	Mutual Monogamy Safe Practices Condom Use	Low-Risk Partner Safe Practices No Condom Use	Low-Risk Partner No Condom Use	High-Risk Partner
		REALAGE		
35	33.9	34.9	36.1	40.2
55	53.8	54.9	56.2	62.4
70	68.6	69.8	70.8	73.6

FOR WOMEN:

Casual Sex Practices

CALENDAR AGE	Mutual Monogamy Safe Practices Condom Use	Low-Risk Partner Safe Practices No Condom Use	Low-Risk Partner No Condom Use	High-Risk Partner
		REALAGE		
35	34.1	35.0	36.3	42
55	53.9	55.0	56.3	62.9
70	68.5	69.9	70.9	73.1

for the presence of any STDs, as these can sometimes be harmful for the developing fetus or newborn. An STD doesn't usually interfere with pregnancy, but extra precautions should be taken to prevent the mother from infecting the child.

Wear It, and Wear It Right

Sexually transmitted diseases that may not produce symptoms are nonetheless causes of chronic inflammation. And chronic inflammation is one of the major agers of our arteries and immune system. Thus, I'm a true believer in making sure you use a condom every time, until you decide on making it mutually monogamous and having only one partner. In my opinion, the two essentials for preventing chronic inflammation are flossing your teeth and using a condom every time you have sex.

Studies of condom use consistently show that people just don't get it right. Don't assume you know how. Although most people perform only three or four steps correctly, there are six essential steps to using a condom properly:

1. Buy only latex condoms, and use a new condom for each episode of intercourse, even if there isn't ejaculation each time. Make sure you use condoms that say they protect against STDs. Joke or novelty condoms may not provide protection. Make sure that the condoms have not passed their expiration date, that the foil pack is intact, and that they have not been left too long in a place where they could get damaged (for example, in the sun—or in a wallet!).

2. Open the package carefully, being sure to avoid damaging the condom with either fingernails or some other sharp object.

3. Place the condom on the erect penis prior to any intimate contact (some STDs, such as gonorrhea, can be transmitted even without penetration). Roll the condom down to the base of the penis, where the penis connects with the body. Make sure the fit is snug.

4. Leave a space at the tip of the condom and remove any air pockets from that space.

5. Use only water-based lubricants such as KY jelly or spermicidal foam or gel. Never use oil-based lubricants such as Vaseline, petroleum jelly, lotions, or mineral oil, as these destroy the latex. Many condoms are treated with nonoxynol-9, a spermicide and lubricant that seems to provide some added protection against HIV and other types of STD infection. It is probably a good idea to use this type of condom, as it gives added protection just in case.

6. Withdraw immediately after ejaculation, while the penis is still erect, holding the condom firmly against the base of the penis.

(Description of these six steps for correctly wearing a condom is modified from the report of the U.S. Preventive Services Task Force, *Guide to Clinical Preventive Services, 2nd Edition.* U.S. Department of Health and Human Services Office of Public Health and Science, Office of Disease Prevention and Health Promotion, 1996, p. 732)

The following are the most common sexually transmitted diseases:

HIV and AIDS

A Two-Stage Disease

While HIV (human immunodeficency virus), the infection that causes or is presumed to cause AIDS (acquired immunodeficiency syndrome), has traditionally been associated with gay men and intravenous drug users, the incidence of the disease is growing in other sectors of the population. Half a million to one and a half million people in the United States are infected with HIV, with six times as many men as women being infected. Infection rates are higher in the African-American and Latino communities, presumably because of other associated risk factors such as higher rates of drug use. And 34 to 43 million people are infected with HIV worldwide. It is a true epidemic.

HIV/AIDS is a two-stage disease. A person infected with HIV can have no symptoms for years, but will still be at risk of passing on the virus to others. Because of recent advances in HIV treatment, people infected with HIV who undergo the proper regimen of medications can remain in this stage for years, and can look and feel healthy and vital. If you suspect you might have HIV, or if you test positive for the virus, seek medical care immediately.

The second stage of HIV infection—the disease stage—is AIDS. By rendering the immune system basically useless, the disease destroys the body's primary line of defense. Infections, cancers, and other immune diseases can then attack the body. A person goes from a young healthy adult to a disease-ridden old person in a matter of months or years.

At first it was not known how the disease was passed along, or how it could be stopped. Now, however, we know that using a condom reduces the risk of infection considerably. No matter what your sexual orientation, choose your partners carefully and always use a condom.

In nine major American cities, AIDS is the number one cause of death for women twenty-five to forty-four years of age. Because women are more susceptible to contracting the disease than men, experts expect AIDS to increase among women.

The Fight Against AIDS

John K., Jr., discovered he had HIV back in 1991. More than a decade later, he still hasn't developed AIDS. In fact, he has a very low level of HIV in his system.

The discovery that John's HIV didn't replicate as it was supposed to led doctors to examine him very carefully. They found that he was born without the genes that create a normal CCR5 receptor on his cells. He is missing an important part of the CCR5 receptor, a protein element that most of us have. Physician scientists then discovered that the entry of HIV into almost all—but not all—cells requires two receptors, and one of these is the normal CCR5 receptor. (A very few cells can still be entered by HIV even without availability of the normal CCR5 receptor.)

This has led to a new therapy and a new approach to therapies that can block replication of the HIV virus, reducing the level of HIV in the system. HIV can still replicate a very small amount in some white blood cells and in cells of the central nervous system, but its major ability to get in, replicate fast, and do its damage quickly is lessened when normal CCR5 receptors are not available. Drugs are now being developed to block those receptors (make them unavailable) and another receptor found necessary for most HIV replication in cells, so that individuals who have HIV will be able to keep the virus at a very low level in their bodies.

Proper disease maintenance can add years to the life of a person with HIV or AIDS. Each year, more effective treatments for the disease emerge, so that the longer an infected person survives, the better his or her odds are for living until a cure is discovered. If you suspect you may have HIV, get tested today.

CHLAMYDIA

Chlamydia is the most common bacterial STD in the United States. The biggest problem with chlamydia is that its symptoms are largely silent: seventy-five percent of those infected show no symptoms. Chronic inflammation with chlamydia is one of the most frequent causes of increased C-reactive protein levels, which correlate directly with aging of the arteries and probably aging of the immune system (see Chapters 4 and 5). Primarily affecting women, chlamydia can cause internal scarring of the fallopian tubes, ectopic pregnancy (a pregnancy outside the uterus), and infertility. Symptoms, when they do occur, include painful urination, vaginal discharge, and abdominal pain. Although men are not usually affected (made ill or permanently scarred) by the disease, they should seek treatment if they are exposed, because they can transmit the disease to their partners. Ask your gynecologist or general physician to include a chlamydia screen as part of your routine battery of tests, particularly if you have recently changed sex partners. Fortunately, chlamydia can be easily treated with antibiotics.

GONORRHEA

"The clap" can affect anyone. As many as two-thirds of women and 40 percent of men infected with gonorrhea have no symptoms. Signs of infection, if they do occur, may include painful urination, unusual vaginal discharge, and menstrual spotting. Gonorrhea is highly contagious and can be transmitted through genital contact, even without penetration. Gonorrhea can cause ectopic pregnancy or infertility in women and seems to increase a person's susceptibility to HIV. Nonoxynol-9, the spermicide most often used on condoms, helps block the transmission of gonorrhea. Untreated, the disease can cause cardiovascular aging. Gonorrhea can usually be treated with antibiotics, although many antibiotic-resistant strains are appearing. Infections from these strains can be cured with a more vigorous and difficult series of treatments.

HEPATITIS B

Hepatitis B is not officially classified as an STD, but its predominant mode of infection is sexual transmission. Hepatitis B can cause severe damage to the liver. There is no perfectly effective treatment, and many people recover on their own. Several treatments are effective in many, but not all, people who are given them. A hepatitis B vaccine is available, and getting a vaccination is a quick, easy way to help yourself stay young, particularly if you are sexually active, and if you plan to have more than one sex partner in your lifetime.

HERPES

Estimates are that one in five sexually active Americans has genital herpes, an increase of 15 to 20 percent since the mid-1980s. This increase has occurred despite safe-sex education and programs encouraging condom use. Many people who have been infected don't have symptoms and are unaware of the disease, but are infectious and spread the disease to their partners. Within the first week or two after infection, symptoms can include fatigue, muscle aches, and itching. Ten days or so after infection, a small blister usually appears in the genital region. The blister can burst and remain for several weeks, causing pain and discomfort. Once the initial outbreak heals, victims remain infected for the rest of their lives and may suffer recurrent outbreaks. Although herpes can be both painful and embarrassing, it does not seem life-threatening.

We now know that herpes stimulates chronic infection that can age both your immune system and your arteries. Specific antiviral medication in topical ointment and pill forms can treat the symptoms and reduce the number of outbreaks and the chance that an outbreak will infect your sexual partner. The medication cannot, however, cure the underlying infection, which remains with a person for life. Although transmission is most common during outbreaks, transmission can occur between outbreaks as well, in a process known as "viral shedding." Women are more likely than men to contract the disease from an infected partner, and herpes can cause more serious consequences if they become pregnant.

HUMAN PAPILLOMAVIRUS

Human papillomavirus is the most commonly transmitted STD. As many as 80 percent of sexually active people are infected with the virus. Surprisingly little is ever said about this disease. For a long time, the virus was believed to be benign, but now we know it substantially increases the risk of cervical cancer, and thus aging the immune system. This STD also produces chronic inflammation and chronic infections that age the arteries. Some strains cause small genital growths or warts which can be uncomfortable; these can easily be removed. If you have had more than two sex partners in your lifetime, or if your partner has had more than two sex partners, chances are you have been exposed to the virus. In general, human papillomavirus infection doesn't do much, and there are no treatments. But once you have it, you have it.

If you do have it, you should make sure you obtain routine Pap smears (women) or urine tests (men). Women should also have yearly gynecologic examinations, or as often as their gynecologist recommends. The importance of routine gynecologic examinations is to detect precancerous cells and prevent cervical cancer from making you older. Women who have been exposed to the virus are more likely to develop cervical cancers. In fact, almost all women with positive results on a Pap smear show evidence of having been exposed to the virus. Positive Pap smear results do not mean you have cancer. Most positive results merely identify an increased risk of developing cancer. If you do get a positive result, you will want to be especially careful about having the condition monitored. Your gynecologist may recommend biannual or quarterly Pap smears or treatments to remove precancerous cells and prevent the development of full-blown cervical cancer.

For men, exposure seems to have little effect, except that exposure is related to rare bladder tumors and rare penile cancers. Men who have been exposed should be sure not to dismiss early warning signs of bladder cancer, such as small amounts of blood in the urine, and should get urine tests. In addition, men who have been exposed can get chronic infections from the virus that are discomforting or that age the arteries. Men who have been exposed can also transmit the virus to their partners, and they can develop growths or warts, sometimes inside the urethra, that cause discomfort.

Recent studies show that the virus may be implicated in some anal and rectal cancers, as well as some oral cancers.

SYPHILIS

If gonorrhea is "the sailor's disease," syphilis is the disease of kings. Famous in the eighteenth and nineteenth centuries because of its ravages on European aristocracy, syphilis is once again on the rise. The incidence of syphilis has more than doubled since the early 1980s. Symptoms include genital lesions, aches, fevers, rashes, hair loss, and skin and mouth sores. If untreated, syphilis can infect the eyes, heart, brain, and other organs, causing irreparable structural damage. In addition, syphilis accelerates the rate of arterial aging. Syphilis is treated with antibiotics and, if eradicated early, leaves no lasting damage.

Sex is a great thing. The more, and the higher the quality, the better, and the younger you will be. There may be no way to get younger that's more fun! Just remember:

Be safe.
Use a condom.
Get tested for STD.
Pick your partner carefully.

What better reason to give yourself a RealAge Makeover than to enjoy sex, as you will be making yourself younger still.

Illegal Drugs: Stay Young Without Them

Just because drugs such as marijuana, cocaine, and heroin are illegal doesn't mean that people don't use them. One out of two Americans age fifteen to sixty admits to having tried an illegal drug at some point in their lives, and over 15 percent of them say they have done so in the past year. Estimates suggest that 5 to 10 percent of the population uses illegal drugs regularly, and many are addicted. The more than three billion dollars spent each year on drug rehabilitation programs is just a small part of the major impact drug use has on our society. Although we tend to associate drug use with teenagers, rock stars, or the inner-city poor, people from all segments of society use and abuse drugs.

Drugs make you older. Drug addiction is a serious physical and mental health problem, and one that has far-reaching sociological impact. However, the complicated problems associated with drug use warrant more discussion than I can provide here. For the purposes of this book, we are only going to look at drugs in terms of what they do to your health.

Most "hard drugs" are illegal for good reason: they're dangerous and addictive. Cocaine, crack, heroin, ecstasy, and a whole array of hallucinogenic (mind-altering) drugs can cause serious health problems. Drugs like heroin and cocaine top the list and can kill a person almost instantaneously. An overdose, if not fatal, is always serious and puts a person's life at risk. Although trying a drug once probably won't do much damage by itself, it may be the first step on the path to drug addiction. Addiction affects a person's physiology, making him or her more likely to suffer real physical aging that is manifested in many ways. Unnecessary aging associated with drug use can be as much as eight years. The mental effects of drug use tend to disrupt our social ties, often causing users to lose their friends, families, and jobs.

Using drugs increases the chances that you'll make bad decisions. Cocaine and crack use is associated with higher rates of transmission of HIV, not because using the drugs increases susceptibility, but because users take risks (unsafe sex, needle sharing) that make them more likely to be exposed to the virus.

Some people think that marijuana—by far the most popular illegal drug—is harmless. That's simply not true. While it may be less immediately dangerous or addictive than other drugs, it can still take a toll on your health, making your RealAge older. Marijuana contains 50 percent more carcinogens and four times as much tar as cigarettes. Studies show that the heavy use of marijuana can cause residual neurologic effects that decrease cognitive functioning (the thought process). Heavy users actually experience aging less from the drug itself than from the behaviors it tends to induce, most notably a lack of motivation. For example, users are less likely to exercise, eat a healthy diet, or maintain the kinds of social networks that help protect against stress. They are also more likely to engage in risky behaviors, such as unsafe sex or driving under the influence.

Methylenedioxymethamphetamine (MDMA, or "ecstasy") is addictive to a sizable number of people who try it even once. Frequent use of ecstasy can cause deterioration of brain function and loss of brain cells, so much so that a CT scan of the brain of a young ecstasy user can resemble that of a person with dementia caused by loss of neurons. We do not know the percent of first-time users so addicted and affected. It's probably a small percentage, but it is still a sobering outcome and unnecessary way to age your brain, fast.

Drug addiction can devastate both the lives of the addicted, and those around them. The best way to safeguard yourself against addiction is to not start. If you already use drugs and find that you can't quit on your own, seek professional help. Although overcoming a drug addiction is difficult, addiction is one of the most pernicious agers of the body, and ending a habit of drug abuse will make you younger and, consequently, make you feel better. It could even save your life.

Stress
Less

The #1 Most Important Way to Grow Younger

A RealAge Makeover Success Story: Maureen K.

We first met Maureen K. in Chapter 1. Her husband was concerned she was too stressed. As you may remember, Maureen K. was a pharmacy benefits manager at an HMO (health maintenance organization), who had to make decisions about drugs based on savings for her company rather than the best interest of the patient. The fact that her choices might potentially harm patients caused her enormous stress. She hadn't done any regular physical activity for a long time and wasn't making healthy food choices, so she was about fifteen pounds over her desired weight.

Maureen was impressed by her husband's return to youth and was willing to give the RealAge program a try. She found friends to walk with at lunch and started lifting weights three times a week. She started playing tennis again, with both Clyde and her own friends. Within six months, she had lost not only the extra fifteen pounds but five more. As she put it, she had become "a babe again at age forty-six."

Maureen K. couldn't reduce her stress at work, though. She was stressed by the decisions she was pushed to make, and stressed from work overload because of a shortage of pharmacists. She tried meditation breaks, yoga pauses, refocusing, and a myriad of other techniques learned from a professional stress-management advisor. She was still stressed. It took two medications plus her healthy eating and her three-pronged physical activity regime (see Chapter 9) to keep her blood pressure in the 120 to 125 systolic and 80 to 85 diastolic ranges. She was not feeling refreshed when she awoke from sleep. She often had to eat on the run between tasks and meetings, and worked such long hours that she skipped some of her exercise schedule. She felt that her work pressures and duties interfered with her ability to keep herself healthy, and rousing her positive attitude.

Maureen and Clyde then arranged their finances so they could live without Maureen working. And with Clyde's support, Maureen made a major decision: to reduce her stress by changing jobs. When I saw her a year after her first visit, just six weeks after she quit her job, she was a new person—a much healthier, happier, and younger one. She now awoke refreshed. Her blood pressure was 115/75 to 80, now with just one medication. She then began a new pharmacy management position, and loved it. She was lucky; she worked in a profession in very high demand so she could choose her new position carefully, and she chose well. Now she felt and was the 15 years younger she looked.

When you're stressed, you don't feel your best. When the phone is ringing, the kids are crying, you've got a stain on your shirt, and you were supposed to have left for work half an hour ago, you might feel that something inside you is about to "snap." While you may have guessed that such a state isn't good for your physical health, the data from scientific studies now prove it. And it isn't only about stress—emotional well-being in general is the most important factor in helping you stay healthy and younger longer. The mind–body connection really does exist, and it plays an important role in preventing and reversing arterial aging, immune aging, and injuries and disabilities from accidents. So for the purposes of your RealAge Makeover plan, how do we put this knowledge to practical use? Which emotional factors help keep you young? Which life events cause age-promoting stress, and what can be done to offset the risk? Learning how to be happier with your life, to be positive, to live as stress-free as possible, and to turn maddening moments into learning or humorous experiences are vital steps in your RealAge Makeover.

■ For years, having a type A personality was believed to be the cause of stress-induced illness. We now know this is not true. You do not age from the stresses you deliberately bring upon yourself, such as pushing yourself to work hard and doing well. Nor do you age from the intermediate stresses you can and do control, such as the flat tire that you get fixed. These Important But Manageable events (I call them IBMs) do not cause us to age, because they are problems we can and do solve. We now know that illness comes only from events that stress *you*—even if they don't seem to stress other people—and do so for a prolonged period. You age from both minor, Nagging Unfinished Tasks (I call them NUTs: We go nuts from NUTs!) and from major life events, which can be as different as the loss of a family member, moving to a new town, or financial troubles that seem beyond your control. Nagging stress seems to wear you out, and persistent stress and major life events are true killers. Reducing stress in your life can give back thirty of the thirty-two years that major life events can take away.

Difficulty rating: Most difficult

■ Being sociable is good for your health. People who live with others, have lots of friends, and stay involved in religious or social activities live longer, healthier lives. Even using a cell phone to keep in touch with friends while walking can make you up to six years younger. During non-stressful times, living with three or more people or having many close friends can make you two years younger than those who don't have this support network. During extremely stressful times, this companionship can keep you as much as thirty years younger.

Difficulty rating: Moderately difficult

■ It doesn't matter how much money you have: if you live beyond your means, you will experience one of the most troubling day-to-day stresses. And worrying about money leads to unnecessary aging. Learn to manage your finances so you don't live beyond your means. Reducing financial stresses can make your RealAge as much as eight years younger.

Difficulty rating: Moderately difficult

■ Doubtless you believe that spending days in the classroom is an activity for the young. What you might not know is that time in the classroom can keep you young. An evening class or a lively book discussion group can be an enjoyable and effective part of your RealAge Makeover plan, because keeping your mind active helps keep your body young. Your mind is like a muscle: you need to exercise it. Even playing games on the Internet (see *www.RealAgeGames.com*) may keep your mind younger. Teaching a course also keeps you young; in listening to life stories, it often fascinates me how much many of us were and are strongly motivated and influenced by our mentors and teachers. So teaching has a double benefit—maybe that's why teaching is one of the longest life expectancies of all professions. Using your brain can make you more than 2.5 years younger.

Difficulty rating: Moderate

- Yes, a positive attitude really does make a difference. Correctly estimating the happiness or unhappiness that certain events cause, and
being happy, interested, and satisfied with your life, no matter what
your circumstances, can make your RealAge six years younger.
Difficulty Rating: Moderately difficult

- Emotional upsets and traumas can be difficult to face, and it's human
nature to cope with deeply upsetting events by taking a head-in-the-
sand approach. But this can make us older. Whether we were
wounded by our parents' divorce when we were children, or are recovering from our own as adults, by not facing these traumas we suffer needlessly, and that affects our health. If your social networks aren't
enough to help you deal with emotional conflicts, seek professional
help (a psychiatrist, counselor, or therapist) and make your RealAge
eight to sixteen years younger than it would be otherwise.
Difficulty rating: Most difficult

If you feel highly stressed a lot of the time, you are not alone. Most of us are
stressed. There is nothing like a day of too many hassles to make you feel yourself aging faster than you should. No doubt, too much stress does indeed age
you. Stress is linked to aging of both the arterial and immune systems. Also,
people under stress are more likely to get into accidents or suffer other hazards
that lead to disabilities which can cause them to age.

Some rare people suffer from stress not because of the pressures of daily life,
but for physiologic reasons. One such person was Harry S., who was seventy-five
years old when he was referred to me. He was going to have surgery for cancer of
the bladder. His surgeon wanted me to make sure Harry was in "optimal shape"
before surgery. I put a blood pressure cuff on him and took a blood pressure
reading every minute as we talked. My goal was to find out what stressed him
and how stable his blood pressure was, because unstable blood pressure makes
surgery and anesthesia more complex and risky for the patient.

As we talked, I found out that Harry had developed hypertension and stomach ulcers in 1967. He underwent an intensive diagnostic study for difficult-to-
control hypertension at the Mayo Clinic eight years later, and again in 1987 at
the Cleveland Clinic. Ten years after that, in 1997 he had a heart attack, and in
2000, a stroke.

Harry had successfully undergone rehabilitation to recover from his stroke.
He still had difficulty controlling his hypertension and was taking four different
medications. As is customary, I had him bring his pill bottles and made sure he
was indeed taking all his blood pressure pills very reliably, and that none of

them interacted with the others. However, as I talked to him, his blood pressure, which was initially 130/85, spiked to 230/130, and his heart rate went from 68 to 98. Talking with me usually is not *that* stressful.

That was a highly unusual and dramatic change in blood pressure. I wondered, "What's the chance that Harry has pheochromocytoma (hypertension caused by a tumor)?" Or was this just a severe case of "white-coat hypertension," the increase in blood pressure many patients have upon first meeting or seeing someone in a white coat in a medical environment. Pheochromocytoma is a rare tumor that causes a great release of catecholamines, a stress hormone. Therefore, the effects of pheochromocytoma are often mistaken for the effects of stress, a much more common condition. As I evaluated him, I saw clearly that his blood pressure was not stable enough for the rigors of surgery. His systolic pressures went from 130 to 230, to 160, to 190, to 130, to 210 in a matter of 8 minutes. At that time I did something very unusual, and very lucky. I had his urine tested for the hormonal products of pheochromocytoma and found that he did indeed have this rare adrenal tumor. It took approximately three weeks to prepare him with medications for surgical removal of his adrenal gland. A large tumor was removed. His bladder tumor was also removed.

That adrenal tumor had done quite a few things to Harry. It had made him nervous and had caused a heart attack and stroke. It also probably contributed to a breakdown in his immune system, allowing the growth of a bladder cancer. Finally, it had made his retirement less happy.

It is possible that stress, or a stress-like substance, could do all that to you? Is that why we need to deal with stress early? Yes, and that's why stress is so important to control right now, starting today. Of course, most of us don't have the rare tumor I was talking about. But we all have stress in our lives, whether it be caused by the neighbor's barking dog, the slew of e-mails waiting to be answered, the traffic jam that holds us up, or the burnt-out lightbulb in the kitchen. Stress is a normal part of modern life, and we can't expect to never have it. But learning how to control and reduce it is entirely possible, and is an important step in our RealAge Makeover plans. The following patient story illustrates this point.

A R e a l A g e M a k e o v e r S u c c e s s S t o r y : N a n J .

In the three years previous, Nan J. had made herself over. After her husband died, Nan started having me care for her. A year after his death, she had a calendar age of fifty-eight but a RealAge that was fifteen years older. In just three years, she had made her RealAge seven years younger. But on this particular visit, Nan seemed troubled and anxious. She also looked fatigued. I asked her what was wrong.

She said, "I'm nervous and don't know what to do. I have 25 percent of all my assets in shares of XYZ Company. I've made a lot of money on this stock since I bought it two years ago, but now I'm worried. I've been reading more and more that this stock is volatile and risky. It's certainly worth far more than when I bought it, but I worry so much about it crashing that I've had a hard time sleeping."

If Nan had been on the brink of bankruptcy, that would have been one thing. But I happened to know that she was a very wealthy woman. Therefore, I knew that the aging she was causing herself by worrying so much about this situation was entirely unnecessary.

I told Nan that, in my professional opinion, nothing is worth losing sleep over, or your peace of mind. That would ruin any RealAge Makeover. No stock profit, no argument with your spouse, and no workplace dispute is worth nights of tossing and worrying. If you find yourself in that position, you must act to either solve that worrisome situation or remove it from your life completely. I don't care if it's a bad marriage, a feared trip to the doctor, a rotten business deal, or a worrisome position in the stock market, you must act—and not care what it may cost financially, because it's better than paying with your health.

I'm a doctor, not a financial advisor, so some could say I overstepped my bounds with what I said next. But I told Nan J. that she had to sell her XYZ stocks to the "sleeping point." I may not know stocks, but I know the aging effects of stress, and she was aging from that investment because it caused her to lose sleep. I told her that until she'd gotten rid of enough of the stock that she could get a full night's sleep, she was making herself older.

Nan took my advice and sold four-fifths of her stock in XYZ a week later. When I next saw her she looked healthier, happier, and more rested; she was back to getting a good night's sleep. And she was still able to get a good night's sleep when the price dropped by over 30 percent in the next year. She was no longer letting unnecessary worry about money undo all the good work she'd done toward her RealAge Makeover.

What lesson can you learn from Nan's story? You can learn an important concept: that we all have a built-in alarm system called the "sleeping point" that signals trouble. If you are so stressed by something that you're not able to sleep, you must come to grips with it. You can tell when you've solved the problem when you get back to your "sleeping point."

Stress is not bad in and of itself. In small doses, it can be good for you, and even necessary. However, too much stress turns normally useful bodily reactions into damaging overreactions. We really do not know all the ways that stress can cause our arteries and immune system to age; on the other hand, we do understand some of the mechanisms. Stress overload can cause the brain to trigger an over-release of "stress hormones" which can lead to aging in the long term. In general, prolonged stress decreases your ability to moderate your cardiovascular responses. That increases blood pressure and ages the arteries. When released on a constant basis, the same neurotransmitter that keeps you alert and able to respond quickly in times of danger causes your body to become overtaxed. Ironically, this constant bombardment actually decreases your ability to sense trouble, prevent accidents, and avoid confrontations. In addition, stress suppresses the immune response, increasing your risk of catching infections or developing more serious diseases. In other words, stress stimulates many of the conditions that cause premature aging.

Almost all of us are juggling too many commitments; that can cause age-inducing stress. You can prevent this needless aging by learning to manage your day-to-day stresses and by developing safety networks you can rely on when a major stress-inducing event occurs. Sociability is a big component in stress management. Companionship and group activities—whether religious, political, business, or just social—can all play a major role in making your RealAge younger.

Sadly, more than one quarter of us will have a "major life event" within any one year: a death, a divorce, a job loss or job change, an illness in the family, financial difficulties, relocation, involvement in a lawsuit, or other trauma. While you can't prevent these unfortunate events from occurring, you can have a stress-control plan already in place when they do. Because stress from a major event has a big effect on your RealAge, having a stress-control plan can make your RealAge substantially younger. Stresses exacerbate one another. Having that first stress makes it more difficult for your body to handle the second, and having the first and second makes it even more difficult to handle the third, and so forth. The occurrence of one major life event makes your RealAge about five years older during the event and for at least one year (and probably two years) afterward. Two major life events in one year can make your RealAge as much as sixteen years older; and three major life events, more than thirty-two years older for at least the following year (see Table 7.1). The question is not whether you will suffer stress, because you know you will, but how you manage it when it happens.

Table 7.1   The RealAge Effect of Stress

"Major life events" cause aging. Twenty-eight percent of Americans will undergo one major life event in any given year. Fifteen percent will have two such life events, and 13 percent will have three or more. A major life event is an experience such as the death or illness of a loved one (especially a spouse or a child), divorce, a major illness, moving to a new locale, being the target of a lawsuit, losing or starting a job, and financial instabilities such as bankruptcy. Recent data indicate that all of the small nagging recurrent problems that chronically bother us (the broken toilet seat that shifts when you sit on it) add up to affect each of us as if one major event had occurred. If you do not habitually deal with small problems and irritations as they occur, add another major life event to your aging burden.

FOR MEN:

CALENDAR AGE	Number of Major Life Events in Past Year			
	0	1	2	3
	REALAGE			
35	27	34	36	42
55	49	54	61	68
70	62	69	77	94

FOR WOMEN:

CALENDAR AGE	Number of Major Life Events in Past Year			
	0	1	2	3
	REALAGE			
35	27	34	38	43
55	49	54	61	67
70	63	69	76	84

The Nature of "Stress"

We often use the terms *stressed* and *stressed out*, and feel we have a general concept of what we're all talking about. But what, exactly, is stress? How does it manifest itself physiologically? Stress is more than just the feeling that there's too much to do, too little time to do it, and too many hassles along the way. Stress is a very complex set of physiologic and psychological reactions. Dr. Hans Selye, one of the earliest researchers to study stress, defined it as "the nonspecific response of the body to any demand made on it." Simply put, stress is the body's reaction when it anticipates the need for extra energy. Almost anything can provoke this reaction: an injury, working under a deadline for a crazy boss, not sleeping enough, or not eating regular meals. Even laughing stresses the body. (Clearly, not all types of stress age you. Laughter may stress your body momentarily but in the long run, it makes you younger.)

It's easy to think—with the feeling of headache or of pressure building in the skull that stress can give us—that stress is a purely mental phenomenon. But it's not. It is also physiologic, affecting many parts of the body. When you are stressed, your body releases a flood of adrenaline, cortisone, and other stress hormones which induce physiologic changes. The heart pounds and blood pressure rises. You start to breathe more rapidly, and you feel more alert. Blood races to your brain and heart and moves away from the kidneys, liver, stomach, and skin. Your blood sugar level rises, as do the amounts of fats and LDL cholesterol in your bloodstream. Unfortunately, there is also an increase in the amount of proteins that cause inflammation and lead to increases in hazardous clotting factors and platelets in the blood. In all, stress causes substantial system-wide changes.

Like almost all other animals, humans have a natural, built-in defense mechanism: the "fight-or-flight" response in which the body primes itself to respond positively to a dangerous situation, and come out alive. The same mechanism that makes a zebra run at the sight of an approaching tiger makes you reflexively pull your hand back when you place it on a hot stove. Or when you reflexively jump out of the way of a car that appears about to hit you. Your reflexive responses are augmented by a massive release of catecholamines (stress hormones). In a situation which your brain registers as a potentially dangerous or fatal situation—such as during an auto accident where you must make split-second decisions to stay alive—this release of hormones at first makes you feel anxious, but also able to react instead of simply to freeze, and later, to feel washed out.

Perhaps surprisingly, these huge but fleeting stresses do not age you. You are simply using one of your body's systems as it was meant to be used. When you have an Important But Manageable life event (IBM) such as a scary near-miss from which you don't suffer an injury, your rate of aging is not affected. The problem arises instead when you are in a "fight-or-flight" state not just occasionally and briefly, but constantly. The important issue is not whether you experience stress, but how much you experience over how long a period of time.

When you allow yourself to suffer from chronic stress, you put your body in a continuous state of siege. The same systems that help you respond to danger for the moment and then shut down are now in overdrive. Imagine a car: when you rev the engine once, no problem. But if you rev the engine continually, the faster you need to replace the engine or its parts. With stress, the faster you rev your body, the more quickly you age. Physically, chronic stress alters the immune responses, causing a decrease in the production of T and B cells, two types of white blood cells essential for fighting virus-infected cells, foreign cells, and cancer cells. Chronic stress also raises blood pressure.

The relationship between stress and aging has been made clear and inarguable through a large body of scientific studies. Recent work published in *The Journal of the American Medical Association* concluded that stress was linked to reduced blood flow to the heart (myocardial ischemia) and to other vital organs. People who had a lot of stress also had more periods of inadequate blood flow to the heart, leading to a correspondingly higher risk of heart attacks and abnormal heart rhythms.

Not only does stress release chemicals that signal the nervous system to raise your heart rate and blood pressure, but it also causes direct aging of the arteries, and this, too, increases blood pressure, driving it even higher. Elevated blood pressure causes the greatest acceleration of arterial aging. Recent research at Johns Hopkins Medical School indicated that people who experienced elevated blood pressure when exposed to mental stress tests (not just the physical stress tests normally used to detect heart strain) were more than twenty times more likely to have heart and arterial diseases. Furthermore, individuals who had "hot" reactions—those more likely to get agitated or frustrated by life events—had twenty times the rate of arterial aging, as measured by the incidence of heart attacks and strokes, than people who had "cool" reactions. Other studies have shown that those who keep anger inside rather than expressing it outwardly (those who are stressed internally) have the greatest risk of aging from the stress.

Three recent studies investigated anger levels in diverse groups: 374 men and women who were eighteen to thirty years old; 13,000 men and women forty-five to sixty-four; and 1,305 men seventy and older. The studies found the same results: those who reacted to situations with anger had arteries that aged 2.5 to three times faster than the arteries of those who reframed the situation (saw the situation in a more positive light). Those who reframed the situation reacted with calmness, tried to learn something from the situation, or used humor. Take the example of the boss who buttonholes you just as you're leaving for home. If you react calmly, you might tell yourself he thinks you can do the task better than anyone else. If you use the situation as a learning tool, you'll ask yourself what this particular episode teaches you: that walking down the stairs instead of passing the boss's office would prevent this situation in the future. Finally, if you react with humor, you might say, "The boss must have seen me drive in this morning and just wants to keep me off the road until after rush hour!" Any of these reactions—instead of anger—will help keep your boss's stressful demand from making you older.

The aging effects of stress are not limited to your arteries. Prolonged exposure to the chemicals released by the body during stress can age the immune system as well. How do researchers measure this type of aging? A study of health-care workers found that those with especially stressful jobs had a lower level of antibody production than those in less stressful positions. Furthermore, chronic stress depletes your body of important vitamins (vitamin C, vitamin D, and the B-complex vitamins, including folate, niacin, B_6, and B_{12}). Stress also increases your rate of bone loss, making you more vulnerable to broken bones and disability if you fall or have an accident. Finally, overexposure to stress hormones, which at first heighten perceptiveness, over time can actually decrease it, thus raising the risk of accidents and acts of violence such as the freeway confrontations called "road rage."

Interestingly, and contrary to popular belief, different stresses affect people in different ways; not everyone is stressed by the same things. Some doctors are completely calm when treating life-threatening problems in the emergency room, but become utterly flustered when tending to the daily tasks of running their offices. Some people love a good argument, and others will do anything to avoid one. Often type A personalities, those who are always pushing themselves to run, run, run, become more stressed when they try to stop those type A behavior; relaxing makes them anxious. Maybe this is why many retired aircraft engineers die soon after retirement. As a group, they may find their precise and difficult work relaxing and non-stressful. Therefore, while you are developing your stress-reduction strategies for your RealAge Makeover plan, your first challenge is to identify what stresses *you*—not your spouse, not your boss, not your neighbor. Then, you can develop a plan tailored to you as an individual for either avoiding stressful situations or, if they can't be avoided, for handling them in ways that reduce your stress levels.

It is surprising that what we think stresses us and what actually does are often two different things. As reflected in the work of Harvard economic psychologist Daniel Gilbert, it appears that our own internal calculations of what brings us happiness and how long that happiness will last are often wrong. Contrary to popular belief, the things that give us the most stress aren't, for example, the broken bones we might suffer, because we learn to deal with the injury and rehabilitate, thereby making it less stressful. These important but manageable events do not age because we deal with them. Instead, aging stress is caused by NUTs—Nagging Unfinished Tasks that you could fix, but don't. This information gives effective ways to deal with stress: fix the small problems before they become stress-causing, and change your perceptions of events that you can't fix, to the lighter side of things.

What is really important is not what happens to you, but how you perceive what happens to you. One person might find riding a rollercoaster exhilarating, whereas another finds it terrifying. Both will feel stress from the event, but one will feel good stress, called "eustress" for the euphoric reaction, and the other bad stress, or "distress." The level of stress you feel has a lot to do with your personality and your subjective interpretation of what is happening to you. While you can't change your personality, you can change many of your perceptions, especially by actively working to cultivate a positive attitude. And that positive attitude can help you stay young by reducing stress and the effects of stress.

Several years ago, I was at a large department store on Christmas Eve. It was closing time, and my son and I were the last ones to get to the register. The mostly-male last-minute shoppers crowded around the register area, pushing and shoving. The cashier was still ringing up purchases an hour after closing time. When Jeff and I finally reached the register, imagining what her day must have been, I said to her, "You must be glad this day's over. Talk about stressful." The woman laughed and said, "I love my job. How many other jobs have this many men fighting over you?!" I had to laugh, and I certainly admired her. She had one of the most stress-inducing jobs, yet she didn't let it get to her. She didn't see the surge of customers negatively but positively: all these men fighting over me! Her ability to see the event with humor meant that she would not age as much from the day's push as she might have.

Measuring the Effects of Stress

Stress has multiple and far-reaching effects on your body and mind. This is reflected in the fact that symptoms of stress are not only physical but also mental, emotional, and behavioral. Physical signs include frequent headaches, difficulty sleeping, sore and stiff muscles, nausea or upset stomach, diarrhea or constipation, a general sense of fatigue, and increased susceptibility to illness. Mental symptoms of stress include an inability to concentrate, confusion, indecisiveness, and loss of your sense of humor. On an emotional level, stress can make us anxious, nervous, irritable, quick to anger, impatient, and depressed. Behaviors indicative of stress include fidgeting, pacing, or restlessness. However, you can also feel sluggish or avoid work because it seems too daunting.

There are three basic kinds of stress. One is ongoing, low-level stress, such as job pressures or juggling work and children. A second is stress from NUTs—the Nagging Unfinished Tasks. The third type comes from those major life stresses that are harder to plan for—the death of a loved one, a sudden job loss, severe financial setbacks, a bad accident, a divorce. Although we know that stress from both the NUTs and the major events age us, it has been much easier for researchers to measure the aging impact of the big one-time events, because there are clear "before" and "after" periods to measure. It is clear, for example, that the death of a spouse has a significant RealAge impact. For more than a year after the death of their spouses, widows and widowers have a reduced level of the important immune system B and T cells, as well as low production of antibodies. Also, both widows and widowers are much more likely to suffer a major health event after such a loss. It is not at all uncommon for a person who has been married for a long time to die soon after the death of his or her spouse, the death of one causing immediate aging in the other.

Natural disasters offer researchers other situations in which to measure the impact of stress, because there are clear sets of dates from which to detect changes in heart attack and death rates. Demographic studies show that the rate of severe or fatal heart attacks increases dramatically in the days after a major earthquake. In the days after the bombings of Israel with Scud missiles in the Gulf War, the rate of heart attacks and strokes surged in that country. So did the rate of accidents. Although the studies didn't investigate the more general impact on aging, we can assume that other aging-related events increased as well. In another poignant example, a recent study published by the National Cancer Institute found that the psychological stress of being diagnosed as having breast cancer caused the levels of immune cells such as T cells and natural killer cells (white blood cells that can kill other cells, such as tumor cells) to plummet, putting patients at even greater risk. In these instances, stress caused substantial aging: One major life event can age you by as much as five years when it occurs, and for at least one year (and probably longer) afterward.

It has been harder for researchers to quantify the impact of long-term ongoing stresses on our aging processes. This is not at all because such stresses are any less real. It is because their starting and stopping points are much harder to define. Further, ongoing stresses seem to be open to a more subjective interpretation. Although everyone finds the death of a loved one stressful, not everyone finds the same aspects of family life or work life stressful. This aspect of satisfaction is what economic psychologist Dan Gilbert's work speaks to. Our happiness may be more adversely affected by recurrent stresses than even by the death of a loved one. We will deal with and manage major stress. But the nagging stresses we never fix are allowed to continue, and these seem to contribute greatly to unhappiness and aging. New evidence makes it certain that ongoing, low-level stress makes us older.

Men are particularly at risk of the aging effects of being unhappy. Recent studies of twins in Finland indicate that predictors of satisfaction in life are major determinants of the death rates for men. These predictors include how happy they are with their lot in life, no matter what it may be; whether or not they are lonely; and whether or not they have a general interest in life. A general dissatisfaction with life predicts not only adverse health behavior (such as smoking, not watching one's diet, and not exercising) but also mortality rates, especially among men. In fact, this appears to be a major difference between men and women. Men who are dissatisfied don't practice healthy habits, whereas women who are dissatisfied with life don't have the same mortality risk. Apparently, women continue to practice healthy habits and do not "give up."

General Habits That Reduce Stress

It's a RealAge truth that a good lifestyle choice that affects one aspect of your life and health will frequently also affect another. I've discussed the health effect of exercise on the arteries. But exercise also happens to be one of the very best ways to reduce stress. Stress causes your body to build up extra energy, preparing it for fight or flight. Exercise burns energy and reduces your stress levels. Exercise metabolizes stress hormones in your blood and increases levels of your body's built-in antianxiety hormones, making you feel calmer. Exercise can make you more efficient and energetic, so that you feel less overwhelmed by the stresses you do face. For example, just walking regularly can increase the level of beta-endorphins and brain-derived neurotrophic factors (both groups are neurotransmitters or hormones that help the body feel pleasure or increase memory) in the brain, to decrease anxiety and tension and elevate one's mood. In addition, all exercise—but especially aerobic exercise—helps divert energy from worrying and anxiety. If you haven't yet added exercise to your Makeover plan, think about the stress reduction benefits you will gain that make your RealAge still younger.

Other effective stress reducers are relaxation techniques, biofeedback, prayer (group or individual), and mental imagery. You may have already instinctively known these would be beneficial, and may be already practicing some of them. If not, consider giving at least one a try. Combination programs like yoga that include both stretching and mind relaxation can be especially effective in easing emotional and physical tensions. One simple technique is visualization. Close your eyes, relax your muscles, and imagine yourself some place far away from the chaos around you. Imagine yourself on a beach or in a mountain meadow, feel the warmth of the sun on your skin, and let your muscles feel soft and heavy. Relax into them. Breathe deeply. Feel the tension dissipate. Dr. Rich O'Neal also taught me another technique that may seem funny at first but really works. Scrunch up every muscle in your face as hard as you can, so that your face is contorted. Concentrate on scrunching up your face. Really concentrate hard on it. Count to ten and then slowly release the muscles of your face. That simple exercise is an effective way to focus your attention and then relieve tension.

A healthier diet and a regular schedule also help lower stress levels, making you younger. Our favorite food vices—sugar, salt, and caffeine—may actually elevate our stress levels. So can cigarette smoking, excess alcohol consumption, and not getting a good night's sleep. Even though you think that you don't have time for a full night's sleep, you will be much more productive if you are well rested. You'll also be more able to adopt a positive attitude, so the tasks and problems you face that day won't stress you as much.

Interestingly, one thing that causes many people stress is not the situation they are in, but how much control they have over that situation, especially when they have many demands on their time. If you're feeling stressed by something that is happening to you, try to figure out what you can do to make yourself feel more in control. How can you make the situation work for you, instead of being controlled by everyone else's needs? At work, be more pro-active in defining your responsibilities. If the boss talks to you only when something goes wrong, make a habit of frequently telling him or her what you've done right. It may change the tone of your interactions and make your job feel less stressful. Remember Maureen K? Maureen went through different techniques trying to make her job less stressful. Finally she realized that nothing she did would the job bearable, and quit. She was then able to transform herself and became more than ten years younger than that stressed person who didn't enjoy her work environment and couldn't find a way to make it less stressful.

Job choice affects the control you have over what you do any one day. So your job choice as well as what you do at that job can affect stress and your perception of stress. And if you think you have too many tasks at home, determine which ones are necessary and which ones aren't. See if you can simplify your tasks. You can also explain your frustrations to your family and ask them to pitch in.

Here are some mental strategies you can add to your RealAge repertoire for stress reduction. Give one a try the next time you feel stressed out.

1. Learn to recognize the conditions that stress you and note your reactions to those conditions. Naming the problem is the first step toward solving it. I usually attach a blood pressure machine to my patient's arm and take his or her blood pressure once a minute as I ask the patient about what he or she does in a daily routine. I can see the spikes in blood pressure from things that stress that person. That gives me clues for helping the patient recognize conditions that stress him or her. When I tell the patient what caused a spike, there is often recognition that the subject being discussed is indeed stressful.

2. Try to think about the situations you find stressful from a different perspective. Is it really that bad? Is there another way of looking at the problem? Reframe the situation just like the salesperson at the department store did on Christmas Eve. She reframed the hassles of men throwing money at her and her register into "men fighting for her." So when people are putting too many demands on you, try to imagine that they're fighting over you, or how valuable they must think your services are.

3. If you can't avoid a stress-producing situation, approach it in a calculated way, taking steps to reduce the stresses. When my mother-in-law's sister was in the hospital, there was no way she could be made comfortable and still remain in control of her mental status. It was sad for my mother-in-law, and stressful. After visiting her sister, my mother-in-law would be in tears. Since it was a situation she couldn't change, she tried to find ways to cope. Having my wife go to the hospital with her was one way to make the visits less stressful. Reassuring herself that she was doing the very best she could helped, too. So did using her cell phone to call others and express her sadness and frustration. Although none of these actions changed the actual situation, they did reduce her stress.

4. If a certain kind of event always makes you agitated, try to think of ways to change the context. What can you do to prepare for that event, so that you don't have to go through the same old thing? If you find Thanksgiving at Aunt Thelma's stressful, don't go, or invite her to your place instead. Just because something's always been done a certain way doesn't mean you have to keep on doing it that way. In other situations that cannot be changed, you can brainstorm with others for coping strategies.

5. If certain individuals are causing you undue stress, whether it's your boss or your teenagers, stop for a moment and try to put yourself in their shoes. If they keep doing something that drives you crazy, ask yourself why they do it. What do they get out of it? By understanding their motivations and perspective, you will be better prepared to develop a strategy for reducing the stresses they cause you.

6. Develop coping skills. Learn to take a time-out when you start to feel your anxiety rise. This is the time to meditate, or take a walk, or do something you know makes you happy. Or just take a time-out by refocusing your attention.

7. If you find that interactions with a particular person are stressing you, talk to that person about it. Don't be accusatory. Take ownership of the problem. Just let him or her know that a certain way of interacting is stressful to you. Together you might be able to find a new way of interacting that's not stressful to either of you, because an interaction that is stressful for one person is usually stressful for both.

Social Networks:
Ties for Life, or Laughing the Years Away with Friends

The RealAge program is all about enjoying the very best that life has to offer. And what could possibly be better than sharing a good laugh with friends? While spending happy times with friends and loved ones is a pleasure and may feel like an indulgence, it's actually a RealAge must. Although for years scientists discredited the effect of social factors on biological health, study after study has confirmed the importance of social connections. Studies have shown repeatedly that the effect of interpersonal relationships on stress responses is not only psychological but also physiologic. These ties can actually affect the number of immune cells you have, which can in turn affects your resistance to disease and cancer. Social connections reduce stress and make your immune system younger.

A RealAge Makeover Success Story: John C.

Three and a half years after they both retired and moved to Florida, John C.'s wife died suddenly. He had seen me yearly on a company benefit for his Real-Age preventive care planning sessions, but not in three years (his wife was not covered by such benefit). He looked twenty years older; his back was hunched over, he had lost tone in his step and sparkle in his face. He was twenty years older. He felt alone, and lonely. He had stopped seeing friends. He had stopped exercising. We talked about what he did enjoy. He visited his two kids once every four months (but felt he was "imposing"), and his two young grandchildren spent some of their Christmas vacation at his home in sunny Florida. But he felt inadequate at times because he couldn't make the cookies Grandma had made. I told him about my new adventures in cooking and suggested he take some cooking classes so he could surprise the grandkids. He looked at me askance—but said, "If you could do it, I can." He not only learned to make great-tasting cookies, he contributed a healthy cookie recipe to the "Cooking the RealAge Way" section of our website. He also found a second love in the cooking class, and now has reversed his aging processes with a great marriage companion. He looks, feels, and is more than 12 years younger thanks to that cooking course, and its associated benefits.

As people age, their social relationships often change in ways they hadn't foreseen. In general, our social supports increase through our lives as we move into our fifties. Then, the neighborhood changes. Friends move away to warmer climates, the kids grow up and start their own lives, and we experience "empty-nest syndrome." By our sixties, our social networks have often begun to decrease. After a lifetime of looking forward to retirement, many people no longer have a daily routine, and feel lonely and isolated.

I have witnessed the experiences of some of my senior patients, who, after much consideration and worry, finally decided to sell the family house and move into a retirement community. This is not a nursing home, but a place that provides not only apartments but also nursing and other care if needed. The new resident goes grumbling off to the "old-age home," complaining about being "turned out to pasture." Suddenly—and I have seen this happen on many occasions—these individuals get a new lease on life. Now, instead of being isolated, they have a whole social world around them, full of activities and new companions to share them with. One friend told me that his ninety-year-old father moved into such a community. He went from being the one who always complained his son never came to see him to being the one who was always too busy. "Sorry, John," he would tell his son, "Saturday we're putting together the community newsletter, and Sunday Madeline's having a brunch. It'll have to be next week." Moving out of an isolated house into a place where there is a social world really can make people younger.

Although such settings are not for everyone, and most of us are happy staying in our homes, I think the example is illustrative. It demonstrates in qualitative terms what we already know in quantitative terms: that having social connections in our lives makes us younger. Norman Cousins claimed that laughter could cure illness. In many ways, you can laugh yourself to youth. Being social isn't frivolous, but vital to our health and youth.

So for the sake of your RealAge Makeover, stop and consider whether or not you have enough social contacts, especially those whose company you truly enjoy, and who live near enough that you can see them when you want to. If you don't have that many and often end up feeling lonely, or don't do an activity because you don't have anyone to do it with, think about building up your circle. How? Become more active in your church or community. Reach out to old friends or new neighbors. Volunteer at your local library. Take an art or cooking class. Join a bridge or a golf club. Anything where you'll meet new people—and make new friends—is good.

Whether they are new friends or old, take the time to cultivate your friendships. It's a give and take—remember, they're getting the same benefits you are. In an Age-Reduction double-dip for both of you, exercise with a friend. Or, if you can't find an exercise buddy, use a cell phone. Then you can walk and talk to friends at the same time. In this way, a cell phone can make you much younger. (Of course, don't talk on your cell phone while driving; this can make your RealAge older.) Learn to use e-mail to contact old friends, and try chat groups on the Internet. The Internet is a way that people who are largely housebound can make themselves younger.

The time you invest making new friends is time invested in your RealAge Makeover. Anything that gets you together with other people on a regular basis can help make you younger. And it's not just a benefit today—it's an insurance policy for the future. Should a major life event befall you, you'll have a support network in place. You won't have to suffer through it alone—the worst ager of all. Find people you care about, who care about you, and learn to lean on them during difficult times. Learn to open up to your family and friends about your problems—it will make your RealAge younger. Don't worry about being a burden; remember, it's a give and take. When their turn comes, you'll be there for them, too.

If you are going through a particularly difficult time, and your friends just don't seem to understand, consider joining a group where the other members are experiencing what you are experiencing. A friend of mine became very stressed when his elderly mother developed Alzheimer's disease. The illness is remarkably unpredictable, and his mother would behave erratically, at times intelligible but at other times incoherent. Sometimes she would be angry for no apparent reason, and other times she would simply start to cry. My friend found the unpredictability incredibly difficult to bear, yet he had to spend an enormous amount of time taking care of her. He also felt isolated. Not only was he watching his mother decline but most of his friends couldn't relate to his situation. (Ironically, sometimes our friends can't relate to our major life events and take a "vacation" from the friendship just when we need them the most. For example, many people who suffer the death of a loved one report that some friends suddenly disappear. They "don't know what to say" and so say nothing. That's why it's doubly important to make sure you have the support you need during trying times.)

My friend's mother's doctor suggested that he go to a program offered by his hospital for relatives of Alzheimer's patients. There he learned what to expect from the disease. More important, he met other people dealing with the same situation. Together they could talk about how it felt to watch a parent slowly lose his or her identity. He found it a great comfort, and it helped him get a different perspective on the disease. When his mother got suddenly angry, he knew that she wasn't angry with him; this was a manifestation of the disease. He learned not to take things she said personally, and this reduced a lot of his anxiety and stress.

One of the books Nancy and I have given to the caregivers of patients who have a chronic disease is called *Share the Care*. This book teaches the caregiver how to bring others in to help so that everyone can share that good feeling of giving care, and so that no single person will be overburdened. Furthermore, when you "share the care," you develop a support network of caregivers that comes to the aid of those needing care. This sharing of care is another RealAge double-dip. Not only are you less stressed by a huge time commitment if someone you know needs care but you also have a support group that helps relieve everyone's stress. Table 7.2 shows the RealAge effect of having social connections.

With all the scientific data to back up what you probably already knew—that spending time with loved ones is good for you—I hope you'll start making more time to build up and cultivate your personal friendships. It's not an indulgence; it's a way to make yourself younger. Learn to value your social relationships and do not sacrifice them to work or other obligations. In addition, do not forget the most important social relationship: the person you choose to spend your life with. How does your partner help keep you young?

Marriage:
Vows to Make You Younger

It goes almost without saying that one of the best social supports can be marriage, and that fact is reflected in health and longevity. Happily married couples live longer. Although there are few data on unmarried people who are in

Table 7.2   The RealAge Effect of Social Connections

Three criteria usually determine the degree of a person's social contacts: marital status; the number of friends seen regularly; and participation in social groups such as churches, community organizations, and clubs. Using this method, this RealAge table assesses the amount of social contact by tallying the number of specific descriptors that apply.

The following RealAge changes occur only if your RealAge is older because of the stress of major life events.

FOR MEN:

HOW MANY OF THE FOLLOWING DESCRIPTORS APPLY?

Is married

Sees at least six friends at least monthly

Participates in social groups

	None	1	2	3
CALENDAR AGE		REALAGE		
35	42	40	31	24
55	60	53	49	46
70	76	73	69	66

FOR WOMEN:

HOW MANY OF THE FOLLOWING DESCRIPTORS APPLY?

Is married

Sees at least six friends at least monthly

Participates in social groups

	None	1	2	3
CALENDAR AGE		REALAGE		
35	41	39	33	28
55	61	59	53	49
70	75	72	69	67

long-term, mutually monogamous relationships, we may assume that the same is true for them, too. Indeed, people who indicate that they are happily married show a RealAge difference of as much as 6.5 years younger than their unmarried counterparts. Widowhood and divorce can have an even greater aging impact than being single.

Although anyone benefits from a loving and stable marriage, marriage seems even more important for men than for women. When comparing the RealAges for thirty-five-year-old men, a man who is married is 6.3 years younger than a bachelor and 5.8 years younger than a man who is separated or divorced. Studies in three countries found that a successful marriage had more of an effect on arterial aging than even total cholesterol or bad (LDL) cholesterol levels. Men who were happily married were less likely to develop cardiovascular disease than unmarried men, even if the LDL cholesterol readings for the married men were much higher. Clearly, being married is enormously beneficial to a man's RealAge.

Women get a RealAge benefit from marriage, too. However, the benefit is not as great as it is for men. Women under fifty show a RealAge benefit of only 2.4 years for being married, and little effect from divorce. Why? The reason may be related to underlying social differences between the genders. Although we don't know for sure, we can presume that contemporary American women are more likely than men to have strong social support beyond their marriages. Also women, more than men, are likely to suffer partner abuse within their marriages. About half of divorced women under the age of fifty seem to show an increase in RealAge, and about half show a decrease. Those who get younger may do so because of the benefits of getting out of unhappy relationships. However, marriage becomes increasingly important to women as they get older. After age fifty, women show a three-year RealAge benefit from being married, whereas divorce can cause 3.5 years of aging.

Thus, in general, marriage prior to age fifty appears to be more beneficial for men than for women. However, our data are imperfect; we just do not yet know enough about marriages and divorces from these large studies, since such studies have no way of discerning the difference between data from an unhappy marriage and data from a happy one. A happy marriage is probably a considerable benefit to everyone, not just young men and older women. The studies show that the benefit of a happy partnership is manifest to a great degree over the age of fifty, when married men and women both have much younger RealAges.

What does all this information mean to you as you plan your RealAge Makeover? Well, if you are happily married or involved in a stable, long-term relationship, know that it is making you younger. If you are single, evaluate your social ties. Do they provide you with support and help? Single people need to make sure that they have adequate social support from family or friends. Many people find themselves suddenly single as they enter their fifties and sixties; if you are in this situation, seek out other avenues of social support. The friendships you find will help keep you younger, and maybe your friends will introduce you to your second "partner of a lifetime."

Remember, too, that RealAge is all about averages: on average, a good marriage helps keep you young; a bad marriage can make you old. Marital stress can be one of the most age-inducing of the social stresses. If you have a marriage that is not working, especially if you are in an abusive relationship, a divorce may be the only solution, the one that will do the most to prevent you from unnecessary aging.

Divorce is a very stressful and difficult process. If you find yourself going through one, don't try to be strong and go it alone. Instead, rely on your friends and family for help, and seek out other possible sources of emotional support. Everyone has different preferences, but ministers, therapists, support groups, and counselors can all help ease the stress of a divorce.

Considering how traumatic the death of a loved one is, it is not surprising that losing a spouse produces results in significant aging for both men and women. Studies show that people who have recently lost a spouse pay more visits to the doctor than the average population, and that the recently widowed have a measurably increased risk of death, of signs of rapid arterial aging such as heart attacks and strokes, of signs of rapid immune system aging such as increased diagnosis of cancer, decreased immune response to vaccination, and an increased rate of automobile accidents and hip fractures, for as long as one year after their loss.

Avoiding the Money Blues: Financial Planning

Money is the subject of the most fights in the average marriage. The issues surrounding money can stir up strong emotions and reactions. In fact, four of the ten most stressful events in our lives are tied to our finances. Declaring bankruptcy, losing a job, changing jobs, and not being able to pay the bills are all financial woes that can cause a tremendous amount of stress. In addition, financial upsets can trigger other events that can also age, such as divorce or major depression.

Because Dennis M. had borderline high blood pressure and was at high risk of arterial disease, he had checkups four times a year. At his April checkup, his blood pressure was through the roof. "Dennis, what's wrong?" I asked. He didn't answer. When I had him return in two weeks just to double-check, his blood pressure was back to normal. Curious.

The next year, his appointment was on April 15, and the same thing happened.

"Dennis, what's going on?" I asked. "Is something bothering you? Taxman got you down?" I said, half-jokingly.

"As a matter of fact, yes," he said, and went into a litany of financial woes.

Dennis owned his own business and paid taxes quarterly. Like many of us, he hated to pay the government so much as a day early. He always skimped on his quarterly payments and then, come April 15, wham! He owed a fortune. Yet as clever as he was at delaying, he never planned very well for actually paying his taxes. So when April 15 came, he owed money he didn't have. Panic set in, and his blood pressure went sky high. He knew that tax time caused him endless worry, but didn't know that needless aging was occurring as well. High blood pressure was aging his arteries and no doubt throwing his immune system out of whack, too.

I said, "Dennis, with the amount of worrying you're putting yourself through, you're giving the IRS something much more precious than dollars. You're giving them years off your life." I convinced him to devise a financial plan that would also serve as a medical plan, keeping him from the needless stress and rise in blood pressure that could cause him to have a heart attack.

Until I met Nan J. and Dennis M., I had never thought that being a good doctor would mean talking to patients about their finances as well as their health! However, I have learned that stress due to money issues is a common, and needless, cause of aging. As a department chairman I would routinely tell residents who were about to leave the poor pay of their residency and take a big jump in income—say, from $20,000 a year to $165,000—that a key to happiness in life is to "pay yourself first, and live below your income." Paying yourself first means putting the first 10 percent of each paycheck into a savings or retirement account first, and living below your income reduces the chance that financial stress will age you. I told residents that if they could live for two or three years as if they were still on a resident's salary and save the rest, the power of compounding would make aging from financial stress much less likely. Many later told me they wished they had listened to that advice. Others who followed my advice told me it was the most important thing I had ever told them. Perhaps the first hour in each preventive medicine course for medical students should describe how to live below one's means.

Although financial blues seem to have nothing to do with your calendar age, the rate of aging does correlate with financial stability. The data aren't precise enough to say with complete certainty that one of the reasons people of higher socioeconomic class have lower rates of aging is that they have greater financial stability, but I think we can assume that to be true. One financial upset is less likely to derail them. Another reason higher socioeconomic status makes you younger, I believe, is the quality of dental care. One of my friends calls it Roizen's Hypothesis: financial solvency leads to better dental care, which thus decreases arterial aging.

Work and Stress: Don't Let Work Age You

If you work, you probably spend more time on average per week with your colleagues than you do with your loved ones at home. Much of your time at home is spent sleeping, so it's not surprising if at some point the break room at the office starts to seem more familiar to you than your own kitchen. Keeping in mind the extent to which work plays a role in our lives, it should not be surprising that our jobs have the ability to make us older . . . or younger.

Even the best job in the world has deadlines, problems, and last-minute snafus—things that stress us. Some people thrive on the stress of a looming deadline (eustress), whereas others feel pushed to the breaking point (distress). What seems to be universal, however, is that the more control individuals believe they have over their jobs, the more likely they are to remain healthy longer. Job satisfaction helps keep you young. This is one reason why health improves as the level of income rises: in general, higher-paid jobs tend to provide people with more flexibility, independence, and choices over their work. If your job makes you unhappy or leaves you unfulfilled, think about what you can do to change that. It may mean looking for a new job, or working with your employer to improve your present working conditions.

Getting fired or laid off ages us even more than work does, no matter how much we may have grumbled about our jobs. Losing a job can make your Real-Age as much as five years older. Such loss is especially significant for men in the middle or late stages of their career; job layoffs and firings seem to have an especially pernicious aging effect on these men, more so than on women. Most likely this gender gap has to do with traditional social roles, in which men are taught to believe that their job is the most central part of their identities. Men who have lost their jobs, and even those who have retired of their own free will, are more than twice as likely to have a major aging event as men who remain continuously employed.

In general, the more freedom you have in a job—the more control you have in decision making—the younger that job makes you. Chicken cutters, for example, have no control. They have to cut so many chicken parts per minute. They can't decide which ones to cut and which ones not to cut. They have time pressures. They also have to use a sharp object that could cause injury. That's a job that makes you older. In contrast, a teacher can decide what he or she is going to teach that day. Even though trying to control unruly kids sounds like a very stressful occupation, teachers tend to live a long time, and without disability. So do people who work excessive hours, but enjoy their work and have control over decisions concerning the work they do. These people have younger RealAges. The goal is to have work that makes us younger. If your job makes you older, you are definitely being overworked and underpaid!

Young Minds:
Become a Lifelong Learner

You know the saying, "Everything you need to know, you learned in kindergarten." Share everything. Play fair. Don't hit. Clean up your mess. Say you're sorry when you hurt somebody. Wash your hands before you eat. Flush.

Well, here is something you probably never learned: going to school and learning make you younger. People who are better educated tend to stay younger longer. In fact, those who don't have a high school education are 30 percent more likely to die prematurely than those who are high school graduates. Mortality rates are lower still for those with some college education or higher. A better-educated spouse makes you younger, too.

There is no direct cause-and-effect relationship between what you studied and your health. Mastering calculus doesn't lower your LDL cholesterol, and failing high school French doesn't put you at greater risk for stroke. Rather, these statistics result from a set of conditions related to levels of education and the way education can affect a person's life trajectory. Some of these reasons are purely economic, because individuals with more education are more likely to have better paying jobs and greater financial stability. Correspondingly, they often have higher socioeconomic standing, less exposure to occupational risks, better access to health care, and a whole range of other benefits that help slow the rate of aging.

In contrast, people with lower levels of education are often poorer, have more dangerous and tedious jobs, live in areas where pollution levels are higher, and tend to choose less healthy lifestyle choices. People who don't have a high school education are eight times more likely to smoke, and are more likely to be overweight, avoid exercise, and eat unhealthy foods. Educational levels are used by researchers to gauge an entire social world, because opportunities, limitations, and social and health behaviors correlate with education.

The effect of education on our health and youth is enormously complex, and no study will ever completely untangle the web. For one thing, the data are too imprecise. Despite the problems in correlating level of education with health, most of the studies try to adjust for confounding variables such as income, social class, and social stresses. However, even when variables are accounted for, a higher level of education still produces a RealAge benefit. All of us probably know people who have high levels of education and don't make a lot of money; think of the people who have spent years training to be actors in the theater, or getting doctorates in theology, despite expecting salaries that won't be commensurate. Such people tend to stay younger longer, because they truly love what they do.

What's behind this correlation between education and health? No one knows exactly, but one theory is that education increases access to information, and part of that information is health information. People who read more are also more likely to pay attention to the news; to think about their health; and to exercise, eat right, and avoid habits that can cause needless aging.

Another reason may be related to the effect of thinking on the active cells in the brain, the neurons. Mental activity is something, like muscular strength, that diminishes with age if we do not use it. However, the variation from one person to another is tremendous. Some people lose that acuity rapidly; others retain a rapier wit and an ability to engage in clever repartee until they die at age ninety. Indeed, it is hard to talk about average trends because so many people defy the trends. The object of RealAge is to learn how to be one of those whose mental acuity doesn't diminish. Education seems to play an important role in achieving this goal. Whether you exercise your neurons or your muscle, you seem to be doing the same thing, making yourself and the cells you exercise younger.

It makes sense that education, either formal or informal, is one of the things that keeps your mind in shape. Jobs that require high levels of education are often the ones that also provide stimulation and variety. They are jobs where you keep on learning while you're working. In doing executive medical planning with individual patients, I found that most chief executive officers work fourteen to sixteen hours a day, five and a half or six and a half days a week. But they thrive on it. What would stress someone else—long hours of hard work—doesn't stress them. Instead, they love their work because they get to choose what work they do, and they keep learning.

What does all of this mean for your RealAge Makeover? It means that you want to make sure you exercise your mind just as you exercise your body.

Chances are, if you are reading this book, you are already doing just that. You have a curiosity about your life. Chances are, too, that you are somewhere past school age. So: how can you make education a part of your adult life?

No matter what your age, consider going back to school, or at least taking an extended learning class. Don't let your calendar age stop you; it's your RealAge you should be thinking about. Not all of us had the opportunity to go to college when we were eighteen. And even if you do have a degree, doubtless you've developed other interests since you were twenty-one. I had a neighbor who obtained her bachelor's degree at age eighty-one. When I asked her what she was going to do next, she told me, "I'm thinking about getting a PhD." She's the best example of what RealAge is all about: someone who takes advantage of the disparity between calendar age and RealAge to do the things she's always wanted to do.

This is a chance to combine having fun (a stress reducer) with learning more (a way to stay young). What you choose to study doesn't have to be academic. Have you always wanted to make the perfect soufflé? A cooking class at a local community center will help broaden your horizons. Also, lifetime learning doesn't always mean you have to be in a classroom. There are many ways to stimulate your mind without attending school: going to museums, reading, taking trips, using the Internet, doing crossword or other puzzles, and developing new interests. If you have an interest in something, explore it. Or, as I like to say, stay young because of it!

A Positive Attitude:
It Makes a Huge Difference

Four studies, all reported in the last five years, have found what many suspected all along: that a positive attitude makes a large difference in how long and how well you live. We all knew that, as it takes a positive attitude to change your habits and do weight lifting, or to take an aspirin, or to take vitamin D or to look at the label to find the real chocolate. But even factoring out all the changes in habits, we now know that the attitude per se makes a difference. The Mayo Clinic study and the study from Duke used personality tests and followed healthy individuals or those recovering from heart attacks for long periods of time. The study of religious orders and the Catholic Nuns' studies used evaluation of essays written sixty or so years before. These studies followed those individuals who were most optimistic or most pessimistic, or who expressed most positive emotions or most negative, and determined the correlation of those with length of life and medical illnesses.

But even with such strong data, we debated whether attitude should be in the RealAge program: how does one develop or adopt a positive outlook, and is the six-year RealAge benefit enough to motivate pessimistic people to change that outlook? We have witnessed enough changes in attitude with such learned habits as focusing on gratitude and keeping a gratitude journal nightly. Savoring an altruistic act, learning good things from a crisis, and feeling gratitude and noting it nightly by writing about the event nightly seem to be methods that can change a pessimist into someone with positive emotions. So we voted to put positive attitude into the program. But no doubt we need to develop methods to experience more positive emotions more often.

And the effect is large: The nuns' study is typical. The nuns who expressed most positive emotions lived about ten years longer than those who expressed the least. When one examines all the studies, it appears that being happy, interested, and satisfied with your life, no matter what your circumstances and irrespective of your other habits, can make your RealAge six years younger. But it is really more than that, as those with positive emotions choose other behaviors that make their RealAge younger more commonly than do those individuals with pessimistic outlooks.

Confronting Your Personal History: Recovering from Serious Emotional Traumas

Sadly, each year a quarter of us will experience a crisis or personal tragedy. A family member may become sick or die, someone may sue you, or you may lose your job. You may have financial worries or be forced to move. Your marriage may fall apart. You may be one of nearly 20 million Americans who have severe clinical depression. Or you may have experienced some trauma in childhood that affects you. See Table 7.3 for the RealAge effect of being a child whose parents divorced. Because more than 50 percent of children are products of subsequently divorced marriages, if the marriage broke up after you were age twenty-one, you are actually younger than the average person in America; so many others would have gone though their parents' divorce before they were twenty-one.

I have talked a lot about what you can do to protect yourself during these tough times, strategies for managing stress and emotional hardship. Nevertheless, what if it's just too much? What should you do when it all seems overwhelming? Or if you have a particular problem that is difficult to talk about with your friends and family members? These topics warrant far more in-depth discussion than I can properly provide in this book. However, numerous books are devoted solely to each of these issues, you should start with those for guidance.

Table 7.3	The RealAge Effect of Parental Divorce		

FOR MEN:

Age of Child at Time of Divorce of Parents

	Never Divorced	Child 21 or Older	Child Younger Than 21
CALENDAR AGE	**REALAGE**		
35	34.1	34.7	38.5
55	53.4	54.6	59.8
70	67.8	69.4	75.7

FOR WOMEN:

Age of Child at Time of Divorce of Parents

	Never Divorced	Child 21 or Older	Child Younger Than 21
CALENDAR AGE	**REALAGE**		
35	34.3	34.9	37.7
55	53.7	54.8	58.6
70	68.3	69.6	74.3

Every person can benefit from being emotionally healthy, and every person has life experiences that affect his or her emotional well-being. Do not hesitate to seek professional help. A therapist, psychologist, minister, counselor, or psychiatrist can provide guidance and insight. The long-time stigma associated with seeking professional help hurt everyone. Thankfully, the past twenty years have seen a marked shift in the way we view mental health. Seeking professional help has become increasingly accepted.

Mental health is a complicated issue because denial can so often play a powerful role, keeping the person from getting the help he or she needs and deserves. That is why those who live with an alcoholic are much more likely to see the problem than the alcoholic himself or herself. Some mental and emotional states have a physiologic component as well as a psychological one. For example, the variations among clinical depressions are defined according to the chemical changes that occur in hormones in the brain. Medications can help these conditions. Common medications include the selective serotonin reuptake inhibitors

(SSRIs), such as citalopram (Celexa), paroxetine (Paxil), fluoxetine (Prozac), and sertraline (Zoloft), and another class of antidepressants, the most commonly prescribed being bupropion (Wellbutrin). One drug may cause side effects in an individual while another drug of a same or similar type will not. Often emotional events will trigger the biological reaction, and, although a pill can change the biochemistry of the brain, it does little to change the emotional stresses that may have triggered the depression in the first place.

Psychotherapy ("talk therapy") can also help. Two forms of this counseling are interpersonal and cognitive/behavioral therapies. Interpersonal therapy tries to help you understand the cause of the depression. Cognitive/behavioral therapy identifies behaviors that perpetuate the depression and tries to design behaviors that avoid further depression. Often talk therapy and medication therapy work best in combination.

Depression

Depression is one of the most prevalent of diseases, and can be one of the most debilitating, in severe cases rendering a person almost completely unable to function. However, because depression is a disease that can be subtle, it often goes undiagnosed. The cause of depression can be physiologic and/or psychological. Although we think of depression as a mental and emotional problem, many depressions actually have underlying organic causes. For example, people diagnosed with clinical depression frequently have low levels of the hormone serotonin in the brain, indicating physiologic origin. Furthermore, there are almost always physiological symptoms, including sluggishness, sleeplessness, loss of appetite, a general sense of helplessness or uselessness, and at times, suicidal tendencies.

People become more prone to depression as they age. It is also a disease that can lead to unnecessary aging. Depression commonly affects women in menopause, both men and women who have recently retired, and anyone who has suffered a major aging event such as a heart attack or diagnosis of cancer. Sometimes the trigger can be biological, sometimes sociological. For whatever reason, depression happens.

What is the relationship between depression and aging? Depression is tied to an increased rate of arterial and cardiovascular aging. In a study done at Duke University, men and women who had heart disease and depression had a 69 percent higher rate of deaths from heart disease over the next nineteen years than those who simply had heart disease and no depression. In the Alameda County study, depressed individuals had a 54 percent increase in stroke rate over twenty-nine years. Other smaller studies have reported similar effects of depression to increase arterial aging events, such as impotence, memory loss, heart attacks, and strokes. Also, women suffering from depression have lower bone density, presumably from increased levels of the stress hormone cortisol, which is found in greater quantities in the blood of depressed people. In addition to causing aging directly, the symptoms of depression—lethargy, sluggishness, a sense that nothing in the world matters—lead to *behaviors* that can accelerate aging. Depressed people are less likely to exercise, to eat a healthy diet, or to make any effort towards healthy living at all.

Women are twice as likely to have depression as men, although no one knows why. Hypotheses run the gamut. Some researchers believe that women face more discrimination and often have to juggle more social roles. Others see the disparity as stemming from biological (largely hormonal) differences. Approximately 10 percent of women suffer from depression during pregnancy, and many suffer with postpartum depression after giving birth. In addition, women tend to have a higher incidence of hypothyroidism, a physical condition also associated with depression.

Social stresses, such as divorce or the death of a loved one can bring on depression. Medications also can trigger depression, as can disease. Individuals recovering from heart attacks and strokes are known to be especially prone to depression. Are the heart attack and its consequences depressing, or is another factor responsible, such as the medications taken? We don't know for sure. However, it is known that those who get depressed after heart attacks have increased risk of further arterial aging. They have over twice the mortality rate in the two years that follow the heart attack as those who get depressed and recover from the depression, and over four times the mortality rate of those who never get depressed. Treating depression with talk therapy and medications, and treating heart disease with medications that reduce arterial aging, such as statins, seems to decrease both the depression and arterial aging.

The good news is that treatment for depression is 98 percent effective within just a few months of its initiation; this means the accelerated aging that depression causes can be avoided. However, the biggest problem is that many depressed people are often unable to seek help on their own. If you suspect that someone you care about is depressed, find out more about the condition and see if you can get help for him or her.

Make sure it's specialized help. Your primary care physician may be terrific, but he or she is probably not the best person for detecting depression. The symptoms are subtle, and because depression was largely misunderstood until the mid-1980s, many doctors were not trained to recognize the disease. One recent study found that family doctors detected depression in only approximately

35 percent of all cases. Thus, if you suspect that you or someone you care about might be suffering from depression, get the right help. Psychiatrists, psychologists, and licensed therapists are all trained to recognize the symptoms of depression and provide many possible treatments.

Other types of emotional distress do not have an organic component at all, but that doesn't mean they aren't true problems. For example, children who experience physical or sexual abuse can suffer the repercussions throughout life. The effects can be both psychological and physiologic.

Following the RealAge program means taking great care of yourself, and that includes great care of your mind. You deserve to enjoy a life of emotional well-being, one that is free from unnecessary stress. It's a better quality of life, and it will help you stay young. A mental health professional can help you develop strategies for dealing with stress and emotional traumas. Just as a financial planner can help you arrange your finances, a therapist can help you evaluate the situations that stress you and develop strategies for avoiding or diffusing them. Sometimes stress can be very subtle and difficult to identify. More and more, we understand that the health of the mind and the health of the body are interrelated. So for the sake of your RealAge Makeover, do not neglect one for the other. Staying well—both physically and mentally—will help keep you young for a long, long time.

Eat Real Chocolate!

The Fifteen Food Choices Proven to
Make You Younger and More Energetic

A RealAge Makeover Success Story: George

Dear RealAge:
I am 50 calendar years old and enjoy the RealAge "tips of the day." About
18 months ago, I was particularly interested in "Thanks for the Memo-
ries," which explained that a pre-diabetic condition can cause memory
loss, and that maintaining a healthy weight can prevent it. Thank you for
making access to important health information in the "tips" so convenient. I have found your science so reliable that I started adopting many
of the healthier RealAge eating choices you sent in your tips, almost sub-
consciously. It's hard to believe, but I have regained the energy I had fifteen years ago when I was thirty-five. And I've lost twenty-five pounds.

Thanks,
George

With the enormous variety of food available in this country, and the often con-
tradictory information in the media about various diets, making food choices
can be confusing and overwhelming. But when it comes to your RealAge Makeover, it's really quite simple. In fact, there are only fifteen food-related habits
that we know affect your energy level and rate of aging:

1. Choose the appropriate total *calories* for your height and build.
2. Limit *saturated* and *trans fats* to less than 20 grams a day.
3. Make sure *healthy fat* makes up about 25 percent of your daily
   calories.

4. Get the right *vitamins* and avoid the wrong ones.
5. Get the right *minerals* and avoid the wrong ones.
6. Get the right *micronutrients* and avoid the wrong ones.
7. Eat four or five servings of *fruit* a day (a serving is about the size of your fist.)
8. Eat four or five servings ("fistfuls") of *vegetables* a day.
9. Eat 25 grams of *fiber* a day.
10. Eat an ounce of *nuts* a day.
11. Eat ten tablespoons of spaghetti sauce or *tomato sauce* a week.
12. Have one to two drinks of *alcohol* a day if you are not prone to alcohol or drug abuse.
13. Get 31 milligrams of *flavonoids* a day.
14. Avoid simple *sugars*.
15. Eat three servings of a variety of *fish* a week.

It should come as no surprise that food plays an important role in overall health and longevity, but too many of us will modify our diets only in order to lose weight. This attitude hurts more than it helps: we get so obsessed with losing weight that we don't eat right. Besides, the preoccupation with weight doesn't actually mean we're getting any thinner. In fact, as a nation, we're getting fatter.

Even though surveys show that the vast majority of Americans know they should eat more carefully and limit unhealthy fat and calorie intake, the overall American diet is getting worse. More Americans are being classified as "overweight" than ever before. In 2001, more than 60 percent of us were classified as overweight, up from 48 percent in 1980 and 20 percent in 1965. Obesity is defined as being thirty pounds overweight for a 5-foot, 4-inch tall woman, or having a body mass index (BMI) of more than 30. In the United States, obesity has doubled from 15 percent in 1980 to 30 percent in 2001. It's not just in the United States, either; it's a worldwide phenomenon.

However, the surprising fact is that just being overweight won't do you much harm if you do not make poor diet choices and do not have the side effects of obesity. That is, if you eat the right foods and are still fat but don't have high blood pressure, arthritis, disordered sleep patterns, a distorted self-image, disordered lipids, or a tendency toward diabetes, and are physically active, the extra weight wouldn't be an aging problem. However, for most people who are overweight, the extra weight will cause complications. Obesity is usually caused by food choices that are less than optimal. Choosing the right foods, even if you are overweight, tends to reduce the likelihood of health complications. So, being fat but fit and eating plenty of fruit, fiber, fish, tomatoes, and healthy fats tends to keep your blood pressure down, normalize your blood sugar and blood lipids, and help you avoid many of the complications of obesity that lead to aging.

A poor diet—one that is full of saturated fats and trans fats (I explain these in detail later) and laden with calories—accelerates aging. In contrast, a diet rich in nutrients, full of fiber, and low in calories can slow the pace of aging. The difference between having a good diet and a bad one can be as much as twenty-seven years in RealAge. A bad diet can make you as much as fourteen years older than the average American; good food choices can make you thirteen years younger. If you like to eat—and who doesn't?—learn how to enjoy foods that taste great and give you energy. It will give a great boost to your RealAge Makeover and buy you added years of good meals.

Let's consider diet from the unique perspective of aging, especially quantifying the ways that eating habits affect your RealAge. I found I was annoyed with my patients. Even after instruction by me and by our nutritionist, they were neither eating the RealAge way nor losing weight. But it was not their fault. I was not explaining it clearly enough for anyone to adopt. But I have learned. My patients are now successful—they are feeling more energy, looking and acting younger. They have learned there are only fifteen food choices they need to know. I have accumulated twenty-four habits (mostly from their tips) that will help you.

It is surprisingly easy with these tips to eat great-tasting food that makes you younger. When coupled with exercise, these food choices will control your weight. I tell you these tips and the fifteen food choices that matter in the pages that follow. Just a few changes in your diet can give you the energy of someone whose RealAge is four to twenty-seven years younger.

- **Don't worry about your weight unless it causes a health complication.**

  The complications of being too heavy are diabetes, abnormal lipid levels, disordered sleep patterns, high blood pressure, arthritis, low back pain, and distorted body self-image. These complications can make your RealAge radically older. Otherwise, a few extra pounds are not as great an ager as we once thought. Although most of us could shed a few pounds, losing weight and keeping it off is no easy trick. Learn how to calculate your body mass index (BMI, the ratio of your weight to your height) and how to combine exercise and healthy eating habits to produce sensible, gradual weight loss. If you have a complication of obesity, any diet that works is a good diet, but most diets, whether the low-carbohydrate Atkins diet or the low-fat Pritikin diet, can be made healthier and better tasting. Maintaining a steady, constant weight can make your RealAge three years younger, as long as you don't have a health complication from being too heavy. If you do have a complication, maintaining a steady, constant weight and reaching your ideal weight will be even more beneficial.

Difficulty rating: Difficult

■ **Eat a RealAge Mediterranean diet.**

The Greeks and Sicilians of the late 1940s and 1950s lived longer than anyone of that era, and their diet was probably the reason why. It contained a lot of nuts, healthy fat, fish, fruits, vegetables, and fiber. They also ate foods that contain the right vitamins, minerals, and micronutrients, including flavonoids, a little alcohol, coffee, and small amounts of cheese (for the intense flavor), and very little trans or saturated fats. If you learn to eat like a Mediterranean person, you can make yourself over fourteen years younger.

Difficulty rating: Moderately difficult

■ **Manage your cholesterol levels.**

Although managing your cholesterol level may not be as important as managing inflammation or some other factors it still matters. Learn how to evaluate your cholesterol levels, what to do if your LDL (bad) cholesterol level is over the danger level of 130 milligrams per deciliter, what to do if it's elevated but not in the danger zone, and what to do if your HDL (healthy) cholesterol level is below 45 mg/dl. The RealAge benefit of managing your blood cholesterol levels is 3.7 years younger.

Difficulty rating: Moderately difficult

■ **Enjoy fish from a variety of sources.**

Three helpings of fish a week (roughly 13.5 ounces) decrease aging of the arteries and probably of the immune system. Is the fat or the protein in the fish the active ingredient? Although we don't know for sure, both appear to have benefits. If you can't tolerate real fish, substitute fish oils. In addition, purchasing your fish from a variety of sources helps you avoid mercury and polychlorinated biphenyl (PCB) contaminants.

Difficulty rating: Moderate

■ **Limit red meat consumption to 4 ounces a week.**

This includes pork, "the other white meat." Use meat as a condiment, not a main course. We don't know whether it's the saturated fat or something else in red meat that is responsible, but we do know that red meat increases inflammation of the arteries and ages the immune system.

Difficulty rating: Moderate

Diseases of the Past Were Not Related to Diet; Diseases of the Present Often Are

The clear correlations between good dietary choices and health and longevity have not always been common knowledge or emphasized. For example, when I went to medical school in the late 1960s and early 1970s, I received just two hours of lecture on nutrition out of more than forty-eight hundred hours of lecture. In the first hour, we learned about diseases associated with vitamin and mineral deficiencies, diseases that are rare except under starvation conditions. In the second hour, we learned—big surprise!—that eating too many calories caused weight gain and that eating too few caused weight loss. Fortunately, this two-lesson view of nutrition is a thing of the past. Increasingly, studies show that the food you choose can greatly affect your rate of aging and substantially alter your odds of being stricken with arterial disease, cancer, diabetes, and other disorders.

That what you ingest into your body affects the health of that body makes such perfect sense, we might even wonder why it took us so long to see the diet–health–youth connection. And what exactly made our attitude finally change toward the importance of nutrition? I attribute the change to what I call the "industrialized society" paradox. From the 1940s through the 1960s, modern medicine really came to the fore. The discovery of antibiotics and safe vaccines helped us control infectious diseases that had ravaged earlier generations, and advances in surgery and internal medicine lowered the rates of other afflictions. Life expectancy increased dramatically. People in the medical community felt a real exuberance, fostering a we-can-conquer-any-disease mentality. As the ravages of some diseases decreased, though, other medical problems became endemic to more affluent societies. Cardiovascular disease and cancer emerged as the new killers, becoming the number one and two causes of death in most industrialized societies. These disease did not fit the old model of disease. Suddenly, issues that had been ignored—diet and nutrition—began to provide some intriguing clues. Only now are we beginning to understand the connections between diet, inflammation, and disease.

Good Health and Longevity Are Principally Related to Lifestyle Choices

How Shedding Pounds Amounts to Shedding Years

Perhaps no health issue is more emotionally charged than weight gain. Oprah has done a series on the emotional causes and underlying issues of weight and weight gain; Dr. Phil did one by himself (with guests) and with Katie Couric. In America, obesity is epidemic. We only need to look at the plethora of diet books and the news stories about eating disorders to sense the concern. Yet, in spite of the abundance of information on emotional causes, diet, nutrition, and the health problems associated with being overweight, Americans have been getting progressively heavier.

Obesity ages us to a great degree only if we have one or more of its side effects: disordered lipid levels, diabetes, sleep apnea (disordered breathing during sleep), arthritis, and the two most common, altered self-image and high blood pressure. Thus, obesity itself is not a great ager unless it comes with the side effects. Unfortunately, over 80 percent of people with a body mass index of over 35 have at least one significant side effect. If you suffer the side effects, losing the extra weight is a great way to give your RealAge Makeover a boost. Let's look at what the benefits would be:

- Reducing blood pressure: up to twenty-five years younger
- Reducing the risk of arthritis: up to six years younger
- Reducing lipids to a normal level: up to six years younger
- Reducing the risk of diabetes: half a year younger for each year you have tight control of blood sugar and blood pressure
- Reducing the risk of sleep apnea: three to nine years younger
- Increasing physical activity: three to nine years younger
- Avoiding negative body image: up to thirty-two years younger

How does one go about losing weight in order to gain the RealAge benefits? Fad diets are not the solution. Losing weight and keeping it off is no easy trick. You must love the food choices you make in order to stick with them for a lifetime. The only way to control your weight and its consequences is to change behaviors at the most fundamental level: weight loss and maintenance of the ideal weight are deeply tied to healthy eating and physical activity behaviors that are practiced for a lifetime. My patients, readers of the RealAge books, and our e-mail subscribers tell us it's not impossible if done gradually and progressively. Here's an unsolicited e-mail about how easy a RealAge Makeover can be:

Dear Dr. Mike,

I just want to let you know how much I enjoy your tips of the day. I appreciate the tidbits of information you send. By reading a little each day, I try to learn something new EVERY DAY, hoping to expand my lifetime little by little.

By the way, I am a school food service manager and should have been very concerned with health and nutrition. But I found myself obese. Nothing worked to keep the weight off. I tried Atkins and lost weight, but then gained more weight back than I lost. But your suggestions are forever. Thanks to the method you shared with us in *Cooking the RealAge Way,* I have lost 44 pounds in the past 19 months. My waist is 7 inches thinner—yes, 7. I feel the energy and the lack of stress—yes, losing weight reduced my stress. I started walking, then retrained my palate, then bought myself the 9-inch plates. And I use the recipes almost every day at home. (By the way, the students love your RealAge Burrito and Smoked Mozzarella and Veggie Stuffed Pizza.)

My friends who live out of town and didn't see the progressive weight loss think I must have had liposuction or plastic surgery or a stomach bypass. I have to tell them I just got RealAge-smart. I have shared *RealAge .com* with the school nurse and the P.E. teacher, and sometimes e-mail your tips to the staff. THANK YOU VERY MUCH!

Karen A.

The customary way to calculate your ideal weight is to determine your body mass index (BMI) or your weight-to-height ratio (see Table 8.1). Although the BMI is one of the best tools we have for assessing whether or not a person weighs too much and is useful for the majority of us as it accounts for variances in body size, giving a standard for evaluating people at a range of heights, it is not very useful in young body builders or athletes. The BMI also does not provide the best possible measure of body fat.

The average BMI for Americans is 27.2 kg/m^2 (kilograms per meter squared). In terms of Age Reduction, the ideal BMI is 23 or less. As long as your weight is not abnormally low because of some health complication, if you have a BMI of 23 or less you can expect your RealAge to be as much as eight years younger than if your BMI were at the national average of 27.2. If your BMI is over 25, you will probably want to consider a moderate weight-loss program

Table 8.1

What Is Your Body Mass Index?

BODY MASS INDEX (KG/M²)*

HEIGHT (INCHES)	19	20	21	22	23	24	25	26	27	28	29	30	35	40
						BODY WEIGHT IN POUNDS								
58	91	96	100	105	110	115	119	124	129	134	138	143	167	191
59	94	99	104	109	114	119	124	128	133	138	143	148	173	198
60	97	102	107	112	118	123	128	133	138	143	148	153	179	204
61	100	106	111	116	122	127	132	137	143	148	153	158	183	211
62	104	109	115	120	126	131	136	142	147	153	158	164	191	218
63	107	113	118	124	130	135	141	146	152	158	163	169	197	225
64	110	116	122	128	134	140	145	151	157	163	169	174	204	232
65	114	120	126	132	138	144	150	156	162	168	174	180	210	240
66	118	124	130	136	142	148	153	161	167	173	179	186	216	247
67	121	127	134	140	146	153	159	166	172	178	185	191	223	255
68	125	131	138	144	151	158	164	171	177	184	190	197	230	262
69	128	135	142	149	153	162	169	176	182	189	196	203	236	270
70	132	139	146	153	160	167	174	181	188	195	202	207	243	278
71	136	143	150	157	165	172	179	186	193	200	208	215	250	286
72	140	147	154	162	169	177	184	191	199	206	213	221	258	294
73	144	151	159	166	174	182	189	197	204	212	219	227	265	302
74	148	155	163	171	179	186	194	202	210	218	225	233	272	311
75	152	160	168	176	184	192	200	208	216	224	232	240	279	319
76	156	164	172	180	189	197	205	213	221	230	238	246	287	328

*To use the table, find your height in the left-hand column. Move across the row to your weight. The number at the top of the column is the body mass index for your height and weight.

Your BMI is the ratio of weight to height expressed in units of kilograms per meter squared (kg/m²). If your exact height and weight are not on the chart, or if you want to calculate your BMI more precisely, the formula for doing so is relatively easy:

1. Convert your weight in pounds to your weight in kilograms by dividing your weight in pounds by 2.2.
2. Convert your height in inches to your height in meters by multiplying your height in inches—not feet—by 0.0254. (For example, if you are 5 feet tall, your height is 60 inches, or 1.52 meters. If you are 6 feet tall, your height is 72 inches, or 1.83 meters.)
3. Square your height in meters (that is, multiply your height in meters by itself).
4. Divide your weight in kilograms (the number you obtained in item 1) by the number you obtained in item 3. The result is your BMI.

that includes boosting physical activity and cutting caloric intake. If your BMI is over 27, excess weight is probably causing you unnecessary aging, and you should also consider a safe and gradual weight-loss plan involving exercise and cutting calories. People with BMIs over 30 should consult a physician or weight-loss professional prior to beginning any diet, to establish a safe and practical weight-loss plan.

Table 8.2 shows the relationship between weight and RealAge.

Another way to determine if your weight is too high is by measuring your waist size, or learning the ratio of your waist to your hip. To measure your waist size, put a tape measure around your body at the belly button level. It's a serious warning sign if you're a women and it's over 35 inches or a man and over 40 inches, because you probably have side effects of obesity. (Abdominal obesity— fat around your middle—is usually associated with increased inflammation of the blood vessels and almost certain aging of the arteries and immune system.)

To determine your waist-to-hip ratio, measure your waist the same way and measure your hips in the area where your hip bones are. Then divide your waist by your hip size. The ratio ages you if it is greater than 0.85 for women or greater than 0.95 for men. For each 0.01 greater than those numbers, your RealAge is about half a year older. The fatter your waist in comparison to your hips, the more aging: the "apple shape" ages more than the "pear shape." We know this relates at least in part to more inflammation and that the fat cells of the abdomen secrete more substances that cause inflammation, but we do not know why this extra secretion occurs.

Despite the well-publicized health problems from obesity, more than 50 percent of all men over age fifty are significantly overweight, 20 percent or more above their desirable weight and having a BMI over 27.8. For a 5-foot, 10-inch man, that would be more than thirty-five pounds over the healthy limit. In 1960, fewer than 25 percent of Americans were significantly overweight. Now it's more than 40 percent. Fifty-five percent of women in their fifties and 42 percent of women age sixty and over are significantly overweight (20 percent or more above their normal desirable weight, with a BMI of 27.3 or higher). From 1980 to 2000, the weight (adjusted for height) of the average American increased by fourteen pounds.

You can see this increase in obesity in America by going to the website for the Centers for Disease Control and Prevention (CDC), *www.cdc.gov/nccdphp/dnpa/obesity/trend/maps/index/htm*. There a series of color graphics illustrates how our waistlines have grown over the years. In 1985, only fourteen states had obesity rates greater than 10 percent, and as recently as 1990, no state had rates higher than 20 percent. Before 2001, no state was in the "most obese" category, with 25 percent or higher. However, our cumulative weight has pro-

Table 8.2 — The RealAge Effect of Weight

FOR MEN:

Effect of Having a Body Mass Index of:

CALENDAR AGE	18.5 or less	18.6 to 21.9	22 to 24.1	24.2 to 26.4	26.5 to 28.7	28.8 to 31.0	31.1 to 33.3	33.4 to 35.7	Higher than 35.7
					REALAGE				
35	35.2	34.7	34.8	35.2	35.4	35.9	36.1	36.2	36.3
55	55.3	54.3	54.6	55.3	55.6	57.6	58.2	58.5	58.6
70	70.5	69.0	69.5	70.4	70.8	73.7	74.7	75.3	75.4

FOR WOMEN:

Effect of Having a Body Mass Index of:

CALENDAR AGE	18.5 or less	18.6 to 21.9	22 to 24.1	24.2 to 26.4	26.5 to 28.7	28.8 to 31.0	31.1 to 33.3	33.4 to 35.7	Higher than 35.7
					REALAGE				
35	34.9	34.6	34.8	35.2	35.5	36.0	37.0	37.5	37.6
55	54.9	54.4	54.7	55.3	55.6	57.4	58.4	59.6	60.0
70	69.9	69.2	69.6	70.6	71.1	73.4	75.0	76.1	76.7

gressively grown. By 2001, thirty-two states had rates higher than 20 percent, and one—Mississippi—had over 25 percent of its population tipping the scales at a dangerous level. Only one state, Colorado, remains in the 10 to 14 percent range.

Some scientists argue that our national obesity stems largely from our food choices. We choose to eat a calorically dense diet, one that is high in saturated fats and trans fats, rich in sugar, and low in fiber and nutrients. Others argue that we are genetically predisposed to obesity. Yet others believe that in our sedentary society, obesity is due to the abundance, variety, availability, and palatability of the food we can eat. That is to say, we overeat. I say it's double trouble. Even taking genetic factors into account, we eat too much, and we eat the wrong things. In addition, we don't get enough exercise, especially strength-building exercise.

What other major factors cause this increase in weight in America? In the last fifteen years, we've learned a lot about emotional and hormonal influences. At least one of these—gherlin, a hormone secreted by the stomach that increases appetite—was discovered accidentally. We learned of the importance of gherlin only by studying people who have had stomach bypass surgery for obesity (bariatric surgery). When you remove part of the stomach, you decrease gherlin levels, which in turn decreases the desire to eat.

Why are some people more prone to being overweight than others? Our genes determine all kinds of influences on height, weight, and metabolic rate, and these vary incredibly from person to person. The study of genetic factors affecting weight gain is a burgeoning field. In 1994, one of the first hormones tied to fat regulation, leptin, was characterized in the now-famous studies of "fat mice:" mice with genetically-created obesity were given injections of leptin and lost weight. Despite the initial belief that a magical new weight-loss drug had been found, the discovery of leptin only proved how complicated the genetics of food metabolism and weight gain are. Subsequent investigation showed that leptin is just one hormone out of many involved in a complicated metabolic pathway. Some people with genetically-caused weight problems have leptin-related disorders, but others don't. Some people clearly have gherlin-related disorders. There will probably be other hormones discovered as well. Weight regulation is a complex genetic trait: many different genes and proteins interact to determine body size. We are still years from understanding the interactions. Good health is not principally a matter of inherited good genes but instead is related to lifestyle choices. When researchers began investigating cardiovascular disease, they found that people who lived in rural Greece and Italy, and even Albania—in communities less "developed" and less affluent than our own—had significantly lower levels of arterial disease. Certain Asian populations also had lower rates. If we Americans and Northern Europeans were so "advanced," why were we so afflicted with these serious health problems?

The first guess was that genetics was the cause: that certain populations just had a bad gene pool. However, studies soon showed that genetic background, while having some impact on the onset of arterial aging and cancer, certainly could not explain the widespread incidence of these diseases. When individuals moved from their rural villages and emigrated to the United States, they developed the same diseases as those around them. The onset of disease correlated with lifestyle. Studies like that of all Danish twins born between 1870 and 1900 showed similar findings; the Danish twins could have much different life spans and could acquire disabilities at very different rates if their behaviors were different. One of the most important factors in the emigrant and twin studies seemed to be diet. Researchers learned that eating a diet rich in nuts, fruits, vegetables, and fish—one that was full of fiber, nutrients, flavonoids, and lycopene, but with a minimum of meat, calories, and saturated fats and trans fat—postponed the onset of arterial and immune system aging to a significant degree. In this healthy diet, the primary fats consumed are olive and nut oils. Both of these oils contain a lot of monounsaturated fat, which decreases inflammation and the ratio of LDL to HDL cholesterol.

The best and simplest way to follow this kind of diet is to eat a RealAge version of a Mediterranean diet. This was first highlighted by Dr. Ansel Keyes, who observed a relationship between heart disease and food intake in certain southern European countries—namely, Greece and Italy.

At least five large-scale epidemiologic studies have now been performed on this phenomenon. The most recent was called EPIC, or European Perspective Investigation into Cancer and Nutrition. EPIC studied 22,043 Greek adults, and its results were published in *The New England Journal of Medicine*. It and the GISSI Prevention Trial, which studied approximately 11,300 Italians who survived a heart attack, as well as a number of other studies (both epidemiologic and randomized controlled trials), have all shown that adherence to a typical 1950s Mediterranean diet reduces death rates and disability rates. In our terms, it makes your RealAge substantially younger. How much younger? The mortality rates indicate that the Mediterranean diet can make you as much as fourteen years younger, with just a little effort, if you enjoy all the right things: fruits, nuts, beans, vegetables, cereal fiber, fish, moderate amounts of alcohol, and monounsaturated fats such as olive oil. What foods should you avoid? Too much red meat, poultry, simple sugars and carbohydrates, and saturated fats, as in full-fat dairy products. In addition, the diet calls for controlled portion sizes and features foods rich in flavonoids, such as onions, garlic, tomatoes, and red wine.

The more closely you adhere to the Mediterranean diet, the lower your chance of having disease or disability, the lower your chance of having a health event like a heart attack, and the younger your RealAge. So while you're enjoying delicious foods such as grilled fish or a tomato and cucumber salad, you'll know that you're making yourself younger. It's not hard to switch to this healthy diet if you do so progressively, instead of all at once. In fact, if you transition smoothly and gradually, you may hardly even notice the new choices. But you'll doubtless notice the effects, as the e-mail from George at the start of this chapter attests.

Small and easy changes in your diet can have transformative effects on your energy, waistline, and RealAge. I learned this because a physician friend of mine took the time to teach me that healthy food can be great tasting. In writing *The RealAge® Diet*, I tried thirteen popular diets, such as Atkins and Pritikin, for two weeks each. I would invite friends over to share the food I'd made. They often told me it didn't taste very good, especially the food from the low-fat diets. Then I learned that a friend who was a physician at the University of Chicago, John La Puma, was moonlighting as a chef at Rick Bayless's great Chicago restaurant, Frontera Grill. I challenged John to use only healthy ingredients and only healthy techniques to make great-tasting food. He in turn challenged the other chefs at the restaurant, and at Kendall College where he was a professor, to do the same. We gave these chefs the ingredients and techniques that make your RealAge younger. They came back with over three hundred fifty great-tasting recipes, or at least the chefs thought they were. We had to find out what other people thought.

I owe my wife a debt of gratitude, because we had eight to twelve people over for dinner four or five nights a week for more than a year to test the recipes. We found one hundred or so recipes that tasted so good that everyone (at least twenty-five tasters for each recipe) agreed they would order that dish again if they went out to a restaurant. All of these recipes also had to be doable in thirty minutes or less by an amateur chef—me. (I specialized in boiling water and toasting bread. I also need to thank others, especially Donna Szymanski, who cooked each of these recipes with me the first time and taught me how to cook.) In addition, each recipe had to be made with only ingredients and techniques that make your RealAge younger. (We cheated just a little, adding cheese because of the intense flavors just a little provides, and salt.) John rose to my challenge and proved that you can have great-tasting food that is also healthy. (You can sample these recipes yourself: twenty-four in *The RealAge® Diet* and more than eighty in *Cooking the RealAge® Way*. Some are also available at *www.RealAge.com*.) So that is how I learned that great tasting food can be healthy and fun to learn about and prepare.

Weight Is a Vital Sign for You

When you arrive at your doctor's office, you usually have your vital signs taken: your heart rate, blood pressure, breathing rate, and temperature. A fifth vital sign has recently been added: your evaluation of how much pain you have. I believe that some other data obtained at this time can be a vital sign for you: your weight (or the BMI that is derived from your weight and height) or even better, your waist size. These vital signs can be used by you to set ambitious but obtainable goals for your weight that will make your RealAge younger.

Studies such as one done at the University of Chicago show that you don't need to follow the latest complicated diet fad to lose weight. What you need to do is simply increase exercise and limit portion size. In this analysis of overweight women, not only did exercise burn calories, it also boosted the overall metabolic rate. In a 2004 study from Duke University, not even changing portion size was needed to maintain weight; just 30 minutes of walking a day was all that was needed to avoid gaining weight (sounds like the cigarette cessation plan that is so successful; see Chapter 6). When you exercise regularly, the body burns more calories per minute even when you are not exercising. Strength-building exercises are especially important, as they build muscle, which burns more calories per minute than other kinds of body tissue.

All too often, when we talk about weight, we are only talking about a cosmetic issue. And to be fair, when it comes to a RealAge Makeover, one goal is to look your best (as well as be younger and healthier). Shedding unwanted pounds will help you do both. However, so far, there are no good and lasting quick fixes.

Strong evidence shows that weight gain between the ages of eighteen (for women) or twenty-one (for men) and forty is particularly dangerous. Weight gain in your early to mid-adult years can make your RealAge one half to one year older for every 10 percent gain in body mass index. Furthermore, every 10 percent increase in relative weight is associated with a 6.5-millimeter rise in systolic blood pressure, and high blood pressure is one of the major factors affecting aging.

Calorie Restriction as a Way of Changing Your Rate of Aging

An intriguing set of experiments started with the Biosphere 2 project ("biosphere 1" being the Earth) by Dr. Roy Walford in the mid-1980s. The Biosphere inhabitants spent two years in a giant, hermetically sealed greenhouse in the Southwestern U.S. desert. They were not able to produce enough food to support their desired weight, so everyone was given only enough food for 75 percent of their usual calories. To their surprise, most of them felt better, and their lipid levels and blood pressure were younger, as was every other intermediate measure of aging of the arteries and immune system. (The one negative side effect was that the inhabitants were constantly hungry and thought about food incessantly. At mealtime, they even scrutinized each others' plates to make sure no one was getting more food than anyone was supposed to.)

The calorie restriction theory that Dr. Walford posed was tantalizing and led to a series of experiments. In small yeast cells, in worms, toads, mice, rats, guinea pigs, and now primates, reducing total calories by 15 to 30 percent of the normal amount extended life by 30 to 150 percent. This effect may reflect the phenomenon, discussed in Chapters 1 and 3, that reducing errors in the energy-delivery part of your cells by not using the energy converting parts of the cell as much, by finding better repair mechanisms, or by finding other chemicals or therapies that protect them, may be a huge benefit in reducing aging.

Resveratrol, a chemical found in grape skins, apparently acts on certain cellular elements to cause the same changes as calorie restriction, and is being tried as an alternative to generate the same antiaging benefits. Whenever calorie restriction without nutrient deficiency has been applied to groups and species of animals, it has almost always prolonged life span. Calorie restriction on humans is difficult to achieve, as we can't even persuade humans to eat just the right amount of calories, let alone 15 percent less than they would ordinarily eat. Investigation is being aggressively pursued to see if the effect of resveratrol can be produced by medicine or another food substance.

Resveratrol may be the prototype for substances that can protect cells and specifically mitochondria, as calorie restriction does, and therefore have benefits greater than just retarding or reversing age-related disease. This type of resveratrol-like substance may reverse or retard the aging process itself. It may be that fish helps you to live to ninety-five at the top of your quality-of-life curve, whereas resveratrol from grape skins—or red wine—may help you live to one hundred twenty or one hundred fifty at the top of your curve. (According to the studies I have read, all grape skins apparently contain some resveratrol, but the amounts vary greatly.)

Calorie restriction may even reduce age-related disease as well. Yes, you have to take nutritional supplements if you are going to live on a highly restricted diet. Nevertheless, the promise of calorie restriction is so intriguing that the National Institutes of Health is spending $20 million over the next seven years to research this topic, and several drug companies are looking for ways to learn how to get the same benefits with pills or other therapies. Unfortunately, Walford himself now has a neurologic disease, so he won't be able to see any of the benefits.

That brings up an important point: if you lose weight you do not want to avoid all fat.

You now need to know a few things about cholesterol—the healthy and the unhealthy—if you are going to lose weight.

Monitor and Manage Another of Your Vital Signs, Your Cholesterol Levels

Your HDL Level Might Be More Important to You Than Your LDL Level

Remember when almost every health story was about cholesterol, and everyone you knew was rushing out to have his or her cholesterol levels checked? Just a few years ago, having a low cholesterol level seemed to ensure long-term arterial health. We now know it's more complicated than that.

There are three basic types of cholesterol in the body: high-density lipoproteins (HDL), low-density lipoproteins (LDL), and very-low-density lipoproteins (VLDL). Because cholesterol tests generally measure total cholesterol, LDL and HDL cholesterol; the VLDL level is rarely measured directly. LDL cholesterol causes aging of the arteries; HDL cholesterol prevents it. HDL is the healthy cholesterol that takes the lousy cholesterol from your bloodstream back to the liver and out of the body as waste products.

While it's generally good to have a low total cholesterol level, and a low LDL and a high HDL cholesterol, many other factors have more of an affect on your aging. In fact, most people who have cardiovascular disease have total cholesterol levels below the high marker of 220 mg/dl (milligrams per deciliter), or LDL levels below 130 mg/dl. Although high levels of total cholesterol and/or LDL cholesterol and low levels of HDL cholesterol can contribute to arterial aging, other factors contribute even more: high blood pressure; inflammation; cigar smoke, cigarette smoke, or passive smoking; lack of exercise; high levels of homocysteine; diabetes; and a diet heavy in saturated and trans fats and poor in nutrients. Nevertheless, you should keep in mind that high LDL cholesterol levels *can* affect your rate of aging.

What Does "High Cholesterol" Mean?

Cholesterol is a type of lipid (a fat-soluble molecule) found in three places: in our cells, in our food, and in our blood. As much as we fear cholesterol, it is a vital component of our bodies. Cholesterol is required for the body to manufacture hormones, build cell walls, and produce bile acids which are essential for the breakdown and digestion of fats. In some parts of the body, cholesterol levels are normally very high. For example, skin cells contain a lot of cholesterol, making them highly water-resistant. This quality protects the body from dehydration by reducing the evaporation of water. The brain also contains high concentrations of cholesterol. (Low cholesterol becomes a problem if the brain doesn't get enough cholesterol for its normal functioning.)

When we measure cholesterol, we measure the amount circulating in the blood. Problems develop not from having cholesterol in the blood—we always need to have some cholesterol in our blood—but from having too much cholesterol in the blood and too much of the wrong type, which can cause damage to the arteries. In general, having a high LDL cholesterol level is bad: excess cholesterol can promote arterial aging. However, even among such high-risk populations as middle-aged men, only 9 to 12 percent of those with total cholesterol readings of over 240 mg/dl will actually have symptomatic cardiovascular disease as a direct result of cholesterol. For each 1 percent increase in overall cholesterol reading in middle-aged men (for example, 202 versus 200 mg/dl), the risk of developing cardiovascular disease increases by 2 percent.

High cholesterol levels affect different population groups disproportionately. High cholesterol seems to have a significant aging effect on young and middle-aged men. The effect is much less significant for older men, and for women of all ages. If you look at the RealAge data and values, LDL cholesterol is less important than HDL cholesterol for women of all ages, and for men over sixty-five. That means that for most of us, it is more important to have high HDL than low LDL. Estrogen (the female sex hormone) generally decreases the presence of cholesterol in the blood, whereas androgens (the male sex hormones) increase blood LDL cholesterol (see Chapter 4).

The Ratio of LDL to HDL

James H. had had high total cholesterol for years. From 1985 until 1996, his total cholesterol ranged from 280 to 340 mg/dl, much too high. He tried everything, but it wouldn't come down. He engaged regularly in vigorous activity, had a thin physique, and avoided saturated and trans fats in his diet. He did both weight lifting and jogging and had a normal BMI (body mass index).

James said his doctor wanted to start him on Lipitor, a statin drug used to control cholesterol. However, he didn't want to take drugs. We obtained a fractionated cholesterol reading (a breakdown), so we could see what his HDL level was. It turned out to be 138, the highest value I had ever seen. He didn't need a statin drug at all. The happy truth was that he had a "trump gene," and he had a wonderfully high HDL level. I didn't refer him back to a specialist in lipid therapy. Instead, I told him to go directly to the National Institutes of Health so they could clone his trump gene. James at first was annoyed that his HMO had not permitted his doctor to fractionate his cholesterol, but was overjoyed he had a trump that made his RealAge much younger.

Of course, this was a highly unusual case. Generally, a total cholesterol reading of 220 mg/dl is too high and can cause arterial aging. In one of the most rigorous examinations of the effect of cholesterol, the Framingham Study, individuals with a cholesterol reading below 200 mg/dl had a 10 percent risk of coronary artery disease over a twenty-year period. Those of the same age with a total cholesterol reading above 240 mg/dl had about twice as much chance (20 percent) of developing the disease.

Most people who have high total cholesterol also have high LDL cholesterol, which causes arterial aging. LDL molecules deliver cholesterol to the cells in the body. When cholesterol rises, excess LDL molecules in the bloodstream can attach to small ruptures or inflammatory lesions in the artery wall. This triggers a process that can lead to the development of arterial plaques and cardiovascular aging.

Like James, some people may have very high total cholesterol levels but arteries in better condition than those of individuals who have lower cholesterol levels. These lucky people have high levels of HDL cholesterol and low levels of LDL cholesterol. Since HDL molecules remove excess cholesterols from the arteries, the more HDL you have, the less arterial aging you will undergo.

When you get your cholesterol tested, be sure to ask for your LDL and HDL levels, your triglyceride level (you must fast for eight hours before that test); and your inflammation number (your hs-CRP [high-sensitivity C-reactive proteins] level). The ratio of total cholesterol to HDL cholesterol—calculated by dividing total cholesterol by HDL—is very important at all ages. The lower the ratio, the better. The average ratio for middle-aged Americans is 5. A fifty-five-year-old man with a ratio of 3.5 (the ratio I try to have my patients achieve) would have only about half the risk of arterial aging as the average man in his age group. His RealAge would be twelve years younger than average.

Having a total cholesterol of over 200 mg/dl suggests a higher risk of aging: Likewise, LDL cholesterol above 130 mg/dl or HDL cholesterol below 45 mg/dl correlates with an increased rate of arterial aging. If your total cholesterol is more than 200, if your LDL cholesterol is higher than 130, or if your HDL cholesterol is lower than 45, you should talk seriously to your doctor about improving your cholesterol levels to retard arterial aging. Having either high LDL levels or low HDL levels can make your RealAge anywhere from three to six years older. Having both high LDL (over 130 mg/dl) and a high LDL-to-HDL ratio (greater than 4) can make your RealAge six to eighteen years older. Even if your cholesterol status is more moderate—LDL levels above 100 but below 130, or HDL levels less than 55 but above 46—you should also consider taking steps to reduce your LDL cholesterol and increase your HDL levels.

Despite all the buzz about cholesterol-free foods, your cholesterol is largely determined by your genetics, weight, activity level, and overall diet. Genetics determine whether or not you will have a tendency toward high LDL levels, and genetics largely determine your LDL-to-HDL ratio. Therefore, genetic factors greatly determine how seriously you will be affected by arterial aging due to elevated LDL cholesterol levels if you don't adopt Age-Reduction activities specifically targeted toward preventing arterial aging. For example, if you are a man with a high LDL cholesterol level or a high LDL-to-HDL ratio, and a number of your close male relatives died early from heart disease, you are at high risk of the premature onset of cardiovascular disease. The great news in the last two and a half decades is that you can control that disease. Weight loss is absolutely key to getting your cholesterol and triglyceride levels into normal ranges. That's one of the real benefits of the Atkins diet for those who lose weight: they normalize their lipid and triglyceride levels. However, to make it a really healthy diet, you should switch from saturated and trans fats to monounsaturated and polyunsaturated fats.

As noted, an HDL level of approximately 60 mg/dl appears to provide tremendous protection against arterial aging. Although statins, especially Lipitor and Crestor, will help increase HDL levels, drugs are not the most effective way to improve your cholesterol ratio. In fact, no technique has been proven to work for everyone. Consumption of healthy fats will increase HDL levels, as will exercise. Women tend to have higher HDL levels than men and are able to improve their HDL levels with exercise to a greater extent than men. A 2001 North Carolina study found that aerobic exercise increased HDL 20 percent in female patients but only 5 percent in male patients. Also, drinking a glass of alcohol at night (half a glass for women) may increase your HDL (see Chapter 11). For most people, losing excess weight improves their HDL readouts. Although the interaction between weight gain and cholesterol levels is still not well understood, the two are strongly related. Remember, if you lose weight you will reduce your LDL cholesterol and triglycerides and make yourself younger. We look at those independently from weight loss, but they are a strong benefit. This effect occurs even if you have gone on the Atkins diet and eaten a lot of saturated and trans fat. But remember, you want to modify that diet so you have healthy fats because saturated and trans fats cause inflammation that will age your arteries.

In contrast, if you have low LDL cholesterol, your genetics are protecting you from arterial aging. There are a lucky few who have both low total cholesterol and high HDL cholesterol. These people also have a genetic trump. All that HDL cholesterol helps protect them from arterial aging. They can have a RealAge as much as twenty-six years younger than those without the trump gene.

Table 8.3 shows the effect of various blood levels of total cholesterol and HDL on your RealAge.

Table 8.3

The RealAge Effect of Blood Cholesterol Levels

FOR MEN:

Total Cholesterol Below 160 mg/dl, and HDL of:

CALENDAR AGE	More than 59 mg/dl	46 to 59 mg/dl	35 to 45 mg/dl	Less than 35 mg/dl
		REALAGE		
35	32.9	34	35.1	35.7
55	51.7	53.2	56.2	57.2
70	66	66.9	71.4	73.4

Total Cholesterol of 160 to 200 mg/dl, and HDL of:

CALENDAR AGE	More than 59 mg/dl	46 to 59 mg/dl	35 to 45 mg/dl	Less than 35 mg/dl
		REALAGE		
35	33.9	34.6	35.2	35.9
55	52.1	54.2	56.3	57.5
70	66.9	66.4	71.6	73.6

Total Cholesterol of 200 to 240 mg/dl, and HDL of:

CALENDAR AGE	More than 59 mg/dl	46 to 59 mg/dl	35 to 45 mg/dl	Less than 35 mg/dl
		REALAGE		
35	34.1	35.1	35.6	36.1
55	52.3	55	56.7	58.3
70	67.6	70.3	72.3	73.8

Total Cholesterol Over 240 mg/dl, and HDL of:

CALENDAR AGE	More than 59 mg/dl	46 to 59 mg/dl	35 to 45 mg/dl	Less than 35 mg/dl
		REALAGE		
35	35.8	37.4	38.1	38.7
55	56.7	58	58.4	58.8
70	68.4	70.6	72.5	73.9

FOR WOMEN:

Total Cholesterol Below 160 mg/dl, and HDL of:

CALENDAR AGE	More than 59 mg/dl	46 to 59 mg/dl	35 to 45 mg/dl	Less than 35 mg/dl
		REALAGE		
35	33.7	34.6	34.9	35.3
55	52.6	53.2	54.7	56.4
70	68.5	68.5	70.2	71.8

Total Cholesterol of 160 to 200 mg/dl, and HDL of:

CALENDAR AGE	More than 59 mg/dl	46 to 59 mg/dl	35 to 45 mg/dl	Less than 35 mg/dl
		REALAGE		
35	34	34.6	35.0	35.6
55	52.8	53.4	54.8	56.5
70	68.5	68.5	70.2	71.8

Total Cholesterol of 200 to 240 mg/dl, and HDL of:

CALENDAR AGE	More than 59 mg/dl	46 to 59 mg/dl	35 to 45 mg/dl	Less than 35 mg/dl
		REALAGE		
35	34	35.1	35.0	35.6
55	52.8	53.8	54.8	56.4
70	68.5	68.5	70.25	71.8

Total Cholesterol Over 240 mg/dl, and HDL of:				
	More than 59 mg/dl	46 to 59 mg/dl	35 to 45 mg/dl	Less than 35 mg/dl
CALENDAR AGE	REALAGE			
35	34.6	36.9	37.1	37.3
55	55.3	55.6	56.5	57.4
70	68.5	69.4	70.5	71.8

mg/dl is the abbreviation for milligrams of cholesterol per deciliter of blood.

How to Treat Abnormal Cholesterol Levels

You may be surprised to learn that eating a low-cholesterol diet is not an especially effective way to reduce LDL cholesterol. Cholesterol consumed in food will increase cholesterol levels for some people but have no effect on others. Only about 15 percent—one in seven individuals—who try a low-cholesterol diet obtain a significant antiaging effect from doing so. Also, some people can get too low an LDL cholesterol level. If your LDL cholesterol goes below 80, you could be at risk of nervous system and immune system dysfunctions, it can go that low if you are both taking drugs and watching your diet. The balance between benefit and risk of what you should do to make your RealAge younger is clear: if you have symptoms of severe arterial aging such as angina or inability to walk more than a block or two without having to stop due to calf pain, you need to get rid of the plaque by reducing your LDL and raising your HDL cholesterol—and not worry about the potential risk of nervous and immune system dysfunctions. But if you do not have such symptoms, I do not believe the potential benefits of trying to obtain a LDL level below 80 mg/dl is worth the potential risk.

Genetic factors largely determine your sensitivity to dietary cholesterol, and people can range from extremely sensitive to completely insensitive. A person who is genetically insensitive may consume as many as 1,000 milligrams of cholesterol daily without negative consequences. In general, though, you should consume less than 300 milligrams a day. People who are particularly sensitive to dietary cholesterol should eat even less, to retard or reverse arterial aging. How do you know your responsiveness to dietary cholesterol? You can judge this only by measuring blood levels before and after restricting dietary cholesterol.

A dramatic decline suggests that you are sensitive; a more modest decrease of 10 to 15 percent suggests that you are not.

For most of us, obesity influences the level of cholesterol in our blood far more than the consumption of cholesterol. Unless you are especially sensitive to dietary cholesterol, your body produces almost all of the cholesterol that exists in your bloodstream. The liver turns the saturated fats, trans fats, and sugar you consume into triglycerides, and then into cholesterol.

Therefore, the best way to reduce high LDL cholesterol is to lose weight and eat foods that are low in simple sugars, saturated fats, and trans fats. If you have high LDL cholesterol, you may also want to consider taking medicine. Talk to your doctor about getting a more extensive lipid evaluation, and about the pros and cons of medication for improving either your overall cholesterol level or LDL-to-HDL ratio. The latest and most effective drugs are the so-called statins, such as pravastatin (Pravachol), atorvastatin (Lipitor), rosuvastatin (Crestor), and simvastatin (Zocor). These drugs lower LDL and increase HDL more effectively than the older generation of drugs, and have improved tolerability and acceptance. Since the statins are relatively new (under twelve years of widespread use), we do not know whether they have negative effects when used over a long period; the longest running study lasted only six years.

Although not conclusive, the data strongly suggest that statins substantially retard arterial aging. As well as normalizing cholesterol values, they somehow inhibit inflammation of and plaque buildup on the valves in the heart, and decrease inflammation in your arteries. If a patient cannot bring his or her inflammation number (hs-CRP, high-sensitivity C-reactive protein reading) into the normal range through exercise, drinking wine, and treating any chronic infections, a small dose of statins can often do the trick. New data also show that statins may inhibit many processes of arterial aging.

We always thought that statins worked by increasing the number of LDL receptors in the liver. This would help the body detoxify the bad cholesterol. We now know that the statins also inhibit the synthesis of LDL cholesterol. Statins are also beneficial for women who have diabetes, arterial aging disease (stroke, coronary artery disease, or peripheral vascular disease), elevated levels of high-sensitivity C-reactive protein, or low HDL cholesterol.

If all the benefits we think statins provide actually prove to be true, perhaps statins should be taken regularly by almost all of us, as aspirin is, and started at about the same time, age thirty-five or forty. At the present time, though, we can't recommend that practice, for two reasons. First statins are so new that we don't know if they have negative effects from long-term use. Second, you don't want too low a cholesterol value, as this may cause neurologic or immune dysfunction.

Low Cholesterol Levels

When we talk about cholesterol levels, we're usually referring to a situation in which your LDL cholesterol level gets too high. But what about the other end of the spectrum? Can your cholesterol level dip too low? Maybe, although we know far less about ultra-low cholesterol than high cholesterol, as very few people without an acute disease or chronic malnutrition have cholesterol levels low enough to be of concern. In a few studies, people with low total cholesterol levels appear to have a higher incidence of cancers, neurologic diseases, and, it's curious to note, suicide. Although very few studies have been done on this subject, and we still cannot say with any certainty how low "too low" is, it appears there is some risk. This effect should not scare you from taking a statin. In the vast majority of patients, preventing arterial aging with statins decreases all arterial aging events, and even decreases the risk of depression. If you have symptoms or signs of arterial aging the benefit of reducing your LDL cholesterol to low levels appears to outweigh any potential risk. If you do not have arterial aging symptoms and signs yet, statins and LDL cholesterol reduction and HDL cholesterol elevation are probably beneficial to an LDL level of about 80 mg/dl. A possible explanation for the relationship of too low an LDL cholesterol level to neurologic disease and cancer may be that cholesterols are necessary components of nerve sheaths (the substance surrounding many of the nerves), cell borders, and vitamin D_3, a proven cancer fighter (see Chapter 10). As for the suicides, no one really understands that apparent cause and effect. Cholesterols are important in brain cell functioning and the production of hormones, so an ultra-low level of cholesterol may affect these two functions.

Nutrition Basics:
Eat Your Way to Youth?

The RealAge plan is all about enjoying the best that life has to offer. And really delicious food certainly can be some of the best of life. Eating should be fun. If your diet is like a prison sentence, you will only end up breaking out. The fact that food really does have to taste great if a person is going to stick to a diet was demonstrated when I was asked to counsel a retired football player. In less than six months after retiring from the National Football League, he had ballooned from 310 to 480 pounds. After six years of yo-yo dieting, he weighed in at 480 to 520, and the extra weight was clearly affecting his life. He was desperate. He chose the best therapy available at the time (the early 1990s): having his jaws

Soybeans as Youth Beans

Recent studies have linked soy protein to a reduction in LDL cholesterol. People who regularly consume soy products—soy milk, tofu, soybeans (but not soy sauce!)—have LDL cholesterol levels that are, on average, 13 percent lower than those who don't. Try substituting soy-based products for animal protein in your diet. Consumption of soy products may have a particularly big impact on those with very high cholesterol levels. It is not clearly understood why or how soy protein helps reduce cholesterol levels, although some experts theorize that soy works as an oxidant on cholesterol. Others think that soy may interfere with plaque formation. To make a substantial difference in cholesterol, you would need 31 to 47 grams of soy protein a day. Soy also contains a natural estrogen that seems to reduce the risk of both breast and prostate cancers, and to provide extra protection for aging of the bones.

wired shut so that he could eat only liquid food. He really gave this diet his best efforts, buying a vegetable juicer and having nothing but vegetable juices and fruit smoothies for eight months. With exercise and resistance training, he was able to lose more than two hundred pounds during that eight months.

Unfortunately, since he hadn't really loved his liquid diet, he abandoned it the first chance he got. I saw him the very first day after his jaws were unwired, at a retirement planning meeting for former football players, where piles and piles of breakfast pastries had been set out for the men. He proceeded to demolish all the pastries—all one hundred fifty or so of them. Single-handedly! It was hard to believe anyone could have that big a stomach or consume that many calories all at once. I estimated he took in over fifteen, maybe twenty thousand calories during that one "breakfast." Clearly, the liquid diet had had no lasting effect on his general attitude toward food.

That taught me once again that a RealAge Makeover is forever. Luckily, the Mediterranean diet with RealAge cooking and spicing modifications is fantastically delicious. You don't have to adhere to it militantly. If you eat something that's not healthy once in a while, it's not the end of the world. What is most important is to retrain your taste buds and develop good general eating habits.

When it comes to eating for weight loss, setting your goal and getting to your goal are crucial factors. Whether it's a modified Atkins diet or the Zone diet, setting a goal that inspires you is the key. I believe that the fifteen food choices listed in this chapter are essential, because they've been shown to slow your rate of aging. Although the Mediterranean diet is best for your health, any diet that helps you lose weight is beneficial, and you can modify almost any diet to make it healthier. In *The RealAge Diet*, we analyzed thirteen of the most current diets, and made each one healthier. For example, you can turn the Atkins diet and other low-carbohydrate diets into a diet that makes your RealAge more than six years younger by doing a few simple things. You can substitute fish for meat, nuts for beef jerky, and olive oil and salsa for cream and butter. You can also add healthy fat and supplements that provide all the vitamins, minerals, and micronutrients specified in Chapter 10.

Changes in your diet don't have to be overwhelmingly drastic. Even small changes can help. With just a little effort, you can gradually shift to low-fat or healthy-fat foods without feeling deprived. Liking saturated fat is not a genetic preference but an acquired taste. In fact, most people who have gone from whole milk to skim find whole milk much too rich when they try it again later. That's because Mother Nature usually made it easy for us: the best-tasting, most colorful, and best-looking food is often the healthiest.

The Fifteen Food Choices That Make a Difference in Your Rate of Aging

Only fifteen items—food choices—in nutrition have been shown by repeated study to make a difference to your rate of aging or RealAge. These fifteen are:

1. Choose the appropriate total calories for your height and build.

The first process of any diet is to decide on what you want to weigh. As indicated by the data above, this can be your weight at age 18 (women) or age 21 (men), or the weight you feel best at. Once you have decided upon that goal, you can calculate the calories you need daily by multiplying your goal weight in pounds by 10.9 (or your goal weight in kilograms by 24). To that number of calories you need to add the number of calories you use by your daily physical activity: for example, a relatively sedentary individual might add 200 calories to this, while a very active individual might add 600 calories. That total is your calorie requirement for that weight, and should be your total calories consumed at maintenance. You can aim to eat 500 calories less a day than that number to reach your ideal weight at the rate of a pound a week.

2. Limit your consumption of saturated and trans fats.

Try to keep your intake of saturated and trans fats (the "aging fats") to less than 20 grams a day. (You'll need to keep track, but don't have to be exact.) Eating more than this amount correlates with arterial aging and cancer, especially breast and prostate cancer. Saturated and trans fats also sap your energy immediately and on a long-term basis. By eating fewer than 20 grams of saturated and trans fats a day out of approximately 60 grams of total fat, you can make your RealAge as much as six years younger. This is a moderately difficult choice, but very important for your health, and my patients learn to do this easily without a feeling of sacrifice. How they do this is to have fewer legs in their fat.

Fewer Legs in Your Fat: Keep the Taste

Fat may seem like a complicated food issue, but there's an easy way to remember which fats are good for you and which aren't. When I was preparing to serve Oprah lunch, I needed a clever way of explaining what healthy fats were and weren't, so I turned to the RealAge scientific team for help. Harriet Imrey, a brilliant epidemiologist on our team, had a great suggestion. She thought I should explain fat in terms of legs: the fewer, the better. Fat from cows and pigs (four legs) is the worst. Chicken (two legs) is better. Fish, nut, olive, and avocado fat (no legs) is best. I thought it was a clever idea and sprang it on Oprah during the show. She looked a little puzzled when I said, "Let's move from four-legged fat to no-legged fat," but when I explained it Harriet's way, she understood instantly.

"Fat" can mean two things: body fat—the fat you have on your body—and dietary fat—the fat you eat. Fat is a chemical compound found in most living organisms, plants and animals alike. Fat is essential. The body cannot manufacture the three essential fatty acids contained in dietary fat, so you must get them from food. You need to eat some fat to absorb vitamins A, D, E, and K, and other age-reducing substances such as lycopene and many other carotenoids and flavonoids. The problem is not so much that we eat fat, but that we eat too much of the wrong kind of fat and not enough of the right kind.

There are four major types of fat: saturated, polyunsaturated, monounsaturated, and trans fat. The first three occur naturally. Trans fat is an artificial version of saturated fat. Although all four types of fat have the same number of calories per serving (120 per tablespoon or 9 per gram), each type affects the body differently. Saturated and trans fats cause aging of the arteries and the immune system. Polyunsaturated fats do not seem to have any substantial aging effects per se. Monounsaturated fats actually appear to make you younger, help-ing to boost the levels of healthy (HDL) cholesterol in your blood.

No matter what kind of fat you eat, remember that fats are "fattening." Fats, whether in our bodies or in the plants and animals we eat, are energy stores and loaded with calories. Fat contains more calories (9 per gram) than either protein or carbohydrate (4 per gram).

The average American consumes 80 to 100 grams of fat a day, which is about 35 percent of his or her total calories. I recommend you limit your total fat in-take to 25 percent of your total dietary consumption. If you go too low on fat, you can develop nerve dysfunction or cancer, or you can lose friends. The nerve dysfunction may be related to the fact that some fat is needed for nerve mem-branes. The immune dysfunction may be related to the need for fat in the membranes of cells that are part of the immune system. The loss of friends oc-curs when you invite them over to eat and give them a tasteless, very low-fat meal. (When I was trying the Pritikin Diet, nobody would accept a free meal the second time.)

SATURATED FATS

Of all the fats, saturated is the worst: just remember "s" for "stay away." Satu-rated fat is found in red meats, full-fat dairy products, palm and coconut oils, and, to a lesser extent, poultry.

No food element has been more closely linked to arterial aging than satu-rated fats and their cousins, trans fats. This relationship was confirmed by a twenty-five-year study that evaluated the development of coronary heart disease and the long-term risk of death. Studies have repeatedly found a strong correla-tion between cardiovascular disease and the consumption of saturated fats.

Apparently, saturated and trans fats turn on certain genes that produce pro-teins associated with inflammation of blood vessels. Foods high in saturated fats promote plaque buildup along the artery wall, which is the first stage of cardio-vascular disease and arterial aging. In addition, saturated fats facilitate the mech-anism that increases LDL cholesterol in the bloodstream.

It's becoming so widely known that fats are bad that even the companies that earn huge profits through the sale of processed food are becoming more willing to change their products, for fear of losing customers. For example, *Time* magazine reported that Kraft is redesigning some of its foods to contain health-ier fats because Wal-Mart demanded it. (You know that when Wal-Mart cries for healthier foods, trans and saturated fats have become a serious public health issue!) What about the Atkins or other low-carbohydrate diets, you might ask, do these not make your cholesterol readings better? The answer is that if you lose weight, your (lousy) LDL cholesterol values will decrease, but your arteries and immune system will still age faster if you eat a lot of saturated and trans fats. The culprit is apparently the inflammation these specific fats promote.

If you do not lose substantial weight on a fat-rich diet, the trans and saturated fats you eat will have a huge effect to increase on our cholesterol levels. Only 20 percent of cholesterol is absorbed from food. The liver manufactures the rest from saturated and trans fats. Contrary to popular belief, for the majority of individuals who do not lose substantial amounts of weight, consumption of saturated fat—not of cholesterol—is the biggest dietary factor contributing to elevated levels of cholesterol in the blood. Excess saturated fat consumption is also linked to elevated triglyceride levels, a reflection of fat in the blood. An elevated triglyceride level makes your RealAge older by increasing arterial aging.

TRIGLYCERIDES

Triglycerides are lipids (fats) that circulate in the bloodstream. Triglyceride measurements are usually taken when cholesterol levels are analyzed, after an overnight fast. The average fasting triglyceride level is 120 to 125 mg/dl. Levels above 209 mg/dl are associated with significant arterial aging, especially with plaque buildup along the artery wall. Because triglyceride levels fluctuate a fair amount, people with high levels (above 190 mg/dl) will want to have their blood analyzed several times to get an accurate estimate. If your fasting triglyceride level is above 209 mg/dl, reduce total fat and simple sugar intakes. Cutting saturated and trans fats to less than 7 percent of your total caloric intake, eating fish rich in omega-3 oils at least three times a week, reducing simple sugars as much as you can, losing weight, and increasing physical activity are all actions to try before considering possible drug therapies (see Table 8.4).

Saturated Fat and Cancer

Does eating saturated fat cause your body to age in other ways? Yes. Although the link between fat consumption and cancer remains nebulous, several studies show a strong correlation. Some experts estimate that as many as one-half of all cancers may be provoked, or their growth promoted or inhibited, by our dietary choices. Apparently, saturated and trans fats promote the growth of cancer cells and the progression of cancer tumors. The Iowa Women's Health Study indicated that postmenopausal women who have been diagnosed with breast cancer have a better survival rate if they keep their weight down and consume a diet low in saturated fats. Other studies have noted a connection between fat intake and a higher incidence of other types of cancers (including lung cancer, lymphomas, and ovarian and prostate cancers).

Table 8.4 — The RealAge Effect of Triglyceride Levels in the Blood

FOR MEN:

Concentration of Triglycerides in the Blood (mg/dl)

CALENDAR AGE	Less than 90	90 to 123	124 to 209	More than 209
	REALAGE			
35	33.2	35.3	35.5	35.7
55	41.6	55.7	56.7	60.9
70	65.7	71.0	71.9	78.2

FOR WOMEN:

Concentration of Triglycerides in the Blood (mg/dl)

CALENDAR AGE	Less than 90	90 to 123	124 to 209	More than 209
	REALAGE			
35	33.9	35.2	35.3	35.5
55	50.1	55.5	56.5	65.9
70	66.8	70.7	71.7	74.8

mg/dl is the abbreviation for milligrams per deciliter.

The Food and Drug Administration (FDA) mandates that product labels list the percentage of saturated fats. Companies now advertise their products as being "low in saturated fat." However, that isn't enough. The food might also contain a type of fat that is just as bad, if not worse: trans fat.

TRANS FATS

Recent research suggests that trans fats are at least as dangerous as saturated fats. Trans fat (also called trans fatty acid) is created when unsaturated fats are hydrogenated (combined with hydrogen), a chemical process that causes fats that would normally be liquid at room temperature to become solid. Any fat we eat that is liquid when heated but that hardens when cooled to room temperature is either saturated or trans fat. Here's a good rule for remembering if a fat is good for you: if it's solid at room temperature, it will age you. Stick margarine is a trans fat. Trans fats, like saturated fats, alter basic metabolic pathways, causing a rise in overall cholesterol levels, particularly the lousy (LDL) cholesterol in your bloodstream.

Studies show that the more trans fat a person consumes, the faster the cardiovascular system ages. In one study of more than 85,000 participants, women who consumed more than four teaspoons of margarine a day had a 70 percent higher risk of cardiovascular disease than those who rarely consumed margarine at all. That makes those fifty-five-year-old women 2.7 years older than if they used olive oil. Some researchers have attributed as many as 50,000 deaths a year to trans fat consumption.

Trans fat is also dangerous because it is very difficult to tell exactly which foods have it. In previous years, food producers were not required to list trans fat on the nutritional labels, so trans fat was called "the hidden fat." Luckily, that will soon change. In 2005 all food companies will be required to list the amount of trans fat on the labels, and many are listing it already.

Many packaged foods—cookies, crackers, and potato chips—contain trans fats because they give food a longer shelf life. A lot of cookies and crackers claim to be "baked, not fried" or to have no cholesterol, implying they are healthy when they are, in fact, chock-full of trans fat. It doesn't matter if a food is baked or cholesterol-free; if it contains trans fat, it will damage your arteries.

Many fast-food restaurants cook food in trans fat to produce the flavor of food cooked in lard, the ingredient used before consumers became concerned about saturated fats. Although the move away from animal fats was supposed to be good for our health, most french fries at your local burger joint contain as much or more artery-clogging fat as if they had been fried in animal fat. Even the chicken at most fast-food restaurants, an option you might think would be healthier, is almost always high in fat, often containing more fat than a full steak dinner. Have a look at the numbers in Table 8.5, keeping in mind that your goal is a limit of 20 grams a day. These numbers mean that a "Happy Meal" should make you anything but.

How do you know if a food contains trans fat? In 2005, food manufacturers will be required to list the trans fat content on the label. Until then, you can figure it out with a little detective work. On the information label, find the total fat content. Then, subtract the saturated fat and the mono- and polyunsaturated fats. This leaves the trans fat. For example, if chocolate chip cookies have 12 grams of fat per serving and the label lists only 4 grams of saturated fat, the cookies also have 8 grams of artery-aging trans fat.

Another way to tell is to look at the list of ingredients. A food label must list the ingredients in order of quantity, from most to least. If hydrogenated or partially hydrogenated oils are listed early on the list and before polyunsaturated or

Table 8.5	Saturated and Trans Fat Content of Some Popular Foods	
	GRAMS OF FAT	DAYS' WORTH OF TRANS AND SATURATED FATS
Outback Bloomin' Onion	100	5+
Arby's Ham Platter	89	4+
Cheesecake Factory Carrot Cake	83	4+
Red Lobster's Rib Eye	82	4+
Cinnabon frosted cinnamon bun	75	4
Denny's Ultimate Omelet	75	4
Dave & Buster's Cheeseburger	69	3.5
Cheesecake Factory Cheese Cake	63	3.1
Taco Bell Taco Salad	61	3.0
McDonald's Big Mac	26	1.3

Much of this information comes from the companies' own websites, so I can guarantee its accuracy only to the point each company's website or the nutrition information they hand out at their stores accurately reflects what is in their products.

monounsaturated fats, you know the product contains lots of trans fat. If the label lists unsaturated or monounsaturated oils, olive oil, or canola oil first, the fats are probably okay. Some experts contend that trans fats make up 25 to 60 percent of all fats contained in processed foods, and 15 to 30 percent of the total intake of dietary fat. Others disagree, saying the numbers are much lower.

The full effects of trans fats are still not understood. Some scientists believe that the artificial molecular structure of trans fat actually causes more harm than naturally occurring molecules of saturated fat. Stick margarine might be even worse for you than butter. We can't say for sure; the research still needs to be completed.

The best advice is to cut out as much saturated fat and trans fat from your diet as possible. Use liquid vegetable oils in recipes that call for butter or margarine. Make substitutions. If you decide to eat margarine, buy "liquid" or soft margarine. The first ingredient listed should be water, vegetable oil, or a vegetable oil blend.

3. Make 25 percent of your calories healthy fat.

You need healthy fat for normal nerve and immune cell function, and to make food taste great. The unsaturated fats in olive oil, canola oil, avocados, flaxseeds,

nut oils, fish, and some legumes have healthy fats. And real chocolate is a wonderful fat. Real chocolate has cocoa-butter fat that is metabolized in the body
into a healthy fat. The correct amount of healthy fat to aim for in your diet is
about 25 percent of calories from these unsaturated fats.

UNSATURATED FATS

The other two types of fats are the unsaturated fats: monounsaturated and
polyunsaturated fats, found in nuts, fish, vegetables, and fruits. These fats are
naturally "unsaturated" because they do not contain the maximum number of
hydrogen atoms, and usually remain liquid at room temperature. The prefixes
"poly" and "mono" refer to the number of the unsaturated hydrogen bonds.
Polyunsaturated fats appear neither to promote nor prevent premature aging. I
remember them as "p" for "passable:" they're okay, but not great.

Monounsaturated fats, in contrast to saturated fats, help reduce the amount
of bad cholesterol in the blood and boost the amount of good cholesterol, causing LDL levels to sink and HDL levels to rise. All oils contain all three kinds of
fat—saturated, polyunsaturated, and monounsaturated—but in varying propor-
tions. For example, olive oil is higher in monounsaturated fats than almost any
other oil but still contains some saturated and polyunsaturated fats as well. At
the other end of the scale are palm and coconut oils, which contain a small
amount of unsaturated fat and have even more saturated fat per gram than red
meat. In between are corn, vegetable, and soybean oils, which are predomi-
nately polyunsaturated fats. The oil with the highest ratio of unsaturated fat to
saturated fat is canola oil. Canola oil has the most monounsaturated fat per
ounce than any other oil except olive, and is the lowest in saturated fat.

Olives and olive oil are key sources of monounsaturated fat. Avocados are also
rich in monounsaturated fat, and high in fiber and potassium. Avocados are also
one of the few dietary sources of vitamin E. If you wish to eat fat, an avocado is a
good choice. Remember that one whole avocado can be as much as one third of
your daily fat allowance, with nearly 20 grams of fat. Florida avocados, while not
as creamy tasting as California avocados, contain significantly less fat.

When you buy oil, buy canola, olive, or walnut oil. (Walnuts are the nuts
with the most omega-3's per ounce, 2.5 grams; most other nuts have less than 0.5
grams of omega-3's, and more omega-6's.) Use each sparingly, because like all
fats, they are still fattening. If the "s" in saturated stands for "stay away," the "t"
in trans fat is "terrible," and the "p" in polyunsaturated is "passable," then the
"m" in monounsaturated means in "moderation."

In my opinion, the healthiest fats are in olive oil, canola oil, fish oils, nut oils,
flaxseeds, and avocados. These have the highest content of omega-3 or monounsaturated fats; and fish and walnuts have the highest content of these oils.

A RealAge Makeover Success Story:
John D. and Linda D.

It's not hard to get out of the habit of eating unhealthy fats—really. Just how easy it is to make the switch is illustrated by our friends John D. and his wife Linda D. (John and Linda are such a model RealAge couple that I requested they join me on an appearance on the *Today Show*.) Linda successfully substituted healthy fat for the unhealthy fat John normally consumed, and that one simple change had a huge effect on his RealAge. She understood that all your genes do is make proteins or control other genes. When John ate saturated or trans fats, he was turning on genes that produce proteins that contribute to inflammation of the arteries. These proteins caused him to feel and actually be older. Linda substituted olive, sesame, peanut, or some other healthy oil for butter or margarine whenever she could. This simple substitution reduced inflammation in their arteries, making them younger and more vigorous. John did not even know Linda had changed anything. It was that simple and easy. He just knew his blood pressure was reduced and he felt more energy. Extra years were added to their lives, all in exchange for a simple switch in ingredients during meal preparation.

4. Eat an ounce of nuts five days a week.

Eating an ounce of nuts (and we do not mean donuts) before dinner is a great way to start the meal with a little healthy fat. This great habit decreases arterial and immune aging.

5. Avoid simple carbohydrates and simple sugars.

Carbohydrates were meant to be complex. Simple sugars in food are absorbed quickly in the intestine, and increase the level of sugar in the blood for one to two hours. A high concentration of sugar in the blood eradicates the natural protective control your body has over the usual, everyday variations in blood pressure. High blood sugar levels also increase the amount of triglycerides in the blood. Furthermore, your body reacts to a high blood sugar level by then causing you to have a low blood sugar level; these swings definitely age the arteries. Avoiding white foods—carbohydrates that are white, cream, and white sauces—is a basic tenet of age-reducing nutrition.

What about honey and natural sugars? Unfortunately, these are not healthy substitutes for white sugar. So avoid foods that are laden with brown sugar, corn sweetener, dextrose, fructose (especially as high fructose corn sweetener), glucose, corn syrup, honey, invert sugar, lactose, maltose, malt syrup, molasses, raw sugar, sucrose, syrup, and table sugar.

In addition, sugar consumption is linked to weight gain. Simple sugars tend to be more concentrated, meaning that you consume more calories per mouthful. Cutting sugar intake is a quick and easy way to make extra calories disappear from your diet. Foods containing lots of refined sugar are high in calories, and most of those calories are empty nutritionally.

What about fruit—doesn't it have a lot of "fruit sugar" (fructose), you might ask? The answer is yes, but it is otherwise so beneficial that fruit overcomes this problem. And if you want to keep that sugar from getting into your bloodstream where it can do harm, have some healthy fat, like a few nuts, a few minutes before you eat the fruit. And remember that although fruit juices count as a serving of fruit, most lack the fiber found in whole fruits, so don't make juice your main source of fruit.

Finally, although it is not true in all cases, many people find that a diet low in simple carbohydrates and simple sugars can help provide a more stable blood glucose (sugar) level, and a slightly lower risk of diabetes. Eating sugar in large doses tends to cause peaks in a person's metabolic level. Lots of people find that eating less sugar gives them more energy without sleepiness after big meals.

6. Remember to add fiber.

Fiber is a key reason that diets high in fruits, vegetables, and grains are good for you. People who eat a lot of fiber have significantly lower rates of aging. The person who eats at least 25 grams of fiber a day has a RealAge as much as three years younger than that of the person who eats only 12 grams of fiber a day, the national average.

Fiber is found solely in plant foods and is largely indigestible, passing through the digestive tract intact. Therefore, it contains no calories but makes you feel full sooner and helps control overeating. *Insoluble fiber* does not readily dissolve in water and is not broken down by intestinal bacteria. This form of fiber can be found in many foods: grapefruit, oranges, grapes, raisins and dried fruit, okra, sweet potatoes, peas, zucchini, whole-wheat bread, granola, papaya, and peaches. While this type of fiber is not as effective as soluble fiber at decreasing your lousy (LDL) cholesterol levels, it still makes your RealAge younger. *Soluble fiber* does dissolve or swell in water. It helps regulate metabolism and digestion, and stabilizes blood glucose levels by moderating the rate of nutrient

Table 8.6	The RealAge Effect of Fiber				
FOR MEN:					
	GRAMS OF FIBER (SOLUBLE IS PREFERABLE) EATEN PER DAY				
	Less than 5.2	5.2 to 11.1	11.2 to 17.1	17.2 to 24.9	More than 24.9
CALENDAR AGE			REALAGE		
35	35.6	35.2	35.0	34.6	34.2
55	55.8	55.3	55.0	54.2	53.6
70	70.9	70.4	70.0	68.9	68.2
FOR WOMEN:					
	GRAMS OF FIBER (SOLUBLE IS PREFERABLE) EATEN PER DAY				
	Less than 5.2	5.2 to 11.1	11.2 to 17.1	17.2 to 24.9	More than 24.9
CALENDAR AGE			REALAGE		
35	36.6	35.6	35.0	34.2	33.6
55	57.2	55.9	55.0	53.7	52.9
70	72.6	71.0	70.0	68.2	67.3

absorption. Soluble fiber is found in grains such as oats, barely, and rye; legumes such as beans, peas, and lentils; and some breakfast cereals (see Chart 8.1). Fiber in your breakfast will make you less likely to want a large afternoon snack.

In a study of forty-three participants at Northwestern University, a 10-gram increase in the daily intake of cereal fiber decreased the risk of heart attack by 29 percent (making a fifty-five-year-old's RealAge 1.9 years younger). It does not take much cereal to produce a definite effect: in the 2003 evaluation of the National Health and Nutrition Follow-Up Study, a 5-gram increase in cereal (soluble) fiber—an easy addition to breakfast—reduced all-cause death rates by 12 percent. That alone makes your RealAge about 0.8 year younger. Individuals who eat less fiber also tend to have worse overall diets and to be more sedentary.

A high-fiber diet also helps reduce the incidence of a quality of life problem, hemorrhoids. Hemorrhoids can be provoked by excess pressure on the bowel walls caused by the forced bowel movements that often accompany a low-fiber diet.

Chart 8.1 **What's Your Fiber Intake?**

To calculate a rough estimate of your daily fiber intake, write down the number of servings of each food you eat on average per day, multiply by the fiber content per serving, write the resulting number in the Total column, and add all of the numbers in the Total column.

FOOD	SERVING SIZE	SERVINGS PER DAY	FIBER CONTENT PER SERVING	TOTAL
Buckwheat cereal	1 cup		10 g	
Cereal, Cheerios	1 cup		3 g	
Instant oatmeal, Quaker	1 packet		3 g	
Instant oatmeal, Nature's Path	1 packet		4 g	
Breakfast Pilaf, Kashi	½ cup		6 g	
Wheatena	⅓ cup uncooked		5 g	
Strawberries	1 cup		0.75 g	
Broccoli	1 stalk (medium)		0.9 g	
Onions	1 cup or one small		0.4 g	
Grapes	2 cups		0.6 g	
Tomato	1 medium		0.5 g	
Apples	1 cup		0.6 g	
Artichoke	1 large		10 g	
Oranges and tangerines	1 medium		0.2 g	
Tomato sauce (varies by brand)	1 cup		0.5 g	
Peaches	1 medium		0.6 g	
Popcorn	3 cups, popped		2.2 g	
Coleslaw/cabbage	1 cup		0.1 g	
Green peppers	1 cup		1.7 g	
Green leafy vegetables (average)	1 cup		0.6 g	
Peas	1 cup		1.5 g	
Lima beans	1 tablespoon		4.3 g	
Almonds	12		2.6 g	
Cashews	14		1.4 g	

FOOD	SERVING SIZE	SERVINGS PER DAY	FIBER CONTENT PER SERVING	TOTAL
Peanuts	15		2.7 g	
Bread, pumpernickel	1 slice		1.3 g	
Bread, rye	1 slice		0.4 g	
Bread, wheat	1 slice		1.5 g	
Kombu	¼ cup		6.7 g	
Soybeans (mature)	½ cup		10 g	
Tofu	1 piece 2½ × 1 × 2¾ inches		0.1 g	
			TOTAL: _____	

Don't go on a high-fiber diet all at once. Increase your fiber intake gradually. Make sure to drink lots of water, as fiber tends to absorb water. Eat breads and cereals that contain whole grains. Even healthy-sounding breads made of "wheat flour" have had their fiber removed by the refinement process. Check the labels on processed foods, which are now required to indicate the overall fiber content.

Table 8.6 shows the effect of daily fiber consumption on your RealAge. Use Chart 8.1 to determine your current fiber intake; then you can decide what to eat to increase your daily fiber.

7. Be a savvy snacker and try fruit.

The lengthening of the average life span in America has paralleled the availability of fresh fruits. Even though this is a correlation and not a proven cause-and-effect relationship, the data suggest that increased fruit consumption may contribute to longevity. Fruits are rich in vitamins, fiber, carotenoids, and other nutrients. Eat fresh, well-washed fruits that are unpeeled, so that you retain the fiber (unless of course the fruit is meant to be peeled, like an orange). Although fruit juices count as a serving of fruit, most lack the fiber found in whole fruits, so don't make juice your main source of fruit.

Carotenoids—there are over six hundred different types—are vitamin-like pigments found in many fruits and vegetables. For a long time, scientists did not know whether carotenoids had any nutritional benefit, but now it is increas-

ingly clear that many of them have antioxidant and anti-inflammatory properties. You can spot carotenoids by the red, orange, and yellow color they impart
to foods such as tomatoes, carrots, and apricots—basically, any fruit or vegetable
with these hues contains carotenoids. Also, carotenoids are plentiful in leafy,
dark green vegetables such as spinach and kale and in broccoli. Lycopene, the
red stuff in tomatoes, is also a carotenoid that helps prevent prostate and breast
cancer, and probably arterial aging as well. Carotenoids are one of the reasons
eating a diet rich in fruits and vegetables can help keep you young.

8. Be sure to get your flavonoids.

Flavonoids help you fight arterial and immune aging, and are plentiful in cranberries, cranberry juice, tea, tomatoes, apples, applesauce, strawberries, broccoli,
onions, red wine, and the more colorful fruits and vegetables. Thirty-one milligrams a day makes your RealAge substantially younger.

Flavonoids are another reason a diet rich in fruits and vegetables will help
you stay young. Like carotenoids, flavonoids are an antioxidant and anti-
inflammatory substance found in plants. Thirty-one milligrams of flavonoids a
day can decrease aging of your arteries and immune system (see Table 8.7).
(One of the reasons red wine has an antiaging effect is that it is rich in
flavonoids, including resveratrol, which has antiaging and anticancer effects in
animals.) The richest sources of flavonoids are cranberries, onions, green tea,
strawberries, broccoli, celery, apples, and grapes (see Chart 8.2).

Because most fruits have only thirty-five to sixty calories a serving, they are
low-calorie alternatives to cookies or candy. Dried fruits contain considerably
more calories per mouthful, so be careful not to overindulge. If you are tired of
common fruits such as apples, oranges, and bananas, then diversify. Buy exotic or
seasonal fruits. I find it easier to have bite-size fruit—grapes, cherries, or small
plums—to munch on. I keep a big fruit bowl in my office. That way, I can grab a
piece when I feel hungry, and everyone else in my area can grab a piece, too.

9. Eat ten tablespoons of tomato (or spaghetti) sauce a week.

Try marinara sauce on pasta, and eat more ketchup. Salsa is also good, although
the data shows that cooked tomatoes are better than raw, especially when they
are cooked with a little healthy oil. The carotenoid found in tomatoes, lycopene,
may be the active ingredient. Lycopene provides an immune-strengthening

Table 8.7	The RealAge Effect of Eating Flavonoids Every Day		

FOR MEN:

	MILLIGRAMS OF FLAVONOIDS EATEN PER DAY		
	0–19	19.1 to 29.9	30 or more
CALENDAR AGE	REALAGE		
35	36.1	34.3	33.8
55	56.6	54.0	53.1
70	71.8	68.4	67.6

FOR WOMEN:

	MILLIGRAMS OF FLAVONOIDS EATEN PER DAY		
	0–19	19.1 to 29.9	30 or more
CALENDAR AGE	REALAGE		
35	36.1	34.2	34.0
55	56.2	53.8	53.5
70	71.6	68.6	68.0

antioxidant, anti-inflammatory flavonoid that seems to inhibit growth of cancers (prostate, lung, breast, and other types) and may also make your arteries younger (see Chapter 5).

10. Eat five fistfuls of strengthening vegetables a day.

Vegetables contain many healthy phytonutrients and lots of fiber. Learning to cook and eat vegetables enjoyably is a key habit to great eating, my patients say. An important part of having more vegetables is retraining your digestive system. Slowly increase your intake so your digestive system can adjust. A "fistful"—an amount the size of your fist—is just right for one serving.

Chart 8.2   What's Your Flavonoid Intake?

To calculate a rough estimate of your daily flavonoid intake, write down the number of servings of each food you eat on average per day; multiply by the flavonoid content per serving; write the resulting number in the Total column, and add all of the numbers in the Total column.

FOOD	SERVING SIZE	SERVINGS PER DAY	FLAVONOID CONTENT PER SERVING	TOTAL
Cranberries	1 cup		13.0 mg	
Cranberry juice	8 ounces		13.0 mg	
Tea (not herbal)	8 ounces		7.2 mg	
Tomato juice	8 ounces		7.2 mg	
Apples	One medium		4.2 mg	
Applesauce	1 cup		4.2 mg	
Strawberries	1 cup		4.2 mg	
Broccoli	1 cup		4.2 mg	
Onions	1 cup or one small		3.0 mg	
Red wine, or 2 cups of grapes	One 5-ounce glass		3.0 mg	
Tomato	One medium		2.6 mg	
Orange juice and blends (e.g., pineapple-orange)	8 ounces		2.4 mg	
Oranges and tangerines	One medium		2.4 mg	
Tomato sauce	1 cup		1.8 mg	
Peaches	One medium		1.4 mg	
Vegetable soups (minestrone, tomato)	1 cup		1.3 mg	
Coleslaw/cabbage	1 cup		0.9 mg	
Green peppers	1 cup		0.9 mg	
Green leafy vegetables	1 cup		0.9 mg	
Peas	1 cup		0.9 mg	
Ketchup or salsa	1 tablespoon		0.45 mg	

TOTAL: _____

11. Enjoy a little alcohol every day.

If you or your family members are not prone to alcohol or drug abuse, one half to one drink of alcohol (beer, spirits, or wine) a day for women, and one to two drinks a day for men, makes your RealAge over two years younger (see Chapter 11).

12, 13, 14. Take the right vitamins, minerals, and micronutrients twice a day, and avoid the wrong ones.

See Chapter 10 for the vitamins you should take, the ones you should avoid, and the right amounts.

15. Eat nonfried fish three times a week.

Any fish, not just fatty fish, makes you younger. Salmon, white fish such as cod or bass, and other fish contain lots of omega-3 fatty acids, a type of fat that actually reduces triglyceride levels in the blood and appears to lower blood pressure. Fish can be very easy to cook, too. The key to great fish dishes is starting with great fish. Fish shouldn't smell fishy at the market; it should smell pure. Ask to smell the fish before it's wrapped up. If it smells fishy, ask for a fresher piece. The best fish are those caught from the wild (as opposed to farmed fish), such as salmon from the wilds of Alaska. Ask if the fish is "line-caught" or "wild" at your supermarket or restaurant.

Eating fish at least once a week may cut the risk of heart attack in half, making a fifty-five-year-old man's RealAge more than 2.7 years younger. Although no one knows precisely how omega-3 fatty acids work to prevent heart attacks, some experts believe that these substances prevent plaque buildup along the artery walls. Other data suggests that omega-3s help stabilize a person's heartbeat, cutting down on the irregular heart rhythms associated with heart attacks. Omega-3s also appear to make platelets less sticky, decreasing the risk of clotting. Recent data showed a 52 percent decrease in sudden death when fish is consumed at least once a week. Omega-3s may also reduce blood pressure. Although you can buy fish oil supplements, it's best for your RealAge to eat the fish itself. By the way, fish doesn't provide iron, so if you're on a mostly vegetarian diet and eat only fish,

Table 8.8	Choice of Fish (Go for the Bold)				
FISH	MERCURY: AVERAGE (RANGE) IN PPM	PCBs	CONCERNS ABOUT DWINDLING SUPPLY	PREDOMINANTLY HEALTHY FAT	CHOICE
Bass, freshwater	**0.00 (0 for 1 sample)**	**No data**	**OK**	**Yes**	**Enjoy**
Bass, saltwater	0.49 (0.10–0.91)	None	Some concern	Yes	Once a week at most
Bluefish	0.30 (0.20–0.40)	None	Some concern	Yes	Once a week at most
Catfish	**0.07 (0–0.31)**	**None**	**OK**	**Yes**	**Enjoy**
Clams	0 (0 for 6 samples)	No data	Depends on harvesting method	No	Once a week at most
Cod, Atlantic	0.19 (0–0.33)	None	High concern	Yes	Once a week at most
Crab, blue	0.17 (0.02–0.5)	None	OK	No	Once a week at most
Crab, Dungeness	0.18 (0.02–0.48)	No data	OK	No	Once a week at most
Crab, king	0.09 (0.02–0.24)	No data	OK	No	Once a week at most
Crab, tanner	0.15 (0.0–0.38)	No data	OK	No	Once a week at most
Croaker	0.28 (0.18–0.41)	No data	No data	Yes	Once a week at most
Flounder/ sole	**0.04 (0–0.18)**	**None**	**OK**	**Yes**	**Twice a week at most**

FISH	MERCURY: AVERAGE (RANGE) IN PPM	PCBs	CONCERNS ABOUT DWINDLING SUPPLY	PREDOMINANTLY HEALTHY FAT	CHOICE
Grouper	0.43 (0.05–1.35)	None	Some concern	Yes	Once a week at most
Haddock, Atlantic	0.17 (0.07–0.37)	None	Some concern	Yes	Once a week at most
Halibut	0.23 (0.02–0.63)	None	Some concern	Yes	Once a week at most
Herring	**0.15 (0.02–0.28)**	**None**	**OK**	**Yes**	**Enjoy**
Lobster, Northern Atlantic or canned, American	0.31 (0.05–1.31)	None	OK	No	Once a week at most
Lobster, spiny, canned	0.13 (0–0.27)	None	OK	No	Once a week at most
Mackerel, king	0.73 (0.3–1.67)	None	OK	Yes	Avoid
Mahi-mahi	**0.19 (0.12–0.25)**	**None**	**OK**	**Yes**	**Twice a week at most**
Marlin	0.47 (0.25–0.92)	None	Some concern	Yes	Avoid
Moonfish	0.60 (0.60 for 1 sample)	OK	Some concern	Yes	Once a week at most
Orange roughy	0.58 (0.42–0.76)	OK	High concern	Yes	Avoid
Oysters	0.0 (0–0.25)	Some concern	Depends on harvesting method	No	Once a week at most
Perch, freshwater	0.11 (0.10–0.31)	No data	OK	Yes	Once a week at most

FISH	MERCURY: AVERAGE (RANGE) IN PPM	PCBs	CONCERNS ABOUT DWINDLING SUPPLY	PREDOMINANTLY HEALTHY FAT	CHOICE
Perch, ocean	0.18 (0–0.31)	None	Some concern	Yes	Once a week at most
Perch, freshwater	0.10 (0.10–0.15)	None	Some concern	Yes	Once a week at most
Pollock	0.20 (0–0.78)	None	OK	Yes	Once a week at most
Red snapper	0.60 (0.07–1.46)	None	Some concern	Yes	Once a week at most
Sablefish (black cod)	0.22 (0–0.70)	None	OK	Yes	Once a week at most
Salmon, Atlantic or Alaskan, line-caught	**None**	**None**	**OK**	**Yes**	**Great**
Salmon, farm-raised	None	Some concern	OK	Yes	Choose line-caught, if possible; once a week at most
Scallops	0.05 (0–0.22)	No data	OK	No	Once a week at most
Shark	0.96 (0.05–4.54)	None	High concern	Yes	Avoid
Shrimp	0.0 (0 for 22 samples)	Some concern	OK	No	Once a week at most
Sole/ flounder	**0.04 (0–0.18)**	**None**	**OK**	**Yes**	**Twice a week at most**
Swordfish	1.00 (0.10–3.22)	None	High concern	Yes	Avoid

FISH	MERCURY: AVERAGE (RANGE) IN PPM	PCBs	CONCERNS ABOUT DWINDLING SUPPLY	PREDOMINANTLY HEALTHY FAT	CHOICE
Tilapia	0 (0 for 3 samples)	None	OK	Yes	Enjoy
Tilefish	1.45 (0.65–3.73)	None	OK	Yes	Avoid
Trout, freshwater	0.42 (0.3–1.22)	None	OK	Yes	Avoid
Trout, saltwater	0.27 (0–1.19)	No data	OK	Yes	Once a week at most
Tuna, canned	0.17 (0–0.75)	None	OK	Yes	Once a week at most
Tuna, fresh or frozen	0.32 (0–1.30)	None	OK	Yes	Once a week at most
Whitefish	0.16 (0–0.31)	None	OK	Yes	Enjoy

Abbreviations: ppm = parts per million; PCBs = polychlorinated biphenyls. If a fish variety is not listed, I could not find enough data on that variety. If you want to choose that variety, just make sure you purchase it from more than one source.

you could end up iron-deficient; be sure to eat enough foods such as spinach, oysters, cereal, and clams, that contain a lot of iron.

Shellfish contain omega-3s, but not as much as finfish. High in cholesterol, shellfish do not make a particularly good diet option. Since cholesterol from food is not actually that big a factor on cholesterol in the blood, shellfish isn't a terrible diet option, but it's not the best, either. Finally, be especially careful about eating raw seafood, which is more likely to carry disease-causing germs than cooked seafood.

People are often worried about mercury poisoning or PCBs (polychlorinated biphenyls) from fish. Eating a variety of fish from a variety of sources reduces the chance of ingesting a specific contaminant. Mercury appears to be highest in bottom-feeding and scavenging fish (shark, swordfish, tilefish, and tuna can have high concentrations), but is less in fish such as salmon, sea bass, or tilapia. Furthermore, it isn't even clear that mercury from fish causes toxicity. In the Seychelle Islands, where people eat a huge amount of fish, the children of mothers who ate fish twenty-one times a week had the same neurologic function or IQs over an extended period of time as did the children of mothers who ate no fish. One study has shown that the form of mercury in most fish—methylmercury sulfate—is much less toxic to human cells than methylmercury chloride. Thus, the mercury content of some fish and the methylmercury chloride poisoning that occurred in Japan may not have as much relevance to human disease and nerve functioning as many believe.

Table 8.8 summarizes what I think about fish choices. (I've used boldface type to indicate my preferences.) I have included a column for "Concerns About Dwindling Supply"; that column pertains to the possibility of overfishing in 2003 and 2004, and the worry that these fish may become extinct.

As we avoid eating such fish, their numbers may return toward plentiful, and the data in this column will change. For a summary of which I consider the best, enjoy salmon (Atlantic or Alaskan, line-caught), freshwater bass, catfish, flounder/sole, herring, mahi-mahi, tilapia, and whitefish.

Twenty-Three Tips to Help You Make Choices

To help you start incorporating new dietary choices into your RealAge Makeover plan, let's consider twenty-three more tips that my patients have found help them and will help you shed pounds and years deliciously.

*1. Make every calorie you eat delicious and
    nutrient-rich.*

Don't eat foods that taste only "okay." If they're not really delicious, don't eat them at all. You deserve to treat yourself well.

*2. Eat breakfast, preferably one containing whole
    grains and a little healthy fat.*

You'll start the day off with energy, avoid hunger pangs that lead to unwise food choices, and have more stable blood sugar levels (see Chapter 11).

3. At every meal, eat some healthy fat first.

One of the best things I ever learned about eating came from my daughter, by accident. To spend time together in spite of our busy schedules, Jennifer and I arrange father-daughter evenings. We do something fun—watch a movie, see an exhibit, or have some kind of adventure. Then we go to dinner, just the two of us. One time, when Jennifer was about eleven, we spent the early evening playing squash. By the time we got to the restaurant, she was famished. She just couldn't wait for an entrée. I suggested, "Let's eat dessert first." Jennifer couldn't believe it. Dad was suggesting what she'd always dreamed of!

"Really?" she asked, "Can we?"

"If you don't tell Mom." I added, "They'll bring it to us quickly. We'll eat a small amount of dessert first, get lots of calories, sugar, and fat, and you won't feel so hungry. Then we can take our time with the rest of the meal and eat right."

Jennifer thought I'd lost it but didn't complain. In what was to become a tradition for us, we shared a small dessert first. Only later did I learn that not only was it fun, but it was also good for us! We still share the joy of that tradition but I make sure I eat less than 20 grams of saturated and trans fats a day.

Switching from saturated and trans fats to healthy fats or less fat is one of the most difficult things we face when trying to improve our diet. For optimal aging, our diet needs to be no more than 25 percent fat. However, most Americans get much more than that. One way to cut back on saturated and trans fats and calories is to eat them in a certain way. Try to eat a little bit of fat—perhaps a little whole grain bread dipped in olive oil or even better, a few nuts—at the beginning of the meal. It will help you feel full faster, and you will end up eating fewer calories. The little bit of fat prevents your stomach from emptying (see Figure 8.1). The ideal amount represents approximately 60 to 75 calories: one-half tablespoon of olive oil or canola oil, six walnuts, twelve almonds, twenty peanuts, or half an ounce of real, cocoa butter-based chocolate or avocado spread.

4. Read the labels for serving size.

Determine exactly how many servings you will be eating, and how many grams of saturated and trans fats that amount contains.

Figure 8.1. Eat a Little Fat First and Gain Four Benefits

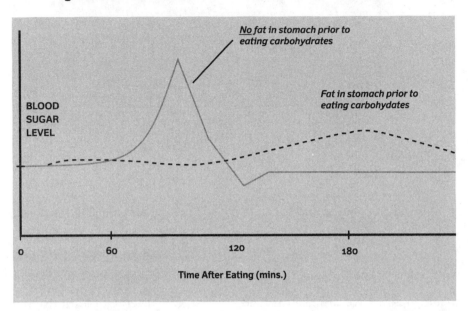

If you eat a little fat before eating carbohydrates, your stomach won't empty its contents into the intestine as quickly. This slowing of stomach emptying has four RealAge Age-Reduction effects. First, you feel full faster and stay full longer, so you eat less. Second, because sugars are largely absorbed in the intestine, the amount of sugar in the blood rises less rapidly and peaks at a lower level. Third, eating fat helps the absorption of fat-soluble nutrients. Finally, healthy fat has its own health-giving properties: it increases your healthy (HDL) cholesterol and decreases inflammation in your arteries.

5. Read the labels for whole-grain content.

Look at the first six items on the label. The first item that names grain should say "whole wheat," "oats," "oats, unprocessed," "brown rice," or "corn." Choose products that have more whole-grain than processed-grain content.

6. Keep a steady weight.

The skeletal body type we see in fashion magazines is not attainable—or even desirable—for almost all of us. Instead, you should be the right weight for *you*. Your aim should be to keep your weight as close to what it was at age eighteen for women, or twenty-one for men. Having a low and stable body mass index— (weight-to-height ratio) is one of the things that will help keep you young. The most important thing is to avoid yo-yo weight loss and gain, which is worse for you than simply being overweight.

7. Make the foods you eat healthier.

Assess your foods and meals in terms of how they could be made healthier by additions, subtractions, or substitutions. A few substitutions can make a big difference in your rate of aging. They also make food taste great! Try substituting olive oil for butter or margarine on bread, or prune purée or drained applesauce for one to three tablespoons of butter in recipes; fruit for cookies; real, dark, cocoa butter-based chocolate for milk chocolate; nuts for chips; and cooked garlic salsa or marinara sauce for a cream sauce. Cocoa butter-based chocolate is a wonderful, age-reducing fat—a saturated fat that is miraculously turned into a healthy fat by your body, that provides age-reducing flavonoids for your body; milk or trans fat-based chocolate is an aging fat, so choose the youth and great taste of real, dark, cocoa butter-based chocolate. You will have to read the label to find it, but that will allow you to really enjoy its magnificent flavor.

8. Take a thirty-minute walk every day with a friend.

I call this a RealAge double-dip. Not only do you get the antiaging benefit that physical activity and exercise give you, but you also build the strong social networks that help prevent needless aging during times of stress.

9. Be a smart shopper, plan menus, and learn to cook.

Cooking can be a true pleasure. When you make a dish yourself, you know what's in it. You can also have the fun of learning how to use herbs and spices to make food taste fabulous. Finally, if you don't *buy* food that's bad for you, you won't *eat* food that's bad for you.

10. Diversify your diet.

Everyone thinks he or she eats a balanced diet, but that's usually not so. Forty percent of Americans don't eat fruit daily, even though four servings are recommended for each and every day. On average, Americans get less than half of the 25 to 30 grams of fiber they need every day. And 30 percent do not eat even one ounce of nuts a week.

Why is diversity in your diet so important? Diversity helps ensure you obtain all the nutrients you need and helps you avoid too much of any one contaminant. There are probably other reasons we do not understand, but no matter what the mechanism, choosing a diverse diet can make your RealAge younger. If you eat from all five food groups daily, you can be as much as five years younger than if you eat from only two. (The five groups are breads and cereals; fruits; vegetables; low-fat dairy products or dairy substitutes; and meats, poultry, fish, nuts, and other proteins.) It is also important not to choose just one item from each food group but to eat diversely within each food group. Any good food might contain lots of one nutrient but virtually none of another. Try to eat four servings of fruit, five servings of vegetables, and two to six servings of whole-grain breads, cereals, or other whole grains a day. These amounts will give you the vitamins and fiber you need without excess calories. Eat one to three servings of low-fat dairy foods or dairy substitutes and a serving or two of protein (nuts, beans, meats, fish, or poultry) daily.

Table 8.9 shows the effect of diversity in your diet on your RealAge.

11. Add variety to your diet and to the way you cook vegetables.

Add variety to the way you cook. Learn new techniques, as described in *Cooking the RealAge® Way*. Try sautéing, pan roasting, grilling, microwaving, roasting, baking, steaming, or using a blender—all healthy techniques. Variety in technique will make your vegetables taste better, even great. It's fun to try new ways of cooking, and having fun makes you younger.

12. Keep your portions energy-giving, not energy-sapping.

The usual restaurant entrée is much larger than an acceptable meal size. Use your fist or a pack of cards to gauge a proper serving size and ask your server to pack the rest for the next day's lunch.

13. Stop eating as soon as you start to feel full.

Because your stomach is roughly the size of your fist, eating meals larger than your fist can stretch your stomach beyond what's comfortable or healthy.

| Table 8.9 | The RealAge Effect of Diversity in the Diet | | |

FOR MEN:

	Number of Food Groups Eaten Each Day		
	1 to 2	3 to 4	5
CALENDAR AGE	REALAGE		
35	38.3	34.8	34.7
55	59.4	54.8	54.5
70	75.3	69.8	69.3

FOR WOMEN:

	Number of Food Groups Eaten Each Day		
	1 to 2	3 to 4	5
CALENDAR AGE	REALAGE		
35	38.3	34.8	34.7
55	59.4	54.8	54.5
70	75.3	69.8	69.3

Remember to eat a little fat first. Then pause before the rest of the meal. Also, remember to stop eating as soon as you first sense you're getting full; if you keep eating, you'll end up feeling *too* full.

14. Don't eat absentmindedly.

All too often, eating is an unconscious act. We lift the fork, swallow absentmindedly, and lift the fork again. Sometimes we overeat simply because we aren't paying attention. Often, we're not even hungry. Be actively conscious of what you're eating, and why. Use all of your senses to enjoy the color, texture, smell, and flavor of your food. Not only will you enjoy your food more, but you'll also slow down your rate of consumption.

Vegetarianism: Pro or Con?

Only about 5 percent of Americans classify themselves as full-time vegetarians, but increasingly the health-conscious are choosing vegetarian diets. Many people have eliminated red meat from their diet, and more are choosing to eliminate poultry as well. These choices may be good for your RealAge. Study after study has shown that a diet low in animal protein and rich in fruits, vegetables, and fiber is vital to keeping a person young. Decreasing red meat consumption to once a week or less reduces aging of both the cardiovascular and immune systems. However, vegetarians need to be careful. They run the risk of not getting the appropriate variety of foods, thereby missing out on proteins and nutrients that are more plentiful in animal products. (Quinoa, a grain that has all the essential amino acids, is a great food for vegetarians to enjoy.)

If you go on a vegetarian diet, you will need to supplement your diet with vitamin B_{12}, since it is obtained almost exclusively from animal products. If you do not eat any animal products, make sure to take a vitamin containing adequate amounts of folate, B_6 and B_{12} daily. I suggest meeting with a nutritionist to discuss your food-choice plan to make sure you're getting everything you need.

15. Increase the IQ (health-promoting potential) of your kitchen.

Increasing your Kitchen IQ is a reliable and wonderful way to make your Real-Age younger. Get rid of items like cookies and potato chips that make you age faster than you want, and have fruit prominently displayed in your kitchen. If you don't have something in your kitchen, you won't eat it. If you have something displayed, you will often grab it first. Our website *www.RealAge.com* and book *Cooking the RealAge® Way* both contain a test on the IQ of your kitchen. Having the right implements and ingredients, and tossing the wrong ones, can make your RealAge much younger, and it is much easier to do than you think.

16. Drink lots of water.

Drink a glass of water between every glass of wine or other alcoholic drink you have. Also, at events where food is served, carry a glass of water.

17. Make cooking a part of your RealAge Makeover

When you cook at home, you get to regulate everything that goes into your dishes, and you won't unwittingly eat a dish that undoes the hard work you've done on your Makeover. Adding flavor to a dish without merely tossing in a stick of butter is a challenge, but it can also be fun. I learned several techniques to do so from John LaPuma, my co-author of *Cooking the RealAge® Way*. He taught me that nonfat additions like a splash of vinegar or lemon juice can give a dish a low-calorie kick. You can add them to the cooking liquids for grains and to tomato sauces for pasta, and sprinkle them on sautéed vegetables or fresh berries and fruits. Spices and herbs are another great way to maximize flavor. (Perhaps you could start an herb garden. That would be a RealAge double-dip, since hobbies such as gardening keep you younger.) Infusing oils and vinegars with basil or hot pepper or other flavors is another way to bring up taste with little or no added fat. Another is to use flavor-intensive pastes such as anchovy paste or wasabi to pack a powerful flavor punch. They add an instant boost to sauces, dressings, and marinades. They can also add zip to a pizza base or cracker spread.

We explore RealAge methods of cooking in detail in *Cooking the RealAge® Way*, if you'd like to learn more. However, for the purposes of your RealAge Makeover, the most important thing to remember is that simple cooking—without lots of fat—and healthy eating are an integral, joyful part of the Real-Age lifestyle.

18. At home, hide unhealthy food and display the good stuff.

Increasing the IQ of your kitchen is a great way to make our RealAge younger. Simply start to display fruit attractively in the kitchen at all times. The first thing you see is often the first thing you'll grab as a snack.

19. Treat yourself to nine-inch plates.

The key to controlling your portions is having the right size plates. Treat yourself to beautiful nine-inch diameter bone china plates or your choice in your favorite colors. It will help you overcome the American habit of eating much more than you actually need.

20. Make eating, and the place you eat, special.

Eat only while sitting down, and only at one of your special places. (Designate no more than three places as "special," one at home and perhaps two at work.) Eat food only on plates, not out of the container. My most successful patients and their families have a special place in their home that is the only place for eating. Not eating anyplace else is their rule—not the TV room and not in the car. Breakfast is the only possible exception; doesn't matter where you eat breakfast, as long as you eat it every day.

21. Learn some tricks so you can "eat healthy" at restaurants.

Learn to be the CEO (chief executive officer) when you eat out. That means asking questions about how the food is prepared and requesting substitution of healthy fat (such as olive oil) for unhealthy fat (such as butter) in the meal preparation. If you stop eating as soon as you almost feel full and do not eat absentmindedly, your RealAge will be younger.

22. Eat foods that aren't processed; but if you do, read the label.

Choose foods with whole grains, no aging trans or saturated fats, and great texture. Processed baked goods will make you older if they contain lots of trans fats and processed flour; and they usually do. I've been told that one Cinnabon—a big frosted cinnamon roll—contains 75 grams of aging fat. That's not a four-pack, either, but just a single roll. In contrast, a slice of whole grain, cinnamon-flavored bread made by our local Montana Bread Company or by Wegmans Supermarket contains no fat or processed flour, and it tastes great. If you want to make it even healthier, you could add some cinnamon apple butter. Do not fool yourself; label reading is moderately difficult to learn.

23. Finally—and most important—make meals fun and nonstressful events.

The best situation is getting several RealAge benefits at once, and you can do this while preparing, cooking, and eating food. By shopping at specialty markets and culinary shops, and experimenting with imaginative new dishes, you can get the stress-reducing benefit of having fun. If you've never really cooked before, the mental activity involved in learning the new skill will help keep your mind young. (Many people are surprised to discover the pleasure that the creativity and challenge of cooking can bring.) And making mealtime a joyous time when family or friends get caught up on the day's events, and, whenever possible, share a laugh, brings you the benefit of strengthening your social network.

Borrow a copy of *Cooking the RealAge® Way* from your local library to see if those recipes appeal to you, ask a friend what book he or she uses for healthy cooking, or log onto our website. Try out a new recipe one night a week. If you live with someone who shares the cooking, make it a game. See who can make the best-tasting low-fat dishes. If you haven't a clue what to do with that funny new vegetable (like kohlrabi), figure something out. Dare to be bold and adventurous. If you always eat a certain style of food, break the mold. Try new options: Thai food, Italian, or vegetarian. Make healthy eating an adventure, not a chore.

These are general guidelines for Age-Reduction eating. It may take a while to adjust to the changes. Stick with it for a couple of months and see how you do. If you have questions about serving size or the nutrient content of foods, I suggest you buy a nutritional information book. Many good books list the calories and nutrients in a whole range of foods. The better informed you are about what you eat, the better food choices you will make, and the younger you will stay.

Looking Younger and Living Longer

There aren't that many important points to remember about losing weight. They're the fifteen points discussed at the beginning of the chapter. Over 95 percent of my patients who have had the discipline to walk thirty minutes every day have succeeded in losing weight. It's the program that Karen A. used to lose seven inches and forty-four pounds, the program George followed to lose twenty-five pounds, and the program that many of the people who send thank-you e-mails every day use with similar success. Let's reiterate the important points for weight reduction, using five simple steps that you should undertake gradually—say, in thirty-day increments.

1. Walk thirty minutes a day. No excuses. If it rains, walk inside a mall. Although you may drag your feet the first few times, chances are you'll come to love your daily walk, and truly look forward to it.
2. Buy a new set of plates, ones you love, that are nine inches in diameter. Portion control is absolutely key to losing weight.

3. Take up weight (resistance) exercise, ideally with a trainer.
4. Gradually change your food choices to more fruits and vegetables. Avoid simple sugars. Eat colorful food and avoid white food.
5. Begin to have a little healthy fat first at every meal.

Remember, if you're trying to lose weight:

1. Start simple, with thirty days of thirty minutes of daily walking. Every day, no excuses.
2. Second, don't torture yourself. The dieter's mentality of sacrifice and denial leads to failure. Don't punish yourself for occasional slipups. Find a stress relaxation technique you like to use (see Chapter 7).
3. Try to establish good eating behaviors that will last a lifetime. It makes no sense to go on a diet for six weeks. Instead, you need to establish routines that will help you keep the weight off for the long term. Don't do anything dramatic or extreme. After 30 days of walking every day, buy yourself a set of nine-inch dinner plates.
4. Use common sense, and talk to your doctor to deal with the complications and aging effects of weight until you lose the excess. Once you lose the weight, the complications will generally go away.
5. Start by changing one habit—for example, eat only complex carbohydrates and totally (yes, totally) avoid simple sugars. I also believe that if the methods here do not appeal to you, you should see a nutritionist or other weight-loss professional about the most effective and healthy strategies for you for losing aging pounds. Remember, your food choices are for life: you can keep young by choosing to eat well.
6. Don't go it alone. It's too easy to lose your willpower. Find someone who has a similar goal and try to lose weight together. Encourage your spouse or partner, friends, and colleagues to support you—or better yet, to join you. Although a diet sounds like the least entertaining thing imaginable, there are ways of making weight loss fun. For eleven years, I had a running bet with a group of friends. We agreed to lose two to three pounds a month—an achievable goal—until we hit our desired weights. Once a month we met for a weigh-in. Anyone who weighed in higher than his or her goal had to pay each of the others a hundred dollars for every pound over the target weight. Having such a high penalty gave all of us an extra incentive to meet our goal. In eleven years and one hundred thirty-two weigh-ins, only one of us ever missed our target weight.

7. Add another change after you have mastered the first—for example, add healthy fats and nuts or avoid saturated and trans fats.

8. If you're on a diet, reward yourself. When you lose the pounds you want, treat yourself to a new outfit, a night on the town, exercise clothes, a massage, or whatever makes you feel good—anything except an ice cream sundae or something with aging fat! Fat choices are learned and can be unlearned. If you know another dieter, help celebrate when his or her weight-loss goal is reached.

9. Gradually add other choices of the fifteen RealAge food groups and twenty-three tips.

10. You may find professional support to be helpful. Joining a responsible weight-loss clinic, or participating in a program such as Weight Watchers, can help a person lose extra pounds. These diet clinics and programs can teach you simple tricks for eating healthier, choosing foods that are good for you, and consuming fewer calories. They provide handy tips on what to order in a restaurant when no low-fat options are obvious, and how to avoid empty-calorie foods. Also, the social environment really appears to pay off. It encourages a "we're-all-in-this-together" kind of attitude, as you learn how to motivate each other and make healthy food choices together. These groups help you celebrate those pounds-off victories. Part of this tenth point is to learn (either in a group or with a personal trainer) how to do resistance exercises, and do them three times a week.

Whatever you do, see food for what it is: a great chance to make yourself healthier and younger, and one of the most effective tools you have to make yourself over from the inside out.

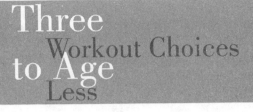

Three
Workout Choices
to Age
Less

How to Reduce Stress, Look Younger,
And Get Measurable Results

A RealAge Makeover Success Story: Cynthia W.

Cynthia W. was forty-three when she became my patient. At 5 feet, 5 inches, she was eighty pounds heavier than she had been at age eighteen. Her body mass index was 38, well over the cutoff point for overweight. The managing editor of a business magazine, she had a chaotic job. She spent every day sleuthing stories, answering phone calls, and making sure that the news got out on time. When deadlines neared, she worked around the clock, living on take-out food. She became my patient after a heart attack scare brought her in for an electrocardiogram. She realized it was time to start taking care of herself.

When I tried to gently bring up the matter of weight, she said, "Dr. Roizen, don't beat around the bush. I know I need to lose weight. And you're the one who's going to help me do it." After fighting with issues of body image and beauty for a long time, her recent heart attack scare had made Cynthia realize that weight loss wasn't about looking good but about being healthy.

Cynthia told me, "One day, I woke up and I was five times the size I always thought I was. I just never made the time to take care of myself. I don't want to haul all this weight around anymore. I need to help my heart. Tell me what I can do."

I explained the importance of regular physical activity, and portion control. She committed to a full range of RealAge strategies to prevent arterial aging, but really wanted to focus first on physical activity.

"I know I should go running, but I never do," she said, looking guilty.

"Don't worry, you shouldn't start with such a strenuous activity, anyway," I told her. "Just start with walking. Walk thirty minutes every day, no exceptions, no excuses, every day. Start with less if you need to, but hit thirty minutes as soon as you can, and do that every day, no excuses"

Cynthia started her first "workout" that day. She walked from her house to the end of the block and back. That was it: short, sweet, and slow. The next day, she did it again. By the end of the next week, she was walking all the way around the block. Within three weeks, she was walking eight city blocks—the equivalent of a mile—each day. Then she began timing herself, increasing her pace a little bit each time. Within three months she was walking half an hour each day. At my suggestion, she rewarded herself by buying a set of beautiful nine-inch plates. She e-mailed me a picture of them. On weekends, she would walk for a full hour.

"Mike," she said to me one day, "I never thought I'd say this, but I actually find myself craving my daily walk. Me, the living paperweight, actually wanting to exercise! I'll be at the office, the phones will be ringing off the hook, the e-mails waiting to be answered, and all I can think is, 'Gee, I really want to take a walk.' "

She had discovered that exercise doesn't have to be painful or exhausting. It can be something to look forward to, a treat. Energy-giving. Cynthia started doing it the easy way, remembering that health should be a priority, a fun priority. She's working gradually toward her goal of eight years younger. Cynthia started by boosting her overall level of physical activity, committing to half an hour a day of moderate activity. Then she started ten minutes of weight lifting a day, working with a trainer for six sessions to get her form right. (It's wise to work with a trainer, since improper weight lifting can cause injury.)

Within two years, she has lost more than forty-five pounds. Her blood pressure dropped, and she feels a whole lot better. "I have more energy, stressful events do not bother me as much—they just aren't as stressful for me—and I actually like the way my body looks and feels," she laughed. Cynthia still hadn't reached the weight she had at age eighteen, but she was getting closer every day, just by walking and weight lifting. Then in addition, she decided to build stamina: strengthening her heart, lungs, and arteries to increase her overall endurance.

She treated herself to a sizable reward after one year of walking every day: a Schwinn exercise bike. She chose that one because it helped her exercise with both her arms and legs. But during 1999, although she was religious in her daily walks and weight lifting, she still wasn't doing a lot of vigorous exercise because she did not enjoy the time on the bike. Then a breakthrough occurred. While on a business trip in November, she stayed in a hotel that had an exercise club with an elliptical trainer in front of a TV (she had not allowed herself to go to a health club or in front of others till then because she had been less than proud of her body, she told me). She loved the elliptical trainer.

She treated herself to a big gift for Christmas in 1999: she bought an elliptical trainer for her home. And she bought a heart rate monitor to go along with the machine. She started by aiming for 70 percent of her maximum heart rate for twenty-one minutes or so, at least three times a week. But within two months she brought that up to 85 percent of the maximum. She continues to do thirty minutes of walking every day, and ten minutes of strengthening and flexibility exercises every day, which are especially important as she builds more stamina, since they help prevent injury.

And she takes an aspirin every day, and eats the RealAge Makeover way. She is now 5 pounds lighter than she was at age 18, and has found the love of her life. She has even talked to me about the risk of becoming pregnant at age 49, with a RealAge of 36. Along with a lot of other items, I told her to make sure she and her fiancé planned to segregate time for herself so she could enjoy any grandchildren rather than having her grandchildren take care of her. She replied that she is now efficient enough at work to have enough time for the exercise.

Her fiancé committed to letting her have at least an hour every evening to exercise; she only needs 30 minutes three times a week, and 10 minutes most days, she told me, because she walks 30 minutes with two of her columnists at work, discussing business as they walk, rather than having "sit down and get old" meetings. In fact, she thinks the columns and ideas are crisper due to these walking meetings.

Her fiancé became a patient, and has started a RealAge Makeover. I have never seen anyone quite as happy to see me as Cynthia at her yearly planning and review session. She could be the "poster child" for RealAge: she has transformed herself from a 43-year-old with the energy and thoughts of a 55-year-old to someone who thinks, acts, looks, and is 36 years old. I almost feel embarrassed to charge her for her once a year, day-long sessions with our program— she really is the expert of her own body now; I'm just a coach.

If you're like a lot of people, you probably feel that you're like Cynthia and you don't have a moment to spare. Between your work and your family life, you may feel that you just don't have the time or the energy to exercise. This is common. But when it comes to exercise, you get back more than what you give, because exercise actually gives you more energy and—since you become more efficient in other aspects of your life—more time. In other words, once you make the effort and take the time to embark on a new fitness plan, you may well find that you actually get more energy and time in return.

Exercise will give a powerful boost to your RealAge Makeover. It not only increases longevity but also, like other Age-Reduction choices, gives you more energy and makes you feel years younger, too. Exercise is the most predictably successful way to manage stress and stave off depression. By adopting a three-pronged approach for boosting your physical activity, you can make your Real-Age 8.0 years younger if you're a man and 9.1 years younger if you're a woman. Integrating a moderate and balanced physical activity routine into your daily schedule is a vital element of your RealAge Makeover. It can also be fun. Exercise is almost always more beneficial and easier to work into your life than you could possibly imagine.

- **First, boost physical activity to boost energy.**
  You don't have to run marathons to benefit from exercise. The first type is just general physical activity: walking, gardening, bringing in the groceries, anything that uses your muscles, no matter what. Just boosting your overall activity level, even without breaking a sweat, can earn you 40 percent of the Age-Reduction effect normally attributed to exercise. Raising your overall caloric expenditure to 3,500 kilocalories a week makes your RealAge 3.2 years younger. (A kilocalorie—kcal—is the same amount of energy as a calorie, except that the custom is to use the term "calories" when we're talking about food and "kilocalories" when we're talking about exercise. Therefore, a donut is said to contain about 400 calories, and swimming is said to burn 400 to 600 kcal an hour.)
  Difficulty rating: Moderately difficult

- **Second, build strength and flexibility.**
  The second type of physical activity consists of building and strengthening muscles and keeping them in top form through weight lifting and stretching exercises. Strength-building and flexibility exercises contribute just 20 percent to the overall Age-Reduction, energy-boosting, and stress-diminishing effects of exercise. However, don't underestimate the value of strength and flexibility exercises: it's a critical 20 percent. These activities provide an insurance policy for the body by helping to prevent injury and skeletal weakening. This allows you to continue your overall exercise routine without the disruptions caused by pulled muscles or broken bones. Strengthening exercises are especially important for women. To protect bone mass and density, women need to lift weights even more than men do. I believe that resistance exercise for ten minutes, three times a week, is the most important thing you can do to get an immediate energy boost and

prevent stress from aging you. Its long-term effect is to create extra (reserve) energy all the time. Lifting weights for just thirty minutes a week makes your RealAge 1.8 years younger.

Difficulty rating: Moderately difficult

■ Third, build stamina

Most people make the mistake of starting their exercise program with sweat-inducing activities. Many Americans use their treadmills, Stair-Master, and exercise bikes as clothes racks because they started with stamina activity before the other two types of exercise, and gave up.

Like Cynthia W., do this only after you have integrated a general physical activity (like walking) and strength activities into your usual routine. I believe you should be doing both thirty minutes of walking every day and ten minutes of strength activities every other day before you even attempt stamina activities. These are activities to raise your heart rate. They are what we usually think of as exercise: jogging, biking, swimming, aerobics, a workout. Through vigorous exercise—anything that makes you break a sweat and causes your heart to beat faster—you can make your RealAge younger. These exercises strengthen your heart, arteries, and lungs; they delay—and may even reverse—arterial and immune system aging, and stress-induced aging. Physical activity also decreases the risk that minor depressions and mental illness will turn into major disabilities. Exercises that cause you to sweat twenty-one minutes at a time have a double benefit: they not only count toward the sixty-three minutes of stamina exercise required per week for optimum Age Reduction, but also burn extra calories toward your goal of 3,500 kilocalories expended per week. Stamina exercises can make your RealAge as much as or even more than 6.4 years younger. Do exercises such as elliptical trainer or exercise bike that do not involve as much up-and-down pounding as running and you'll increase your odds that osteoarthritis will not keep you from continuing your age reduction plan.

Difficulty rating: Moderately difficult

The best fitness plan is one that builds on all three components. Many people would say there are four types, making stretching-flexibility separate from strengthening exercises. But the RealAge scientific team can find no data indicating a separate effect of flexibility exercises on mortality, and all data on disability examines the two—strengthening and flexibility exercises—together, as in yoga. So we group strengthening and flexibility together. I believe there is a RealAge effect that is separate for each of the three physical activities: general, stamina, and strength. One without the other two will provide a substantial but not the maximum Age-Reduction effect.

Exercise and Longevity: The Basic Facts

Exercise is a health and lifestyle issue that seems to weigh on many peoples' consciences. They know they should do more, but they somehow never quite get around to it. More than 90 percent of Americans agree that exercise is an important part of healthy living, but only 15 percent exercise as much as they should. Despite the sports fashion boom of the 1980s, Americans seem to be exercising less and less. As a nation, our fitness level is declining. Fewer people (as a percent of the total) are fit in the 2000s than in the 1990s, fewer were fit in the 1990s than in the 1980s, and fewer people in the 1980s were fit than in the 1970s. In other words, fitness has been in steady decline. More than two hundred fifty thousand deaths a year, 12 percent of the national total, can be attributed to lack of regular physical activity. Although Americans spent more than four billion dollars on fitness equipment in 2000, much of that equipment is gathering dust in the basement. But, expensive equipment isn't what's really needed.

According to a study published in the *Journal of the American Medical Association*, one of the key reasons that most American don't exercise enough is that they think they need to invest an hour or two in a vigorous workout in order to get the health benefits of exercise. Since they can't fit this plan into a busy schedule, they do nothing at all. Luckily, this way of thinking is completely false. The truth is that even modest physical activity can make your RealAge younger, substantially younger. And you don't have to let it disrupt your daily schedule. Just thirty minutes of walking a day—which every one of us can fit into our current lives, given the slightest commitment—can make a world of difference. Even getting just 750 kcal of physical activity a week (about two ten-minute walks every day) makes your RealAge 0.9 to 1.7 years younger than if you did nothing. Three recent studies reported that just twenty minutes of walking a day reduces the likelihood of breast or prostate cancer by 20 to 44 percent. If you get an hour's worth of physical activity a day—and that includes such things as walking up the stairs or taking a couple of ten-minute strolls—you can make your RealAge two to five years younger. For a double benefit, walk while you talk to a friend on your cell phone. (Companionship and exercise are the two parts of the RealAge double-dip; see Chapter 7.) Getting younger doesn't have to mean hard-sweat exercise, just anything that gets you out of the armchair. In fact, I often don't even use the word "exercise," preferring "physical activity." Physical activity, just boosting your overall activity level, is a key component of Age Reduction.

As with so many other health issues, our thinking about physical activity has changed over the years. Just two decades ago, doctors and scientists believed that heredity determined your ability to exercise and to benefit from it. More recent studies indicate that your own desire and resolve to stay in shape determine by more than 70 percent your ability to achieve and maintain physical fitness. The first step is changing your frame of mind.

Being physically active is a magic bullet when it comes to our health, and it costs us nothing. And anyone can do it—even people who have been physically incapacitated. In fact, such individuals actually tend to do more, as they appreciate being able to be active. Even if you have a health problem, you should incorporate physical activity into your life (although you'll want to do so under the guidance of your physician). In fact, if you have a health problem, you should especially start an activity program, because you stand to benefit the most. For those at higher risk of cardiovascular disease and other chronic illnesses, exercise makes their RealAge disproportionately younger. The biggest benefit occurs if you start exercising before a major health problem—an aging event—occurs. However, it's never too late to start.

While we might think of physical activity such as sports as being in the realm of the young, older people who become active actually stand to benefit more. People who start doing even moderate physical activity in midlife age less rapidly. Fitness researchers have even found that encouraging the frailest of nursing home residents—people already in their nineties, and some even one hundred—to lift weights actually makes an astounding difference in the quality of their lives, enabling some to move out of their wheelchairs and back onto their feet. (In fact, I've been told that the nursing home where these studies were done had to close a wing after the studies were finished, because so many of their residents got well enough to go home.) No matter what your age or physical condition, exercise will almost always make you younger. What is most important about fitness is that you continue to exercise. Within five years of stopping exercise, even great college athletes are no more fit and no younger than those who had never exercised. In other words, physical activity keeps you young only as long as you keep doing it.

Exercise will help you look better, too. And although you may think it makes you look better because of "buffed" muscles or because you are thinner, it makes you look better for another reason: any physical activity makes your arteries younger, and that keeps your skin younger.

Finally, exercising is really showing love for your children. You'll be around to help care for their children rather than them having to care for you.

Table 9.1 shows the kilocalories utilized by various activities, and Table 9.2 shows the RealAge benefits of physical activities.

Exercise and Disease: Reducing Risk

Exercise does not affect just one or two parts of your body; it affects all of it. It doesn't just give your muscles more strength and energy, it makes your whole body younger and gives all of your organs more energy. Exercise affects everything: your cardiovascular system, your immune system, your musculoskeletal system, and your emotional well-being. Its effects go all the way down to the cells. Let's consider the scientific research on physical activity as it pertains to various health conditions.

■ **Coronary and arterial aging**

People who exercise regularly have significantly less cardiovascular aging, and are at far lower risk of heart attack, stroke, and impotence, regardless of their genetic backgrounds. By keeping your arteries young, you increase the ability to provide more nutrients to all of your organs, and that makes you less tired, or conversely gives you more energy. Exercise lowers blood pressure, raises the level of protective HDL cholesterol, stimulates weight loss, decreases inflammation, and helps prevent blood clots. The Harvard Alumni Study has found that the incidence of heart attack was inversely proportional to the amount of exercise performed: men exercising less than 2,000 kcal a week had a 64 percent higher risk of heart attack than those who exercised more than that. Exercise significantly decreases the feeling of stress, abdominal fat, inflammation in blood vessels, and blood pressure. Even a little exercise does those good things and more. Studies have also shown that a three-month period of intense physical activity, such as that experienced by military recruits can increase healthy (HDL) cholesterol as much as 33 percent and decrease lousy (LDL) cholesterol as much as 9 percent. Exercise is one way to control cholesterol without medication and to make your RealAge younger. Even non-intense exercise has relatively immediate and long-lasting benefits. In the Cardiovascular Health study, individuals who did any physical activity, even just

Table 9.1	How Many Kilocalories (kcal) Does Each Activity Use?	
INTENSITY	**ACTIVITY**	**KCALS USED PER MINUTE**
Light	Walking for pleasure	3.5
	Bicycling for pleasure	4
	Swimming, slow treading	4
	Conditioning exercises, slow stretching	4
	Home care, vacuuming	4
Moderate	Raking lawn	4 to 5
	Walking briskly	4 to 5
	Home repair, painting	4.5
	Mowing lawn with a power mower	4.5
	Racquet sports, table tennis, doubles tennis	5
	Golf, pulling cart or carrying clubs	5.5
	Conditioning exercises, general calisthenics	6
	Fishing in stream	6
Intensive	Ice or roller skating	7
	Soccer	7
	Moving furniture	More than 7
	Conditioning exercise, stair stepper, ski machine	More than 7
	Singles tennis, racquetball	7–8
	Running	8
	Basketball (game play)	8
	Cycling, fast or racing	10 or more
	Squash	12
	Canoeing or rowing in competition	12

20 minutes of walking daily, had a 19 percent lower risk of heart attacks and strokes, and of all-cause mortality.

■ **Immune system aging**

As mentioned, physical activity affects you even at the cellular level. It reduces the rate at which your cells age, meaning that you are less likely to develop cancers, and that any microscopic cancers you already have are less likely to spread. Exercise also improves the overall functioning of the immune system, increasing the production of "watchdog" cells that seek out and destroy invading disease cells and cancer cells. Those who are physically fit have fewer serious infections, cancers, and even colds.

■ **Colon cancer**

The rate of colon cancer is significantly higher in highly industrialized, affluent societies. Researchers blame our fatty diets and sedentary lifestyles. Several studies, including the ongoing National Health and Nutrition Examination Survey, have shown that individuals who are physically active have much lower rates of colon cancer. A study in Sweden found that those with low levels of activity were three times more likely to get colon cancer.

■ **Breast cancer**

The incidence of breast cancer is more than one-third lower for women who exercise regularly than for those who do not exercise regularly. Studies from Norway, Japan, Canada, and the United States found that women who exercise were 20 to 44 percent less likely to get breast cancer. Some scientists hypothesize that women who exercise more have lower fat stores and, hence, less long-term exposure to impurities stored in fat cells, less storage of compounds that stimulate estrogen receptors, and less inflammation. Others hypothesize that endurance training helps increase the number of immune system cells that are known to kill off potential cancer cells and reduce inflammation. And again, in studies of breast cancer risk, even non-intense exercise has relatively immediate and long-lasting benefits. In a 2003 Los Angeles study, woman who did any physical activity, even only 20 minutes of walking daily, had a 38 percent lower risk of early-stage breast cancer.

■ **Prostate cancer**

Men who exercise consistently have much lower rates of prostate cancer. The Harvard Alumni Study found a significantly reduced risk of prostate cancer among men who exercised more than 4,000 kcal a week, and an increased risk for men who expended less than 1,000 kcal a week. The risk was nearly 50 percent lower for men over seventy and more than 80 percent lower for men under seventy.

■ **Pancreatic cancer**

Several studies, including the Nurses Health Studies (which is studying 117,000 nurses) and the Health Professionals Study (which is studying 46,000 men), have found that walking four hours a week cut the risk of this cancer by more than half.

■ **Weight management**

Strengthening exercises are particularly important, because they build muscle. The more muscle you have, the more calories you burn, even when you're not exercising. Although any exercise is better than none, for weight loss more exercise is better than less. One study published in 2003 observed 202 subjects, half in Minnesota and half in Rhode Island. The group that was encouraged to do more physical activity and at a higher intensity lost more weight by the six, twelve, and eighteen month points than the group that was not. Both groups lost weight, but the group that did 2,400 kcal a week lost about twice as much weight as the group that increased physical activity to 1,600 kcal a week.

■ **Diabetes**

Exercise helps increase the body's sensitivity to insulin. This in turn lowers blood sugar levels and decreases insulin production. Active people, even if they have a genetic predisposition to the disease, are much less likely (by 30 to 70 percent in three studies) to develop adult-onset diabetes (type II diabetes). Furthermore, if symptoms do occur, exercise helps diminish their aging effect. Just thirty minutes of walking a day decreases the aging impact of type II diabetes by almost 30 percent. If you combine tight control of blood pressure, tight control of blood sugar levels, and thirty minutes of walking a day, you decrease the aging due to a chronic disease such as type II diabetes from 1.46 years older to only 1.06 years older for every year you have the disease. In addition, if you do other healthful things, you can actually age less than one year for every year you have the disease, even if it's type II diabetes (see Chapter 12).

■ **Arthritis**

Practically everyone over the age of sixty-five begins to show some sort of arthritic symptoms. A study published in 2003 in the *Journal of the American Medical Association* found that people who had osteoarthritis can and should exercise. Moderate to vigorous exercise, in conjunction with strengthening exercises, eliminated many of their symptoms and made their joints younger. Adding an anti-inflammatory supplement such as glucosamine and chondroitin sulfate and/or aspirin plus vitamins C and D, calcium, and magnesium in the proper amounts to a physical activity routine greatly diminishes the risk of progression of osteoarthritis.

■ **Osteoporosis and loss of bone density**

Any resistance activity—walking up a hill or lifting groceries— strengthens muscles and just as important, increases bone density, making bones stronger and less likely to fracture. Indeed, resistance activity actually increases the calcium content of bones. A study of over 9,500 women found that those who walked three days a week had a 30 percent lower risk of hip fracture than those who walked less than three days a week; more walking, and more walking up hills were associated with even lower risks of hip fracture. Although strengthening (or weight-bearing) exercises are the best for improving bone strength, new evidence shows that exercise such as riding a stationary bicycle and water aerobics may also increase bone density. Take note, however: some new studies warn that people who exercise vigorously need to get proper amounts of calcium—1,000 to 1,600 milligrams a day—to ensure that enough calcium is available for the bones to build density. During intense training, large amounts of calcium are lost through perspiration. For every hour of exercise you do, add 200 mg (milligrams) more calcium that day. And for every 12-ounce can of caffeinated beverage such as Diet Coca-Cola, and every 4-ounce cup of coffee you drink each day, add 20 mg more calcium.

- **Falls and broken bones**

Each year, approximately 35 percent of individuals over the age of sixty-five fall down, and fifteen percent of those who fall suffer serious injuries, including about 330,000 hip fractures and 200,000 other bone fractures a year in the USA. Falls are also the leading cause of traumatic brain injury. More than 6 percent of all medical care dollars spent on populations over sixty-five involve fall-related injuries. Hip fractures and other bone breaks age a person significantly. It's not just the bone break that ages, but the long period of immobility that often follows. Studies of elderly populations found that those who exercised, particularly those who did balance-building exercises such as tai chi or yoga, were much less likely to fall or to sustain an injury if they do fall.

- **Sleep-related disorders**

Sleep research studies done at both Stanford and Emory Universities found that adults who exercised fell asleep more quickly and slept better than their sedentary counterparts. Sleep is best when the exercise is done more than two hours before you go to sleep. Proper sleep is a great age reducer (see Chapter 11). Furthermore, physical activity provides an extra benefit by decreasing your weight, and this decreases sleep apnea, and acid reflux (heartburn) and other conditions that involve obstruction of the airway.

Sleep apnea—a pause in your breathing during sleep—is usually due to obstruction of the airway by soft tissues. As you age, the muscles near your breathing tube become less firm. With the increased fat inside your jaw—such as the fat in a double chin—you're at increased risk of having your airway close. This airway closure is often what occurs when people snore heavily. When a person who is snoring heavily suddenly stops snoring, total obstruction may be occurring, with no air flow. This is followed by more snoring when the airway opens again. Physical activity decreases the fat in your throat, thus decreasing this form of sleep-related disorder (see Chapter 12).

■ **Depression and anxiety**

Doctors have known for years that exercise, particularly when done in a social environment, helps relieve clinical depression. Exercise also reduces anxiety disorders and improves mental health in other ways. Even for those who have not been diagnosed as having a mental health problem, exercise is a known mood lifter, and those who exercise feel happier and more upbeat.

■ **Stress management**

Regular exercise decreases the stress response, meaning that you are more relaxed, feel better, and are better prepared to cope with life's stressful events. That element of stress reduction is especially true of sports that require intellectual focus as well as muscular focus, such as basketball or squash. However, any exercise helps you deal with stress. We all experience stressful life events at one point or another, but by staying fit you can be better equipped to avoid their aging effects.

■ **Long-term memory**

Performing physical activities (particularly when you do all three kinds) helps improve long-term memory and brain function. This is logical, as memory and all cognitive functions depend on the health of the arteries. Not surprisingly, physical activity helps prevent the arterial aging that contributes to the early onset of Alzheimer's disease, as does playing games that make your mind work.

■ **Tobacco use**

Increasing the amount of exercise you do will help you quit smoking. I routinely ask patients who want to quit smoking to walk for thirty minutes a day prior to initiating pill, patch, and coach therapy. This has produced a success rate of more than 95 percent in quitting cigarettes for at least two years (see Chapter 6). Regular exercise of any type diminishes nicotine cravings, and it is as easy as simply walking.

Having seen the wonderful benefits of physical activity, perhaps you're ready to embark on your own exercise plan. But how to start? The rule is to start with small, consistent steps, and then build up slowly. Cynthia's story at the start of this chapter is typical of my patients (not the fiancé part, but the physical activity part). Like Cynthia, if you want to start the key is to commit to it each day, no excuses. In the beginning, a simple walk around the neighborhood is better than a five-mile run—suddenly demanding rigorous exercise from your body can lead to injury or, more likely, can lead you to abandon your new program just as abruptly. Once you've taken a daily walk for thirty days, add strengthening activities. After sixty days of daily walking and thirty days of resistance exercises, then and only then can you go for stamina. So walk, then lift, and only then sweat for fun and youth. The more you sweat, the fewer wrinkles you'll have.

By far the most common excuse for not exercising is that a person doesn't have the time. Working women especially feel that between driving their kids to school, grocery shopping and preparing meals in addition to their "real" jobs, the thought of trying to do yet more is overwhelming. However, most of my patients who have adopted the three-pronged RealAge physical activity plan tell me, as Cynthia did, that they save more than an hour a day when they exercise for thirty to forty minutes a day. They are more energetic and more efficient in all the other things they do. And it's no wonder. They're 8 to 9.1 years younger.

Physical Activity:
The Antiager

Most Americans lead extremely sedentary lives. We work at a computer. We get around in a car. We sit and watch television. The first goal of any fitness plan is simply to boost your level of activity. The more sedentary your lifestyle, the greater the RealAge benefit from even small changes.

In a 2003 study by Harvard's Department of Urban Planning and Design, approximately five hundred metropolitan areas were ranked for the ease of physical activity for their residents. Higher rankings were given to areas that had sidewalks and bike paths where residents could walk to the places they needed to go during the day, such as grocery stores. The areas ranked as the easiest for physical activity in everyday life had the healthiest people.

Boston, Chicago, New York, and San Francisco were some of the areas that made physical activity easiest. In contrast, those places with urban sprawl—where you had to drive to get to the grocery store or post office and where sidewalks were uncommon—ranked the lowest, had the highest mortality rates, and the highest percentage of obese people. In fact, going from the highest ranked area to the lowest represented a weight increase of about ten pounds for the average person in that area. Future archeologists may label us "The-Sit-Around-and-Get-Round-Society."

The decision to get in shape may seem like a big decision, but it's the commitment and the small steps, like thirty minutes of walking every day, that really matter. Walking to the neighborhood grocery store instead of driving. Pedaling an exercise bike while watching the football game instead of kicking back in the La-Z-Boy. Lifting weights instead of chips during the commercials. Actually walking the dog, instead of just shoving him out into the backyard. As it says on our sister website *www.DogAge.com*, "If your dog is fat, you are not getting enough exercise." Every movement you make improves your physical fitness. Housework, gardening, mowing the lawn—not to mention fun things, like dancing and sex—are all activities that burn extra calories. The point is to get your muscles moving. The more active you are, the younger you are.

At rest, your body burns 1,400 to 1,900 kcal a day. This is your resting metabolic rate: the energy your body spends just keeping you alive, the energy it uses to keep your heart beating, to keep your blood flowing, to digest your food, and to breathe. Your resting metabolic rate is approximately one kilocalorie per kilogram (kg) of body weight per hour. (To find your weight in kilograms, divide your weight in pounds by 2.2.) If you weigh 132 pounds, or 60 kilograms, you will burn 60 kcal an hour. Then multiply this hourly number by 24 hours to get your expenditure per day. A person weighing 60 kilograms would burn 1,440 kcal a day even doing nothing. Likewise, a person weighing 90 kilograms, just about 200 pounds, would burn 90 kcal an hour and 2,160 kcal a day. Ideally, you should expend 3,500 kcal of energy a week in exercise above and beyond your resting metabolic rate. Getting that much physical activity gives you the maximum health benefit with none of the drawbacks of over-exercising. Just as examples, brisk walking burns 300 kcal an hour, and jogging burns 400 to 500 kcal an hour (see Table 9.2).

When you're planning a RealAge Makeover, it's a good chance to look at your current lifestyle and get creative. Try to think of little ways to add extra movement throughout the day. Put on your favorite record and dance to a couple of songs—go on, no one's watching. Instead of hiring a neighborhood kid to rake the leaves, do it yourself. Ride your bike to work instead of driving, and always take a walk at lunchtime. In the middle of the afternoon, take a ten-minute break and instead of having another coffee, walk around the block. It will give you an energy burst without the caffeine. Or you can do it with the caffeine. One study organized at a popular coffee company in Champaign, Illinois, reported that walking for forty-five minutes as people consumed their coffee yielded a sizable weight loss, a considerable increase in healthy (HDL) cholesterol, a sizable decrease in abdominal fat, and a higher mental status in six-month and two-year periods. It's amazing what walking with coffee will do. (Walking and talking with a friend may have also been a factor, but the effect of companionship was not reported in this study.)

Walking a city block burns 9 kcal. Walk short distances instead of driving. Instead of spending ten minutes looking for the perfect parking spot, park a bit farther and use those ten minutes to walk to your destination. Find a companion or a colleague to walk with you. You can even plan a business meeting around a walk. I call it the "walk-and-talk." (I wear an inexpensive pedometer, and try to walk ten thousand steps a day. If you'd like to do the same, start with three thousand steps a day as a goal and then keep increasing it gradually. Five thousand steps a day is probably about right for most of us.)

Buy a stationary bicycle, treadmill, or rowing machine and put it in front of your TV. That way, you can catch the evening news, expand your mind, or watch a classic film, a taped version of last night's Leno or Letterman monologues and burn 300 to 600 kcal in an hour.

You don't have to allot large blocks of time out of your daily routine. Just thirty minutes of physical activity a day, in eight- to ten-minute bursts, is all you need. As with so many elements of a RealAge Makeover, it's not what is required of you that's difficult, it's changing your familiar routine and habits. It may feel odd the first couple of times you deliberately park far away from the mall so you have to walk to get there, but the great changes you'll see from just a little effort will make it worth it.

Remember, every little bit of physical activity helps you become younger. Studies have found that people who begin exercise programs by doing several small workouts in a day are more likely to stay with the routine than those who try to do an extensive workout all at once. And that's good, because your goal is not just to do it today, but to keep doing it, even enjoying it every day. And don't take a "what's the use?" attitude because you've been sedentary for so long—you stand to benefit the most. If you are now relatively sedentary, burning just 750 kcal a week beyond your daily average can make you one year younger in three years' time.

And you'll get more than a physical benefit: you'll also see positive emotional effects. You will feel younger and more vigorous, you feel more able to tackle the ordinary challenges of daily life, and you'll probably find that you laugh more. Exercise provides a "dose-response" relationship: the more exercise you get, the better you feel. Thirty minutes every day should be your commitment to yourself and your RealAge Makeover.

If you are at risk of cardiovascular disease or other kinds of chronic disease, physical activity is even more important for your RealAge Makeover than it is for the average person. An important study by fitness researcher Steven Blair at

Starting to Exercise

ere's what I recommend my patients do to start Age-Reduction exercising:

1. *Start slowly.* Don't overdo it. Just go for five or ten minutes, and then build on that. Even a walk around the block is a place to begin. Build up to thirty minutes of walking a day.

2. *Exercise a bit more, and only a bit more, each week.* Try to increase your workout by a couple of minutes each week. Aim to increase your workout by 10 percent a week, but no more than that: too much too fast can lead to injuries or abandonment of the entire program.

3. *Warm up first and stretch afterward.* Save your muscles from pulls and tears. Notice how good your body feels when your muscles are warm beforehand and stretched afterward. (Some trainers and other professionals advise stretching before the start of exercise, but the studies on this practice do not show a reduction in injuries. Nevertheless, I still advise stretching before starting the vigorous part of any workout, even though the data do not support this recommendation.)

4. *Treat yourself right.* If it hurts, slow down. If it feels good, do more than you planned, but just a little more. Remember, you don't want to overdo it.

5. *Cross-train.* Try to plan your workout so you're doing a number of different activities such as walking, resistance exercises, biking, and swimming on different days. Rotate them.

6. *Reward yourself.* Set goals and treat yourself when you achieve those goals. After thirty days of walking thirty minutes a day, buy a set of nine-inch plates or a new pair of shoes or get a massage. Celebrate your successful RealAge Makeover!

7. *Drink water.* Every ten or twenty or thirty minutes, take a break and drink half a cup or more of water. Don't let yourself get dehydrated.

8. *Find an accomplice.* For an extra RealAge double benefit of friendship and relief of stress, exercise with a friend. You'll encourage each other and push yourselves to meet your goals. Get the whole family involved.

9. *Take a lesson.* Even if you don't normally work out with a trainer or a pro, treat yourself to an hour with an expert who can show you how to maximize your workout and avoid needless injuries. Or how to triumph over a long-time opponent whom you'd really love to beat. It's a great way to get started.

10. *Vary your workout pace.* Do more on some days and less on others.

11. *Consider whether you need a medical exam before you start.* Most adults do not need to talk to a doctor before beginning an exercise plan of moderate intensity, especially if you start with walking. However, if you have a chronic disease or some other health problem, you should talk to your doctor first. Also, if you are a man over forty or a woman over fifty and you are planning to start an intensive fitness program, you might also want to ask your physician to help you design a workout routine. If you don't have a regular doctor, ask your clinic or health maintenance organization (HMO) if anyone on its staff specializes in fitness.

the Cooper Institute for Aerobics Research in Dallas showed that people who were physically fit, and even those who first became physically fit later in life, had significantly lower death rates regardless of cause of death and regardless of any other risk factors, such as a family history of cardiovascular disease or previous heart attacks. The Harvard Alumni Study found that people who smoked, had high blood pressure, and didn't exercise had more than seven times the chance of having an arterial aging event like a heart attack or stroke. Having two of these three factors meant a person's risk was only twice as high as the norm. If you are a smoker, have high blood pressure, or any other major risk factor that ages your arteries, exercise is especially important to retard or reverse aging. (Although it seems logical that any physical activity could decrease heart disease or even arterial aging, it seems magical that physical activity also makes your immune system younger, which means you are less likely to get cancer or serious infections. Also, both exercise and sex seem to magically decrease the risk of and disability from accidents.)

Two factors are crucial to the success of your new physical activity plan. One is that you truly enjoy the activities that you do. There are enough choices that everyone can find an activity he or she genuinely loves. The second is that you have the support of your family. Talk to your spouse or partner about the need for physical activity and its importance for both of you. Each of you can set physical activity goals. When one of you reaches a goal, have the other cook a really tasty, saturated-fat-free celebratory meal or give some other reward. It may sound corny, but encouraging someone to stay in shape is the best way to say "I love you." It means you want that person to be around for a long time. Use physical activity as a way to be together in spite of busy schedules. You can tell each other about the day's events just as easily walking together or exercising on bikes at the gym as you can in front of the TV at home.

Lack of time is only one excuse people use to avoid starting and sticking to a physical activity routine. Another is the weather. Many people begin an exercise regimen in the spring, work out in the summer, reach their fitness peak in the fall, and then, as winter approaches, give up altogether. Then they start from scratch all over again the next spring. This disruption to the routine is completely unnecessary, since it's so easy to come up with alternatives to exercising outdoors. Joining a gym or a club, or buying equipment for an at-home gym, can fix this cause of unnecessary aging. Even shopping malls provide great indoor walking routes, as do hospital corridors. (Hospital corridors can certainly help remind you how important it is to do all you can to stay healthy.) More than 4 million Americans over sixty-five now mall-walk regularly to burn an average of 2,000 kcal a week. That makes their RealAge as much as four years younger.

Find a sport you love that can be played indoors in the winter such as badminton, squash, or racquetball. You could swim in an indoor swimming pool. If you really prefer being outdoors but get stopped cold by winter, learn how to dress for the weather. The proper gear can mean the difference between suffering and enjoyment. Advances in exercise wear in the past ten years have produced new fabrics that make exercise clothing both warm and lightweight. To really make the most of the cold weather, learn a winter sport. There are few sports that provide the complete body workout of cross-country skiing. Ice-skating, downhill skiing, and snowshoeing are other fun sports that can turn those gray winter months into something you actually look forward to.

Once you've gotten started doing activity regularly you'll probably find that you enjoy exercise a lot more than you thought you would. However, if this isn't the case for you, and even if you do love it, there will be days you do not feel like doing it. On such a day, you might try considering it your job. As Hillary D. said to me, "Sometimes I don't like aspects of my job, but I always show up for work. Sometimes I just don't feel like exercising, but just like my job, it's something I simply have to do, every day, no excuses. On trips or vacations, I try to have fun planning for exercise. I get maps of the areas, ask questions about safety, and plan to walk to sights I would otherwise miss."

It may be tempting to let your routine slide when you travel, but there's no reason to do so. I do a lot of traveling for work, and I always try to stay at a hotel that offers fitness facilities. It's a great way to start the morning off right or to unwind after a long day of meetings. If I can't find a hotel with a gym, I pack a jump rope and resistance bands. Twenty minutes of jumping rope done in the right shoes on a low-impact surface is a great workout that you can do anywhere with a little bit of elbowroom. (Jumping rope also helps clear your sinuses, an

Table 9.2	The RealAge Effect of Physical Activity				

FOR MEN:

Kilocalories Expended Per Week

CALENDAR AGE	Less than 500	500 to 2,000	2,000 to 3,500	3,500 to 6,500	More than 6,500
			REALAGE		
35	36.7	35.0	33.1	31.4	32
55	57.7	55.0	53.3	49.6	52
70	72.9	70.0	69	66.7	68.2

FOR WOMEN:

Kilocalories Expended Per Week

CALENDAR AGE	Less than 500	500 to 2,000	2,000 to 3,500	3,500 to 6,500	More than 6,500
			REALAGE		
35	36.7	35.0	34.1	32.4	33
55	57.7	55.0	54.3	55	53
70	72.8	70.0	69	67.2	68.2

extra benefit if planes and travel cause yours to get congested.) The resistance bands can also be used in a small space. Put the "Do Not Disturb" sign on the door of your room, so your exercise routine won't be disrupted.

Your basic exercise sequence should be:

- *Warm up*
- *Strength or stamina exercises, or both strength and stamina*
- *Flexibility exercises and cool down*

Let's get started!

Strength and Flexibility:
Strengthen and Stretch It to Your Limits

Once you have started your physical activity plan and become more active, you will have more energy. At that point, it's often tempting to dive into an aerobic workout such as running. However, before you do, there's an important second phase to master that will provide benefits that aerobic activity can't: building muscle and bone. For this, you need strength and flexibility exercises. If you try to skip phases one or two and jump to aerobics (stamina), you are more than twenty times more likely to abandon your entire physical activity program than if you start with walking and then add strength before going to stamina. Although our data on aging indicate that strength and flexibility exercises produce only 20 percent of the RealAge benefit attributable to exercise (1.7 years younger), these exercises help protect joints, muscles, and tendons from strains and tears. Strength and flexibility exercises also help prevent osteoporosis (the loss of bone density) and fractures. In addition, they improve balance and help prevent fat gain. Strength exercises increase the efficiency of oxygen use by your muscles, reduce arterial aging, and improve immune function, thus decreasing the risk of early onset of chronic diseases such as arthritis.

In contrast to the extensive amount of research on aerobic exercise, relatively few studies have been done on the benefits of strength and flexibility exercises. Nevertheless, data do show that those who are strong and flexible are better able to perform everyday activities, are less likely to develop back pain, and are better able to retain mobility through old age. In 1995, a review in the *Journal of the American Medical Association* analyzed eight studies on the benefits of strength and flexibility exercises. Such exercises were important in preventing falls and increasing bone density. Some studies even show a huge RealAge benefit of 2.7 to four years with just ten weeks of strength and flexibility training. However, when the RealAge scientific team analyzed all recent and past data, keeping yourself strong and flexible makes your RealAge about 1.8 years younger. The RealAge benefit from strength-building exercises increases as you get older (see Table 9.3).

As you get older, you are more prone to stiffness and orthopedic injuries. Your muscles become stiffer, and your tendons and joints become weaker and less elastic. Studies show that when you do strengthening exercises and become stronger, you are more likely to begin doing other exercises as well. We all lose muscle from our twenties on. That's one reason we gain weight as we age. On average, a pound of muscle uses 75 to 150 kcal of energy per day, whereas a pound of fat uses only 1 to 4 kcal of energy per day. Even marathoners lose muscle if they don't do strengthening exercises. If you do strengthening exercises

Table 9.3	The RealAge Effect of Strength-Building Exercises				

FOR MEN:

Minutes Per Week of Strength-Building Exercises

	None	1 to 5	6 to 20	21 to 30	More than 30
CALENDAR AGE	REALAGE				
35	36.5	35.0	34.2	33.8	33.5
55	57.1	55.0	54.4	53.6	53.2
70	71.7	70.0	69.3	68.6	68.1

FOR WOMEN:

Minutes Per Week of Strength-Building Exercises

	None	1 to 5	6 to 20	21 to 30	More than 30
CALENDAR AGE	REALAGE				
35	36.6	35.0	34.1	33.9	33.6
55	57.0	55.0	54.3	53.5	53.2
70	72.1	70.0	69.0	68.4	68.1

regularly, you will counteract this attrition, and your body will burn more calo-ries all day long, even when you're at rest. Strength exercises thus prevent aging from fat accumulation and weight gain. (Stamina exercises, in contrast, don't build muscles.) At age fifty-five, doing just twelve weeks of strength training six times a week for ten minutes at a time will increase the number of calories you burn by 15 percent.

Strength training involves working your muscles in opposition to a force of resistance, such as free weights. Remember, the muscle you are using needs to work the weight perpendicular to the earth, against gravity. If you are working the weight other than perpendicular to the earth, you're probably not getting the benefit in that muscle, but just stressing a different muscle. One four-year study showed that lifting weights regularly led to increased bone density, up to one third more than any other activity. Another study found that post-menopausal women who began weight training preserved bone density, gained muscle mass, and significantly improved their sense of balance. Yet another study found that ninety-year-olds living independently increased strength at least 20 percent and some as much as 90 percent within six months of starting a weight-lifting program that consisted of three thirty-minute sessions a week. If you are ninety or younger, you can and will increase your muscle strength by at least 20 percent within three months of starting a weight-lifting program, making you about one year younger. Weight training can also help improve performance in other sports; one study found that runners who began doing leg lifts regularly increased their speed by as much as 40 percent.

It's very important, if you have never lifted weights before or have never done any strengthening exercises, to get instruction first. It's easy to get hurt from lifting weights incorrectly, and just a little guidance can ensure that you will get the most out of your weight-lifting time and avoid injury. One way of combining weight training and stamina training is to begin circuit training, in which you lift weights in rapid succession, walking briskly between sets.

If you join a gym, it will probably have a Cybex or Nautilus circuit already set up. If you are going to buy weights to use at home, consider free weights. All-in-one weight machines are much more expensive and take a lot of time for readjustment between each maneuver, meaning you spend a lot of your workout time fiddling with the equipment.

There are several safe ways to increase resistance in your stamina-building exercises. Many aerobic exercise machines allow you to set a particular level of resistance. On treadmills, you can raise the angle of the track. Also, many stationary bicycles can be adjusted to increase the amount of force needed to pedal.

I do not advise walking with weights. It's too easy to injure yourself, and that will make you older, not younger. I've seen too many upper-arm joint injuries and subsequent need for surgery in people who walked with weights.

You should always do flexibility exercises (stretches) after any vigorous workout. You can do strengthening exercises either before or after your stamina workout or on the days in between.

There are many kinds of flexibility exercises. Many gyms offer stretch classes. And of course, there are the gold standards of flexibility exercises: yoga and Pilates. Although no data show that yoga and Pilates are better than other stretching techniques, most yoga and Pilates routines provide comprehensive, full-body stretches as well as strengthening of all the muscle groups in one workout. Personally, I think they are great and better than any other strengthening and stretching or flexibility program. We just do not have the data to prove it.

A Personal Trainer: The Benefits of Professional Instruction

The term "personal trainer" probably conjures images of celebrities and the Hollywood lifestyle. However, the truth is that we can all benefit from some time with a personal trainer. It's not that expensive to have two or three sessions with a professional trainer, and it can provide in return a big payoff for your RealAge Makeover.

When my daughter Jennifer needed rehabilitation after a knee injury, at first she refused to work with a trainer. Once she started, she quickly realized the value of having a trainer. The trainer taught her how to focus on her workouts and how to visualize her muscles actually getting stronger. She learned how different muscle groups worked, and how best to strengthen them. This process helped strengthen the muscles around the knee, and she recovered more quickly.

The best way to choose a personal trainer is to get suggestions for good trainers from friends or colleagues. Then, ask that trainer for his or her references, and call one or two. While this may seem like a lot of work, remember that your health is in that trainer's hands; it's worth the effort to do a little research. Another place to start is with the director of personal training at the club you use—ask that individual to whom he would refer a good friend with your characteristics. If you do not like the way that person works with or teaches you, ask for another referral. There are several certifying organizations for personal trainers. I would insist that your trainer have a degree—a BA or BS with a specialty in exercise physiology or sports medicine—or is certified by one or more of the following organizations: ACSM (American College of Sports Medicine), ACE (American Council on Exercise), NSCA (National Strength and Conditioning Association), NASM (National Academy of Sports Medicine), or AFAA (Aerobics and Fitness Association of America). Each organization has specific requirements for certification. Certification is a minimum to insist on.

When referring a patient of mine to a trainer, I always ask a friend who is a master exercise physiologist—Tracy Hafen—and use her website, *www .affirmativefitness.com*. Her website has a form for you to fill out, asking what you want from your trainer, where you live, and what medical conditions you have; then it tries to match you to a personal trainer near you. You can try that too. Start heavy on instruction, with a number of sessions in a row, and then taper off. A good trainer will focus closely on technique, so you learn how to do each exercise properly. See the trainer several times in the first two weeks. Having a number of sessions close together reinforces what you learn—you won't forget as easily. After the first two weeks, go for a refresher once a week for a month and then monthly after that, or as needed. If hiring a trainer seems like too much of a splurge, consider a weight-training class. Even one lesson will help you improve your form and will lessen the risk of injury.

One of the things that Jennifer liked best about going to the trainer was that she learned several exercises for each muscle group. Now she can alternate between them or simply do the ones she likes best. "What my trainer really taught me is that you should do the exercises you love to do," she told me. "If you don't like one, there's usually another way to get the same effect."

Flexibility Exercises: The Basics

When it comes to flexibility exercises, do them twice: at the start and end of your exercises. A good warm-up first is essential, because warm muscles stretch more readily than cold ones. Each stretch should be done with slow and gentle movements. Extend into each stretch, feeling the pull on your muscles, for thirty seconds. Do not bounce, as this can strain or tear muscles.

You do not have to do these in this order; any order will work. Do not do any stretches to the point of pain, and do not do any stretches by yourself until you have received instruction and are judged capable by your instructor of doing them with correct form. Doing any stretch with incorrect form can cause injury.

- **Achilles tendon and calf stretch**
  This exercise stretches your lower leg and helps prevent damage to your Achilles tendon. Face a wall. With both hands against the wall, place one foot well behind you and the other foot flat on the floor with toes touching the wall. Keeping the rear leg straight and your heel on the ground, slowly lean in toward the wall. Keep your back straight. Hold it. Then switch and do the other leg.
- **Gastrocnemius stretch**
  This exercise stretches your lower leg (calf) muscle. Move the back leg closer to the wall and tilt the front foot upward along the wall, with the toes propped up against the wall. Lean in toward the wall. Repeat with the other leg.
- **Quadriceps stretch**
  This exercise stretches the long muscle that runs down the front of your thigh. Face a wall. Put your left hand on the wall for balance. Bend your right leg up, behind you. Reach your right hand behind your back and grab your ankle, pulling it gently toward your buttocks until you feel tension along the front of your thigh. Then do the same

thing for the left leg: place your right hand on the wall and grab your left ankle.

- **Hamstring stretch**

  This exercise stretches the muscles running down the back of your thigh, as well as the muscles in your lower back. Stand on one leg. Prop the other leg straight out on a chair or table so that the entire leg is as close to parallel to the ground as possible (do not lift it to the point where you have pain). Bend over so that you bring your face over your knee. Slide both hands toward the propped up ankle as far as they'll go. (Doing this stretch eventually protects your back, but initially can be hard on it. So go slowly and do not let yourself experience pain.)

- **Chest and triceps (back of the upper arm) stretch**

  Find something taller than you to grab onto, such as the top of a door-frame, or an overhead pole designed for pull-ups or stretching. Reach both hands over your head and grab onto the doorframe or pole. Lean forward and stretch out your upper torso. Another way to stretch the same muscles is to stand about four inches from a wall, with your back to the wall. Gently lean your back into the wall, tilting your head upward so you're look at the ceiling. Arch your back, shoulders, and arm away from the wall (still with your head arched into the wall). Then return to a straight standing position and walk away. (Do not do this stretch without your physician's approval if you've ever had neck pain.)

- **Biceps (front of the upper arm) stretch**

  Stand along a wall, facing the wall at an angle so you are facing a little forward, with your back arm (if you are looking to your left, with your right arm) straight out at shoulder height and slightly behind you with fingers and palm against the wall. Lean forward, so that your arm is stretched out behind you. Then stretch the other arm. (Many people have problems visualizing this stretch from the description—you may want a trainer to show you this one—I cannot describe it better.)

- **Back and abdominal stretch**

  Lie down on your back. Put a rolled-up towel under the small of your back. Place arms on stomach. Relax for five minutes.

Building Stamina:
Getting Fit for the Long Run

Now, finally, you're ready for the third element of your exercise routines: stamina-building (aerobic) exercises. Jogging, swimming, biking, and even brisk walking are all fun activities that will raise your heart rate, make you sweat, and at the end of the day really give you that satisfied feeling of accomplishment. Realistically, if you plan to get 3,500 kcal of activity a week, you will need to do something that really gets you moving. Start slowly and work your way up. Stamina-building, like strength-building, is a RealAge double-dip: you boost your overall physical activity—burning kilocalories—plus build stamina and aerobic capacity. In the Harvard Alumni Study, those who expended 3,500 kcal a week had half the rate of aging as the least active people. In RealAge terms, individuals who were fit—those who reached overall activity levels of 3,500 kcal a week and included stamina-building exercises in their weekly routine—were at least 6.4 years younger than those who did less than 500 kcal a week in physical activity.

Aerobic exercise increases the body's uptake of oxygen. An increase in oxygen boosts your overall metabolic rate, so the more you exercise, the more calories you burn, even when you're sitting still. Elevating your heart rate to 65 to 90 percent of its maximum for twenty-one minutes three or more times a week will give you a stronger heart, arterial system, and lungs, and will help your body increase its resting metabolic rate. Why twenty-one minutes you might ask? We do not know, that is just what the data show. If you do stamina activity, you also will reach your 3,500-kcal-a-week goal faster. To judge if you are in that 65 to 90 percent range, all you need is a cool room. If you are sweating continuously in a cool room, you are at 70 percent of your age-adjusted maximum heart rate.

Contrary to what is often commonly believed, the goal of aerobic exercise is not simply to burn calories. Instead, the goal is an increase in the maximum "metabolic equivalent units" (METs) you can do, meaning an increase in your metabolic rate, or the amount of oxygen your muscles consume during exercise. One MET is your metabolic rate at rest, sitting quietly or lying down. When doing a vigorous workout, your goal should be to increase your metabolic rate to 10 or 11 METs. That is, you're trying to boost your metabolic rate to ten times its rate at rest. Increasing the work you do to even four METs decreases your risk of serious adverse events after a surgical operation by 50 percent. That's the equivalent of being six to nine years younger at the time of that operation; pretty amazing for just 4 METs of training activity. And virtually everyone I've worked with preoperatively can do that within 60 days.

Whereas kilocalories measure the total amount of energy burned, METs measure the intensity, or rate, at which you burn that energy. The higher your metabolic rate (the higher your METs), the more kilocalories you burn in a period of time. The goal of the third prong of your exercise plan—the stamina-building prong—should be to reach 10 METs for sixty-three minutes a week if you are a woman, and 11 METs for sixty-three minutes a week if you are a man.

The peak METs you can achieve is considered your exercise capacity. If a man can do 11 METs and a woman can do 10 METs, his or her RealAge is more than four years younger.

Unfortunately, you really can't measure your METs, at least not easily, unless the machines you use are calibrated for them. METs can only be measured accurately at a sports medicine clinic or some other place equipped to monitor METs. However, there are three other pretty good ways to estimate your metabolic rate: estimating the kilocalories burned per hour (see Table 9.1), estimating "sweat time," and determining your heart rate (see Table 9.4). Use these guidelines to measure the intensity of your workouts. Look at "calories-per-hour rates" to get a rough estimate of your MET level. If you walk briskly (300 kcal per hour), you will reach a metabolic rate of six to seven METs. If you do something that burns more than 600 kcal an hour, then you are somewhere close to 10 METs. Another good way to estimate METs is by "sweat time:" try to sweat for twenty-one minutes or more three times a week. This amount of sweat time is a relatively reliable indication you have reached 70 percent of your maximum heart rate and metabolic rate. The third way to estimate METs is by measuring your heart rate, the number of times your heart beats per minute. During bouts of vigorous exercise, your heart rate should reach 65 to 90 percent of the maximum.

How many beats per minute is "the maximum?" It is *your* maximum. To calculate your maximum heart rate (the number of times your heart beats per minute when pushed to the limit), subtract your calendar age from 220. If you are forty, your maximum heart rate should be about 180 beats per minute. If you are sixty, your maximum should be about 160 beats per minute. As I've gotten more fit, I challenge myself by subtracting my RealAge from 220. When you first start this part of your physical activity program, the goal is to raise your heart rate to at least 65 percent of the maximum for twenty-one consecutive minutes, at least three times a week. As you get in better shape, you should initially try to reach 80 percent. For example, if you are forty, you should initially try to raise your heart rate to 117 beats a minute $[(0.65) \times (220 - 40)]$ for twenty-one consecutive minutes each time you do a stamina-building exercise. As you progress, try to increase to 144 beats a minute $[(0.80) \times (220 - 40)]$. Another example would be if you are sixty and just beginning to exercise, you should raise your heart rate to 104 beats a minute and later aim for 128 beats a minute (see Table 9.4).

These are general guidelines that describe ideal heart rates for the average person in a particular age range. Remember, however, that there are individual variations in heart rate levels.

If you want to measure your heart rate, do so when you are well into your workout. Stop exercising, place the finger of one hand on your opposite wrist,

Table 9.4

Boosting Your Heart Rate During Stamina Exercise: What Should You Aim For?

This table gives the range of heart rates for each age group, as percentages of the maximum. To get a good aerobic, stamina-building workout, you should initially aim for 65 percent of your maximum heart rate, and later for 80 percent of your maximum heart rate.

	YOUR CALENDAR AGE OR REALAGE								
PERCENTAGE OF MAXIMUM HEART RATE	**20**	**30**	**40**	**50**	**60**	**70**	**80**	**90**	**100**
	HEARTBEATS PER MINUTE								
100	200	190	180	170	160	150	140	130	120
90	180	171	162	153	144	135	126	117	108
80	160	152	144	136	128	120	112	104	96
70	140	133	126	119	112	105	98	91	84
60	120	114	108	102	96	90	84	78	72
50	100	95	90	85	80	75	70	65	60
40	80	76	73	68	64	60	56	52	48

100 percent	Reaching your maximum possible heart rate is a very hard thing to do and impossible to maintain. Also, it may not be a safe thing to do.
90 percent	Only high-level athletes can achieve and maintain a heart rate this high.
80 percent	This should be your goal on the days you have a really strenuous workout.
70 percent	If you can get here and maintain it, you will be getting the benefit of a real stamina-building workout, this is the level to start if you are over sixty calendar years of age.
60 percent	This should be your goal when you first start working out if you are sixty calendar years of age or younger. It's a good place to start.
50 percent or below	You're slacking off. If you want to get the benefits of stamina exercise, you need to boost your heart rate higher than this.

and find the pulse point. It lies on the spot on your wrist just below the base of your thumb. Make sure to use a finger, not your thumb, to feel for the pulse, as the thumb itself has a pulse point that can distort your reading. Then count the number of heartbeats in fifteen seconds, subtract one, and multiply by four to get your heart rate for a minute. Remember, a heart beat has two parts to it: an "in" and an "out." You should feel both. If you find it difficult to get this down, or if you want a more exact measure of your heart rate, buy a heart rate monitor—usually two pieces of equipment, a monitor watch, and a heart rate detecting and transmitting strap that goes around your chest. Your heart rate signals are transmitted to the monitor watch which displays your heart rate. These devices can be found at sporting goods stores or on the Internet ("sports heart rate monitors") but can be expensive.

When you begin a sport, it is more important to build your duration up to twenty-one minutes, rather than intensity. Run farther but at a slower pace. Bike farther, rather than going all out for a short distance. Begin slowly and build, as Cynthia did. Each week, increase your workout by at most 10 percent. Soon you will start to sweat; that's the sign that you're getting an aerobic workout. Remember, quantity matters most. And variety is important, too. Do stamina exercise every other day or switch between sports.

An Easy Test of Your Fitness (RealAge)

Are you curious about how fit you are right now? There are three factors that reveal a lot about a person's risk of death and disability—his or her RealAge. They all focus on the body's reaction to vigorous exercise. (These tests have resulted from studies done at the Cooper Clinic, The National Lipid Clinic Trial headquartered at Johns Hopkins, the Cleveland Clinic, my own clinic, and several other sites.) Do these tests only if you routinely do vigorous activity, or with a physician's supervision.

1. *The ability to achieve 80 to 90 percent of the age-adjusted maximum heart rate with exercise for three minutes (see Table 9.5).* When you are performing the maximal exercise you are capable of, does your heart rate reach 80 to 90 percent of the maximum heart rate desirable for your age group?
2. *The maximum exercise capacity in METs (see Table 9.6).* How strenuous an activity can you perform? That is, what is your exercise capacity in terms of METs? We convert that number of

Table 9.5	The RealAge Effect of Achieving 80 to 90 Percent of Age-Adjusted Maximum Heart Rate with Exercise for Three Minutes		

FOR MEN:

Ability to Achieve 80 to 90 Percent of Age-Adjusted Maximum Heart Rate with Exercise for Three Minutes

	Less than 80%	80 to 89.9%	90% or higher
CALENDAR AGE	REALAGE		
35	36.1	34.0	31.4
55	57.7	52.9	49.6
70	72.9	67.0	63.7

FOR WOMEN:

Ability to Achieve 80 to 90 Percent of Age-Adjusted Maximum Heart Rate with Exercise for Three Minutes

	Less than 80%	80 to 89.9%	90% or higher
CALENDAR AGE	REALAGE		
35	36.7	34.0	31.4
55	57.7	52.4	49.0
70	73.1	66.2	63.2

METs to kilocalories per hour and per minute, because kilocalories are the unit listed on many exercise machines such as treadmills, bicycles, elliptical trainers, stair steppers, and rowing machines.

3. *Heart rate recovery two minutes after maximum exercise (see Table 9.7).* Two minutes after stopping strenuous activity that pushed your heart rate to its maximum, how much of a return (in beats per minute) to the normal rate at rest occurred in your heart rate?

Each of these tests can predict your risk of dying and disability in the next ten years from all causes (not just heart disease or arterial aging). Use the result

Table 9.6	The RealAge Effect of Your Maximum Exercise Capacity in METs

FOR MEN:

Maximum Exercise Capacity in METs

	Less than 4.5	4.5 to 7.6	7.7 to 8.9	8.9 to 10.9	11.0 or more

or Maximum Exercise Capacity in Kcals Per Hour

CALENDAR AGE	Less than 400	400 to 550	551 to 650	651 to 750	751 or more
			REALAGE		
35	36.1	35.0	34.0	32.8	31.4
55	57.7	55.0	52.9	51.3	49.6
70	72.9	70.0	67.0	65.3	63.7

FOR WOMEN:

Maximum Exercise Capacity in METs

	Less than 4.4	4.4 to 7.3	7.4 to 8.5	8.6 to 9.9	10.0 or more

or Maximum Exercise Capacity in Kcals Per Hour

CALENDAR AGE	Less than 400	400 to 520	521 to 600	601 to 680	681 or more
			REALAGE		
35	36.7	35.0	34.0	33.7	31.4
55	57.7	55.0	52.4	50.7	49.0
70	73.1	70.0	66.2	64.7	63.2

from only one table: the table that makes you the youngest; the results are not to be added together.

Let me explain how to determine your RealAge with the following simple test. You will need to have a method of measuring your heart rate, and the information on Tables 9.5, 9.6, or 9.7. Right at the end of the most strenuous workout you do, note your heart rate and the rate of kilocalories you are burning per hour at peak. Then stop all exercise (this one time, and one time only, do

Table 9.7	The RealAge Effect of Heart Rate Recovery Two Minutes After Maximum Exercise

FOR MEN:

Heart Rate Recovery (Decrease in Beats Per Minute) Two Minutes After Maximum Exercise

	Less than 22	22 to 52	53 to 58	59 to 65	66 or more
CALENDAR AGE			REALAGE		
35	36.1	35.0	34.0	32.8	31.4
55	57.7	55.0	52.9	51.3	49.6
70	72.9	70.0	67.0	65.3	63.7

FOR WOMEN:

Heart Rate Recovery (Decrease in Beats Per Minute) Two Minutes After Maximum Exercise

	Less than 22	22 to 52	53 to 58	59 to 65	66 or more
CALENDAR AGE			REALAGE		
35	36.7	35.0	34.0	33.7	31.4
55	57.7	55.0	52.4	50.7	49.0
70	73.1	70.0	66.2	64.7	63.2

not cool down) and check your heart rate two minutes later. Then do your normal cool down and your usual stretches.

If you achieved at least 90 percent of the maximum heart rate desirable for your age group, 751 kcal per hour peak maximum exercise, or your heart rate declined by 66 or more beats per minute in the two minutes after you stopped, your RealAge is at least five years younger than your calendar age. If you are not there yet and want to make your RealAge younger, follow the program recommended near the end of this chapter to gradually and progressively achieve a RealAge Makeover.

Forget the saying, "No pain, no gain." Instead, remember "Pain is the messenger," and in this case, the message is that you're overdoing it. Physical activity shouldn't be painful. True pain is your body's way of telling you to back off. If you hurt, slow down or try a different regimen.

However, when you first start exercising, you may feel one kind of pain—a slow, burning ache in the muscles that is normal and not a cause for concern. This "normal" burning indicates you are reaching your anaerobic threshold, meaning you're at the limit of your endurance. The pain is believed to result from the buildup of lactic acid in your muscles, which occurs when your muscles are not getting enough oxygen (anaerobic means "in the absence of oxygen"). This burning is not an indication of an injury, but that you're reaching your fitness limit. (Some world-class and professional athletes believe that a massage—after stretching—removes the lactic acid from their muscles before their muscles have cooled down and lets them achieve peak performance again the next day.) The more you work out, the higher your anaerobic threshold (limit of endurance) will go, and soon you will be able to work out for longer periods and at a more vigorous rate.

Feeling sore after a workout does not mean that anything is necessarily wrong, especially if it occurs the next day. Unless you've actually sustained an injury, the pain will probably go away within a day or two, eventually producing lean muscle in place of flab. That's why you should space your workouts and rotate your activities, so that different muscle groups get worked on different days, getting a day off in between.

Setting new goals and then feeling pride in achieving them is a great way to build your regimen. Don't be satisfied with the same workout day after day—try to increase length and intensity, but very gradually. Start small but be consistent, and you will do wonders for your body and your health. The body has a remarkable ability to get younger—to achieve a RealAge Makeover—and physical activity is one major choice for that makeover. (For most people, exercise becomes enjoyable after ninety days.) Stamina-building exercise can give you 6.4 years or more of youth.

Hitting the Maximum:
Can You Overdo It?

Because less than 15 percent of Americans exceed the 3,500-kcal mark that is the RealAge optimum, most of us need not worry that we are overdoing it. Nevertheless, it is possible to get too much of a good thing, and exercising too much will make you older instead of younger. For example, one of my patients, Mary, took up jogging in her early thirties. Within a few years, she was running road races and had even run several marathons. Her times were good. She often finished in the top twenty, and she began to take her training more seriously. Her goal was no longer merely to run a marathon but to win one. Soon she was running three ten-mile runs a week and a fifteen-mile run on Sundays. She was in fabulous aerobic shape. Yet the longer her runs, the more pressed for time she got. Despite my advice, she did not do strengthening exercises before she started the stamina exercise of running. (Running on a flat course, as she did, is an aerobic exercise and does not build strength.) To run in the morning and still get to work on time, she began to shorten her warm-up time. She also quit stretching afterwards. Then the inevitable happened: she tore a ligament in her leg. She was on crutches for months and was never able to run seriously again. In the end, she gave up exercising altogether. At forty-five, her RealAge had been close to thirty, but one year later it was over forty.

The keys to a good exercise routine are balance and consistency in all three of its aspects. An extreme exercise plan can make you older. Exercising too vigorously (more than four hours a week at a top rate) can produce three major problems: oxidant buildup, inflammation, and subsequent aging; destruction of muscle tissue; and injuries from overuse of tissues.

If you exercise more than 6,400 kcal a week, or if you exert more than 800 kcal an hour for two hours in any one workout, you are overdoing it. This much exercise overwhelms your system. The body cannot dispose of free radicals fast enough, and they build up in your tissues. Exercise increases cellular metabolism and, hence, oxidation and inflammation. And oxidant buildup can damage cells, particularly the DNA. Small-scale studies have shown that oxidation damage, inflammation, and the aging it causes can be reduced. Although the findings are still preliminary, vitamins C and E taken together appear to decrease this effect in people not taking statin drugs. I recommend taking these two vitamins together about an hour to two before exercise, just as a precautionary measure. You should be taking C and E anyway (see Chapter 10). I also recommend (after gaining approval from your physician) taking a 325-mg aspirin or another NSAID such as ibuprofen (for example, 200 mg of Motrin) with plenty of water one or two hours before exercising, to help prevent the swelling and inflammation that often result from exercise.

Muscle damage is another thing you risk when you overexercise. Muscles need time to repair themselves and rebuild after a workout; if you overexercise, they don't have the chance. A successful RealAge Makeover requires resting between workouts, plus cross-training by switching between activities on different days.

The third and most obvious problem associated with exercising is injury caused by overuse of muscles and joints. The wear and tear that results can cause real problems.

Avoiding Injuries:
Basic Guidelines

It's important to learn how to avoid exercise-related injuries, and what to do if you get one. Just because you pull a muscle doesn't mean you should stop exercising altogether. By staying in shape, you are more likely to avoid future injuries. Just lay off the sore muscle for a while. Try a different exercise that doesn't stress the pulled muscle. For example, if you injure a muscle in your leg, consider swimming, relying mainly on your arms to do the work. Or, use a rowing machine. If your ankles or knees ache, try something with no impact, such as a cross-country ski machine, an elliptical exercise machine, or a stationary bicycle. If your aerobics class has you hurting, consider taking a water aerobics class; you'll get the same workout with none of the impact.

You'll quickly learn the difference between the pleasant ache that follows a good workout, and the sign of a real problem. If you tear a muscle or do something particularly damaging, the pain will make it obvious. For pain or swelling remember "RICE"—rest, ice, compression, and elevation. Don't use the muscle; ice the injury for twenty minutes every eight hours for forty-eight hours; wrap (and slightly compress) the injury with an ACE bandage or similar; and keep the injury elevated to reduce swelling. If the pain doesn't begin to subside, or if you suspect a more significant injury, see your doctor.

When injuries aren't as drastic, however, it's easier to ignore the possible problem. For example, the tendon in your elbow might ache or burn, but if it's not really that bad you might keep on playing tennis every day anyway. Or you might feel the throb in one knee and favor the other leg, upsetting your balance and doing more long-term damage. You will make your RealAge older, not younger, this way. You keep running, despite the shin splints or the dull ache of the stress fracture. For any injury that bothers you for more than a few days, consult your doctor. Most clinics and health maintenance organizations now have doctors who specialize in sports medicine. Such doctors, in conjunction with physical therapists and other injury rehabilitation staff, can help you when you do get injured, or when you want to devise a workout plan to stay in shape and prevent injuries.

Injury prevention is another area in which time with a personal trainer can be valuable. He or she can teach you the proper movements to help keep you injury-free. Knowing what to do and what not to do to get the most out of your workouts and avoid injury-provoking mistakes can save you days, if not weeks, of pain and grief.

Again, I cannot say it enough: if you are planning to make exercise part of your life—that is, if you plan to adopt an active lifestyle—there is no need to rush into it. As Eddie E. said when he started walking and losing weight: "I'm in no hurry, this is a lifetime plan." You, like Eddie E., have time to work into it gradually. That way, you'll be less likely to have an injury and more likely to make it part of a manageable, lifelong routine.

Here are some general guidelines to avoid getting hurt and to get the maximum Age-Reduction benefits:

1. *Vary your exercise pattern.* Don't do the same activity every single day, and certainly not more than two days in a row. If you go jogging three days a week, consider swimming on the other two. Or rotate between the different aerobic machines at the gym: do the StairMaster one day, the treadmill the next, and then the bicycle. Try to use all of your muscles, working both the upper and lower body.

    Also, it is often better to do a variety of exercises that complement a training routine rather than just one activity. For example, when I played competitively, it took me years to learn that my squash game actually improved and that I was less prone to injury if I did a number of unrelated activities that built strength, flexibility, and stamina rather than just play squash every day.

2. *Do strength and flexibility exercises before you start your aerobic workouts.* Combinations like biking and weight lifting, running and yoga, or aerobics and stretching exercises are mutually reinforcing. They help ensure against a damaging injury.

3. *Warm up.* Start by doing something that gets your muscles moving. Walk briskly or jog at a slow pace for a few minutes. (If you exercise at a club, consider walking to the club if you live or work within a mile of it, a double-dip). Don't think that you will save time by skimping on the pre-workout. Beginning a strenuous workout with tight, stiff muscles is the most likely way to damage or injure a muscle. Remember, too, to cool down by stretching your muscles at the end of each workout.

4. *Use equipment designed for your sport.* You don't need to go crazy buying sports equipment, but it is important to have equipment that is fitted to you and your particular activity. Wear shoes that are expressly made for your exercise program and replace them when they show signs of too much wear and tear (about every three hundred miles of workouts). You don't need expensive shoes, but they should provide good support for your feet and ankles. Be particularly careful about having good shoes if you do aerobics or any

sport that involves lots of running, jumping, or bouncing, as you will be more prone to ankle and leg injuries. Replace shoelaces frequently, because they get stretched out quickly, losing their support. If you bike, get a bike that fits you. Always, always wear a helmet (that keeps you younger, too!). Likewise, if you roller-blade (in-line skate), make sure to wear a helmet, knee pads, shin guards, and wrist guards, especially if you are playing hockey or some other game. Go to a specialty store, talk to the salespeople about the advantages of specific equipment, and evaluate what you really need. The people who work in smaller stores are often fairly serious athletes themselves and can be extremely knowledgeable.

5. *Avoid overexertion.* Gradually increase your exercise time by no more than 10 percent a week. Even if you are training to meet a goal like running in a marathon or playing in a tennis tournament, do not overdo it. More than 40 percent of marathoners who run over thirty miles a week will develop injuries within the training year—the quickest way to put the dream of the race to rest. And always do strength training for at least 30 minutes a week—it will improve your times and decrease your risk of injury.

6. *Do stamina exercises without axial (up-and-down) motion on your hip, knee, or spine joints.* Osteoarthritis affects over 95 percent of us by age 85. In Chapter 12 you'll learn how to make living with it and keeping it from progressing more likely. One way is to do exercises that do not involve pounding on your cartilage; so avoiding running on pavement, and preferably use exercises machines such as a bike or elliptical trainer that does not involve pounding up-and-down shocks to your hip, knee, or spine joints.

7. *Take vitamin C, vitamin D, calcium, and magnesium in appropriate doses, and avoid vitamin A in too great a dose.* In Chapter 10, I describe the appropriate doses of these to help maintain bone, muscle, and joint health. They will help you continue to make yourself younger by enjoying physical activity for a long time.

Strengthening Exercises: The Basics

Strengthening exercises are an essential part of your RealAge Makeover plan. Once you've mastered the basics, and made them a regular part of your routine,

Joining a Gym:
What You Need to Know

Joining a gym or health club can be a great investment, a time-saving and motivational way to get your body in shape. Or it can be a boondoggle: only one in three people who joins a gym works out more than one hundred days a year. Before sinking a lot of money into a membership, make sure that you will actually use the gym.

Before you join a gym:

1. *Try it out.* Most reputable clubs will allow you to work out free at least once before joining. That way you can test the equipment and the atmosphere. Do your workout at the time of day that you normally plan to work out to see how crowded the club gets and how long you would have to wait for machines.

2. *Find out about classes.* Ask to see a class schedule and talk to some instructors. Find out if classes are free with your membership.

3. *Find out if someone is regularly on staff to answer questions about your workout.* Good gyms will have someone available to teach you for free how to use all of the equipment properly. Find out, too, if your gym has personal trainers who can take you through your workout. This usually involves a fee (as we said earlier, be particular about who you choose as your trainer). Although you might not want to use a trainer all the time, having a pro look at your workout every once in a while can do wonders to improve your technique.

4. *Join a gym that is close to your home or work.* Fitness club gurus have what they call the "twelve-week/twelve-mile" hypothesis: most people who join will work out for only the first twelve weeks of their membership, and only if the club is less than twelve miles from their home or office. Find a place that's close and convenient.

5. *Consider the atmosphere.* Pick a gym where you feel comfortable. Look at the individuals who go there and think about how you would feel working out among them. Maybe working out with the "twenty-somethings" makes you strive for more. Or maybe you prefer a place that offers classes designed particularly for people over sixty. Some clubs are geared exclusively or primarily to women, and others are more geared to men. Shop around and decide what best fits you.

6. *Ask about hidden costs.* Before joining, read the contract carefully and ask about extra expenses that might get added in. Remember, too, that if you sign a full-year contract, you will have to pay for the whole year, even if you don't use the gym.

7. *Ask about special discounts for joining.* Gyms may have monthly deals, or offer special rates to first-time members. Ask around for pricing specials at comparable gyms in your area. You might be able to get a lower price from the gym you want to join, especially if you join between March and December (the period when most clubs offer low rates for new members).

8. *Check out the equipment.* Does it look new? Is it of good quality? Is it what you need for your workout? Don't believe promises about new equipment that's "coming in next week." I prefer a club that not only has the equipment I like, but also the equipment I might use if I develop an injury. So if a club does not have several elliptical machines and rowing machines available at the time I am most likely to exercise, I would choose another club.

9. *Determine your workout needs.* Some people like being pampered in upscale gyms that offer the most deluxe equipment and amenities, such as massages, juice bars, and day care. Others are happy in a concrete room with just a treadmill and a set of free weights. Decide what activities and frills you would like, and which ones you are willing to pay for.

10. *Decide if it's the best option for you.* Local park departments may offer free or low-cost access to gyms and exercise equipment. Also, many YMCAs, YWCAs, and YM-WHAs have gyms that cost less than commercial options. Check, though, to be sure that the membership does not include other services that you do not want to pay for.

you'll feel stronger, younger, and better. I remember the strengthening exercises, and the rules for them, by the mnemonic **I-NEED-IT**.

Inner core (center of the body) first. Strengthen these muscles before you work on others. These are represented by the first seven exercises below. Do these for at least two weeks before starting to strengthen other muscle groups.

Never sacrifice form for weight. The weights you use will increase dramatically over the first fourteen weeks (best if under the supervision of a trainer) and then very gradually for as long as you continue to lift weights, which I hope is for life.

Eight to 12 rule: You've got to be able to lift the weight at least eight times to gain the benefit, otherwise it's too heavy a weight. But if you can lift it more than twelve times, the weight is too light. If you can lift it more than twelve times, all you are getting is a stamina benefit in the muscle, not a strengthening benefit. You should strive to exhaust the muscle you are trying to strengthen somewhere between repetitions 9 and 12.

Exhale on the most strenuous portion of the lift of the weight against gravity.

Do walking every day first (on an angle or hill is best, after you have strengthened your calf muscles).

Intensive cardiovascular exercise should be done only after you have done strengthening and walking every day.

Triumph of persistence makes exercise fun after ninety days.

Strengthening Exercises:
The Magnificent Fourteen, and a Bonus

The first seven of these exercises are the ones you should start with. They will strengthen your core. After a month of these first seven, add the other seven, too. These exercises can be done on machines, with free weights, or with exercise (resistance) bands. I describe how I do these exercises with free weights; you can also do them with resistance bands as I describe on our website *www.realage.com/realagecafe/myfitnessplan.* Many other exercises will strengthen the same muscles; I just list the ones I know, teach, and do. Remembering the I-NEED-IT rule, you will want to choose a weight or a resistance band strength that allows you to do each exercise 8 to 12 times; after you have completed one set (gone through the 7 or 14 you are doing that day), repeat the set in full. And remember to exhale on the most strenuous part of the exercise.

1. Bent-Over Back Row
2. Stationary Lunge (most important; you can do them every other day)
3. Squats
4. One-Leg Calf Lift
5. Abdominal Crunch
6. Oblique Crunch
7A and B. Arm and Leg Lifts

You can start doing the next seven exercises after you've mastered the first seven for at least two weeks, although it would be preferable to start the second seven after a full month of doing the first seven every other day.

8. Chest Press
9. Biceps Curl
10A and B. Triceps One- and Two-Arm Overhead Extension

11. Standing Side Lift (use light weights to start this, as the deltoid is a weak muscle)
12. Rotator-Cuff Rotation (use very light weights—1 or 2 pounds or ½ to 1 kilogram weights at first)
13. Overhead Press
14. Lateral Deltoid Lift (use light weights to start, as the lateral deltoid is a very weak muscle)

Doing these fourteen exercises is a joy, as you will strengthen all the different muscle groups. But do not do these exercises by yourself at first. Always learn with a trained partner or preferably a professional trainer. After three training sessions, ask the partner or trainer if he or she feels you are ready to continue on your own.

1. Bent-Over Back Row, Free Weights

MUSCLE GROUPS WORKED: Major back muscles including the latissimus dorsi and lower back muscles.

STARTING POSITION: Find a solid, comfortable bench or chair without wheels. With your back parallel to the floor, put your left knee on the bench and your left arm on the bench. With your right hand, which is hanging at your side, pick up the weight.

ACTION: Lift the weight toward your trunk, keeping the elbow in tight at your side. Exhale as you lift upward. After you've done between eight and twelve repetitions on one side, repeat on the other, remembering to keep your elbow at your side and the weight in.

TIPS:
1. Your body should be anchored, and all the work should be done by your arms and back.
2. Don't allow your shoulder blades to separate between repetitions.
3. Don't lift your shoulders to your ears. Keep your shoulder blades pulled downward as much as you can.

2. Stationary Lunge, Free Weights

PRIMARY MUSCLE GROUPS WORKED: Quadriceps (front of thigh), hamstrings (back of thigh), and gluteal (buttocks) muscles.

STARTING POSITION: Stand with the feet a natural width apart, with one foot in front of the other and both feet pointing directly forward. Your weight should be centered between both legs. As you get stronger leg muscles, grasp equal-size weights in each hand.

ACTION: Keeping focus forward and spine erect, bend both knees and lower your back knee toward the floor, allowing the back heel to lift off the floor. Stop when your back knee is an inch or two from the floor, your front thigh is parallel to the floor, and front knee is bent at a 90-degree angle. Keeping your weight centered, press back up to the starting position. Repeat until you complete the set. Then, repeat on the opposite side.

TIPS:

1. Don't allow your front knee to extend forward past your toes. Drop your weight straight down toward the floor, not forward.
2. Keep both feet pointing forward (the tendency is to angle the back foot slightly out to the side)

3. SQUATS

PRIMARY MUSCLE GROUPS WORKED: Quadriceps, hamstrings, and gluteals (front of thigh, back of thigh, and buttock).

STARTING POSITION: Stand with your feet about shoulder-width apart and your toes pointing forward or slightly out. As you get stronger muscles, grasp equal-size weights in each hand.

ACTION: Keeping your focus forward, chest lifted, shoulder blades drawn together and down, the natural arch in your lower back, and your navel pulled in toward your spine, slowly bend your knees, taking your hips back toward the wall behind you and down toward the floor until your thighs are almost parallel to the floor. Slowly push back up to the starting position.

TIPS:

1. Keep your upper torso lifted but don't lean forward excessively. Focus on lowering your hips, not your torso.
2. Do not allow your knees to extend past your toes. Focus on driving your hips back behind you, not straight down.
3. Keeps your heels on the floor.
4. Keep your knees pointing in the same direction as your toes. Do not allow them to bend toward the inside of the foot.
5. I often do this exercise with a large ball (2 feet in diameter) behind

my back, against a wall. I then move up and down against the ball, which rolls against the wall.

4. One-Leg Calf Lift, Free Weights

MUSCLES WORKED: Gastrocnemius and soleus (calves).

STARTING POSITION: Stand with the ball of your right foot near the edge of a stair. Hold a weight in your right hand and hold onto a railing or wall with your left hand to balance yourself. Lift your left foot up so that it hangs relaxed near your right ankle. Lower your right heel off the edge of the stair as far as you comfortably can.

ACTION: Keeping your right knee straight, but not locked, use your right calf muscle to press yourself up on your toes as high as you possibly can. Slowly return to the starting position. When you have finished all the repetitions in the set, repeat with left side.

TIPS:

1. Keep the ankle and foot aligned so that your weight remains over the center of the ball of the foot. Do not allow the ankles to roll out.
2. Avoid dropping quickly into the starting position, which causes a bouncing or rebound motion.
3. Beginners should start this exercise using both legs and performing the exercise on the floor, without extra weight. Gradually advance to one leg and then to the stair. Finally, add weight.

5. Abdominal Crunch

PRIMARY MUSCLE GROUPS WORKED: Rectus abdominus and transverse abdominus (midsection, stomach, your "six-pack"!).

STARTING POSITION: Lie on your back on the floor with your feet braced against the wall, your hips and knees bent at about a 60- to 90-degree angle. Point your toes outward slightly (10 and 2 o'clock). Place your hands behind your head, keeping your elbows pointing out to the sides, or cross your arms over your chest.

ACTION: As you exhale, curl your head and shoulders up off the floor until your shoulder blades clear the floor and your abdominals are contracted as fully as is comfortable. At the same time, pull your navel down toward your spine so that the abdominals appear flat or hollowed and do not bulge upward. Hold for one count at the top of the motion as you exhale any remaining air. Slowly roll back down, one vertebra at a time, as you inhale. Stop just short of the starting position, so that your abdominals do not completely relax before your next repetition. This is one exercise where you will want to do more than 12 at a time. Do these until you feel the slow burn in your abdonimal muscles. Remember, get instruction first.

TIP: Do not pull on your neck with your hands. Keep your elbows out wide and hands just lightly supporting the head. It is normal to feel some tension in your neck during this exercise. After all, your neck muscles have to lift your chin. Your chin should not be pointed up toward the ceiling, nor tucked excessively. Keep your head in line with your spine.

VARIATION: Your feet may be placed on the floor instead of the wall, with your knees bent. Or, you may place your feet higher on the wall in a straight-leg position.

6. OBLIQUE CRUNCH

PRIMARY MUSCLES WORKED: Internal and external obliques (sides and front of the abdomen).

STARTING POSITION: Lie on your back with your right knee bent and right foot flat on the floor. Cross your left leg over your right, with your left ankle resting just above your right knee. Place both hands behind your head, with elbows out to the side.

ACTION: As you exhale, lift your head and both shoulders off the floor and twist so that your right armpit moves in a line toward your left knee. Contract the abdominals as fully as you comfortably can. Hold for one count at the top of the contraction and exhale the remaining air. Inhale as you return toward the starting position. Do not allow your abdominals to relax between repetitions. Continue the set until you have completed your repetitions. Then repeat on the opposite side.

TIPS:

1. Do not allow your elbow to cave in toward your knee.
2. Keep your elbows back.
3. Keep your head in line with your spine.

VARIATION: For a more advanced exercise, cross your legs more fully, so that one knee rests on the other. For a less advanced exercise, allow one elbow to remain in contact with the floor.

7A. QUADRUPED OPPOSITE ARM AND LEG LIFT

PRIMARY MUSCLES WORKED: Anterior and medial deltoid (shoulders), gluteal muscles (buttocks), hamstrings (back of thigh), and stabilization from abdominals (stomach) and erector spinae (lower back).

STARTING POSITION: Place both hands and knees on the floor with your arms and thighs parallel to each other and perpendicular to the floor. Your knees should be directly under your hips, and your hands should be directly under your shoulders. Keep your elbows soft, not locked. Your head should be in line with the spine, face toward the floor. Your back should be straight but with your natural arch in the lower back.

ACTION: Lift your right arm and left leg slowly off the floor and extend them straight out, so that your leg, back, and arm are roughly in one line. Slowly return to the starting position. Either repeat the exercise all of one pair, then the other, or alternate arm and leg combinations as you go.

TIPS:

1. Do not allow your abdominals to relax and your back to sag.
2. Do not lift your arm and leg excessively high.
3. Stretch as far as possible from your toes to your fingertips.

7B. PRONE OPPOSITE ARM AND LEG LIFT

PRIMARY MUSCLE GROUPS WORKED: Gluteus maximus (buttocks), hamstrings (back of thigh), erector spinae (lower back), and possibly deltoid (shoulder) muscles.

STARTING POSITION: Lie facedown on the floor with both arms extended straight out on the floor over your head. Your legs should be straight. Rest your head in a comfortable position with your forehead on a towel, or with your head turned to one side.

ACTION: Keeping your lower chest and hips on the floor, lengthen your right arm and left leg out away from you as you slowly lift them off the floor. Hold for one count. Slowly return to the starting position. Either repeat the exercise all on one side, then the other, or alternate sides as you go.

TIPS: Do not lift your arm and leg so that it produces an excessive arch in the lower back.

Once you have mastered the first seven and done them for several weeks to strengthen your inner core, then add the following:

8. CHEST PRESS, FREE WEIGHTS

PRIMARY MUSCLE GROUP WORKED: Pectoralis major (chest).

SECONDARY MUSCLE GROUP WORKED: anterior deltoid (front shoulder)

STARTING POSITION: Taking a free weight in each hand, lie on the floor, holding the weights close to your chest. Bend your knees and place your feet flat on a bench or the floor. (If using a bench, you may place your feet on the floor as long as your feet can rest comfortably without causing your lower back to arch excessively.) Press the weights straight up from your shoulders with your palms facing each other. Keep your elbows slightly bent. Bring the weights close together.

ACTION: Keep your shoulder blades drawn together, a natural arch in your lower back, your navel pulled in toward your spine, elbows slightly bent, and wrists firm. Slowly lower the weights out to the side until your elbows are even with your shoulders or the bench. Hold for one count. Exhale while slowly bringing your arms toward each other as you raise them upward until they reach the starting position.

TIPS:

1. Do not lower your arms beneath the level of the bench (not a problem if you are doing this on the floor).
2. Keep the weight on the lighter side for this exercise. Do not use as much weight as you would for the chest press.

9. BICEPS CURL, FREE WEIGHTS

This is one of my favorite exercises for people who are in nursing homes and starting to exercise. They can do this exercise seated, using a can of soup as a weight, or anything else that's light. (I have them choose their favorite soup: keeping it fun makes exercising easier.)

PRIMARY MUSCLE GROUPS WORKED: Biceps brachii (front arm), brachialis (side arm), and brachioradialis (upper-outer forearm).

STARTING POSITION: Stand with your feet approximately shoulder width apart, knees slightly bent, arms down at your sides and palms facing forward.

ACTION: Bend your elbows slowly, bringing your hands up towards your shoulders while keeping your elbows down at your sides and directly under your shoulders. Keep your focus forward, a natural arch in your lower back, shoulder blades pulled slightly together and down, chest up, and navel pulled towards your spine. Exhale as you lift the weights up. Return slowly to the starting position.

TIPS:

1. Keep your upper arms stationary and at the side of your body without excessively pressing against your body.
2. Make sure you do not start with too heavy a weight, as that can strain the upper back.
3. If you have balance problems, sit in an armless chair while performing this exercise.

VARIATION: You can do this exercise seated on a bench or stool; you should do it that way if you have low back problems.

10A. TRICEPS ONE-ARM OVERHEAD EXTENSION, FREE WEIGHTS

MUSCLES WORKED: Triceps (back of arm).

STARTING POSITION: Sitting on a bench or chair, grasp a weight in one hand and straighten your arm above your head, with your upper arm against your ear, elbow facing forward or out to the side. Your palm should be facing forward or to the opposite side. (The way this exercise is done can be varied, so do what is more comfortable for you: have the weight either directly behind your head or to the side.)

ACTION: Slowly lower the weight behind your head, keeping your elbow pointing upward. Straighten your elbow without locking it; then press the weight back up.

TIPS:

1. This "behind-your-head" stance means you risk hitting your head with the weight when it comes down. I know this from personal experience. Once, when I was in a foreign country, I misread kilograms for pounds on the weights. It was too heavy, and I hit myself on the head. So, with this exercise (and all others) take care to protect yourself.
2. Keep your elbows high, never allowing your upper arm to move away from the side of your head.

10B. TRICEPS TWO-ARM OVERHEAD EXTENSION, FREE WEIGHTS

PRIMARY MUSCLES WORKED: Triceps brachii (upper inside of arm).

STARTING POSITION: Lift the weight in both hands and put both arms behind your head. (This exercise uses your strongest muscle group, so you can probably use a heavier weight than you would for the other exercises)

ACTION: With your arms bent and the weight at about shoulder level, extend your arms straight over your head, exhaling as the weight goes up. Then, lower your arms back down to the same position. Remember not to hit your head!

TIP: Keep your elbows high and don't allow your arms to move away from the sides of your head.

11. STANDING SIDE LIFT, FREE WEIGHTS

MUSCLES WORKED: Middle deltoid (side shoulder), anterior deltoid (front shoulder), and supraspinatus (a rotator cuff muscle).

STARTING POSITION: Stand with your feet about shoulder-width apart, and your knees and hips slightly bent. Lean forward slightly from the hips and let your arms hang straight down, with your elbows slightly bent and palms facing each other.

ACTION: Pull your arms up and out to your side, keeping your wrists straight and elbows slightly bent. Continue lifting until your arms are almost parallel to the floor and your hands are slightly in front of you. As with the tubing, the hands should be continuously visible with your peripheral vision. That is, the hands should be in front of your body. Slowly lower them back to the starting position.

TIPS:

1. Your shoulder is not strong in this position, so use light weights (start with 1- to 3-pound or ½- to 1-kg weights). It's crucial that you discontinue the exercise if any shoulder or back pain occurs. If you're using your back to raise the weight to where it should be, use a lighter weight, even if it seems too light. Remember, the goal of these exercises is to strengthen muscles, not to injure yourself.

2. Make sure your shoulders stay down. In this exercise, people typically try to lift with their shoulders, and their shoulders end up practically covering their ears. Have another person look at your shoulders or hold them down while you're doing this exercise, or look in the mirror at yourself, to ensure that you are doing it correctly.

3. I like to do this in a modified-lunge position, and I do two sets, alternating one set with the right leg forward and one with the left leg forward. If you do them in this manner, make sure you split the sets up with another set of exercises in between, so that you don't do two sets in rapid sequence.

4. Women very rarely get past 8 pounds in free weights; men very rarely get past 15 pounds, so I would start with considerably less weight (1- to 3-pound or ½- to 1-kg weights for women, 3- or 5-pound or 1- to 2½-kg for men) unless you're a semi-professional weight lifter or body builder.

12. Rotator Cuff Rotation, Free Weights

PRIMARY MUSCLE GROUPS WORKED: Infraspinatus, teres minor (shoulder girdle muscles and external rotators).

STARTING POSITION: Lie on your side on a bench or the floor with a weight in your top hand. Bend the elbow at a 90-degree angle and hold the upper arm against the side of your body with the forearm down across your body. Lie with your head in line with your spine.

ACTION: Keeping your abdominal muscles engaged, a natural arch in your lower back, and your wrist firm, lift the weight by rotating your top shoulder outward while keeping your upper arm against the side of your body. Continue to lift until your forearm is almost perpendicular to the floor.

TIPS:

1. Don't use a heavy weight; start with 1- to 3-pound or ½- to 1-kg weights. Think of the exercise more as a warm-up exercise than as a strength-building exercise.
2. Stop the exercise before the muscle feels fatigued.

13. Overhead Press, Free Weights

PRIMARY MUSCLES WORKED: Anterior deltoid (front shoulder) and triceps (back of arm).

STARTING POSITION: Sit on a bench or chair with back support. Rest your feet on the floor and hold one weight in each hand. Lift the weights until your forearms are perpendicular to the floor at shoulder level and the weights are above shoulder level, with your palms facing forward and elbows out to the side, bent slightly more than 90 degrees.

ACTION: Keeping the natural arch in your lower back, navel pulled in towards your spine, shoulder blades drawn together and down, and your focus forward, press the weights upward until they almost come together over your head and your elbows straighten (without locking). Exhale as you press up. Slowly return to the starting position as you inhale.

TIPS:

1. Keep your wrists firm and straight.
2. Keep your back erect.
3. Stop this exercise if you experience any popping, clicking, or discomfort.
4. You may also try this exercise with your palms facing each other.
5. Do not lock your elbows at the top of the movement.

14. LATERAL DELTOID LIFT, FREE WEIGHTS

PRIMARY MUSCLES WORKED: Posterior deltoid (back of shoulders), upper and middle trapezius (upper back), and rhomboids (middle back).

STARTING POSITION: Find a solid, comfortable bench or chair without wheels. With your back parallel to the floor, put your left knee on the bench and your left arm on the bench. With your right hand, which should be hanging at your side, pick up the weight.

ACTION: Keeping your shoulder blades drawn in toward the spine and down toward your lower back, your natural arch in your lower back, navel pulled in toward your spine, head in line with your spine, and your wrists firm and elbows slightly bent, pull your arm up and out to the side until your elbows are slightly higher than the level of your torso, and your hand has reached the level of your shoulders. With your shoulder blades squeezed together, slowly return to the starting position.

TIPS:

1. Don't allow your body to move back and forth in a rowing position: Your body should be anchored, and all the work should be done by your arms and shoulder muscles.
2. Don't allow your shoulder blades to separate between repetitions.

Those are the fourteen strengthening exercises I recommend. I also advise all my patients over forty to add one more exercise, and when I tell them that it can makes their sex lives truly magnificent, they are usually willing to give it a try.

A BONUS: PELVIC FLOOR (KEGEL) EXERCISES

The muscles forming the floor of the pelvic cavity act as a sling that supports the pelvic organs (bladder, bowel, and penis or uterus). When muscle tone is poor, the pelvic floor does not support the organs as well; women are likely to develop uterine prolapse and urinary stress incontinence (loss of bladder control). That is why these exercises were originally developed for women. However, when these muscles are toned and conditioned through exercise, both men and women experience increased sexual pleasure, and women also experience a noticeable improvement in bladder control. These exercises should be started around age forty and should be continued throughout your life.

To perform Kegel exercises, you must be seated on a toilet with your legs apart. (Men and women both sit.) The exercises consist of a sequence in which you urinate a small amount, try to stop the flow midstream by contracting the muscles, and then hold the contraction of the muscle for about five seconds. If you can stop the flow, you are doing the exercises correctly. You then release the muscles and again urinate a small amount. Again stop the flow by holding the muscles for five seconds and continue until you have emptied your bladder.

One conceptualization will help you do these exercises. Imagine that the pelvic floor is an elevator. When the pelvic muscles are completely relaxed, the elevator is at the basement. You then contract the muscles to the "first floor" and, without relaxing, continue to tighten the muscles to the second floor. Hold at each level for a count of five. When you reach your limit, don't release suddenly. Gradually release the muscles "floor by floor" until completely relaxed. Some people practice contracting these muscles when they are waiting for the light to change while driving a car. Contract the muscles and relax five to ten times.

All of the exercises in this chapter are just basic stretches and lifts—resistance exercises—you can do at home without any elaborate or expensive equipment. As you progress, you may want to add more to your workout, increase the duration and intensity of your workout, or even take a class that integrates your strength and flexibility exercises into one circuit workout.

Take some time to work with a trainer to learn to do them properly and safely. A great physical activity routine that includes these exercises is a wonderful and enjoyable way to make yourself look, feel, and actually be younger, from the inside out. Doing these for ninety days (the first thirty with walking only, and then walking and strengthening for the next thirty days, and then gradually adding stamina for the next thirty days) will produce a remarkable start to your RealAge Makeover. Try it: you will probably love and enjoy it the way I and many of my patients do. And like Cynthia W., you will crave it—it will become a fun, almost addictive, part of your RealAge Makeover.

Vitamin
Power

Why Just Any Multivitamin Won't Work

A RealAge Makeover Success Story:
A Member of H.M.'s Health Club

Hello RealAge,
My name is H.M. I enjoy getting your tips of the day and I often print them and post them on my bulletin board. Let me tell you about a customer of our health club whose life one of your tips probably saved. Your tip told of the possibility of elevated homocysteine levels causing heart attacks, strokes, impotence, etc., and the easy benefit of folate in decreasing those levels and risk (and making such a person's RealAge as much as 4 years younger). One of our members, a 26-year-old man, read this tip on my bulletin board. He was an avid exerciser and watched his food and weight; in fact, he was on a high-protein diet. He was really worried about his life, and structured activities to prolong it but really didn't believe he would live to 40. His brother had died of a heart attack at age 29, his father had a stroke at age 36, and his uncle died of a heart attack at age 39, so he was really motivated to keep exercising and do the right thing. But his multivitamin had only 200 micrograms (μg) of folate. He read your tip and wondered if that homocysteine problem was one of his problems. He got his level measured and it was off the chart: 29, he told me, and his physician thought that might be the cause of his family history. He added more folate, and his level is now a non-risk-producing 9. Not only was his level sky high, so was his younger brother's, his sister's, another uncle's, and his father's. All have now controlled their levels with simply folate, B_6, and B_{12}. From another tip of

yours, he learned that his high-protein diet was making this worse; he has adjusted his diet to keep his homocysteine level less than 9.

Your tip probably saved their lives. You have remade his attitude on life. He now thinks he may have a future and maybe he can have children, and help see and support them thru college and have a long-term life with his wife. So, thank you for helping save and remake the life of one of my members. But I have a request. I own a health club in Virginia and recently put together my own Web page. I would like to link your website with mine, so my members could access your information. You might save more lives that way. Is this possible, and, if so, what is the process? (By the way, that member was so happy about the bulletin board, he just bought a life membership in my health club. He now feels he will be young enough for a long time to benefit from a lifetime membership, so a double thanks.)

H.M., via e-mail

Can vitamins play a role in your RealAge Makeover? Absolutely. The right nutrients in the proper amounts help protect your body from needless aging. Although we often hear about the recommended daily allowance (RDA), the minimum needed to prevent disease from deficiency, I believe you could think instead about a "RealAge Optimum" (RAO). This is the dose you really need to stay as young as you can be, the dose that maximizes your RealAge Makeover. The RAO varies for each of the different vitamins, depending on your age, gender, and the medications you are taking.

- Hundreds of vitamins, minerals, herbs, and supplements are available from many sources. Learn to take the supplements that can help keep you young and avoid those that make you older. For example, you should avoid taking more than 2,500 IU of vitamin A and beta-carotene in supplements, and you should avoid taking iron at the same time as other vitamins and minerals. Taking the wrong combination of vitamins, or taking needless vitamins, can make you 1.7 years older.
  Difficulty rating: Quick fix
- Despite all the media hype surrounding high cholesterol, there may be something more dangerous to worry about: homocysteine. This amino acid is a by-product of the processes your body uses to metabolize all the protein you consume. High levels of homocysteine correlate with the early onset of arterial aging (heart and vascular disease) more than almost any other factor. But not to fear: by getting adequate amounts of folate (folic acid) as well as vitamins B_6 and B_{12}, you

can lower homocysteine levels, making your RealAge more than 3.75 years younger.

Difficulty rating: Quick fix

■ Antioxidants are all the rage because of their supposed antiaging effect. This chapter will explore those claims. What is oxidation? How does this bodily equivalent of rusting age your body? When taken together, vitamins C and E work as a team to keep your arteries, immune system, and organs young. You have an army of antioxidants in your body which help protect you, and for which vitamins C and E appear to play a crucial additive effect. While we do not know if this is primarily due to an antioxidant effect, we know that when taken consistently, these two vitamins can make your RealAge one year younger.

Difficulty rating: Quick fix

■ Frail bones and arthritis are hallmarks of aging. The danger of these conditions can be reduced by getting the proper levels of calcium and vitamin D. Getting 1,200 mg (milligrams) of calcium (and even more if you are a woman, do stamina exercises, or drink caffeinated beverages) and 400 IU (international units) of vitamin D a day can help make you 1.3 years younger.

Difficulty rating: Quick fix

■ Magnesium is needed to keep the heart rhythm stable, and to balance the effects of calcium on nerve function. Getting 400 mg or so of magnesium a day (one-third of the amount of calcium you take) from supplements or from a magnesium-rich diet reduces your complications from cardiovascular-related problems by decreasing abnormal heart beats and decreasing nerve dysfunction, and makes your RealAge 0.9 year younger.

Difficulty rating: Quick fix

■ We would all like to eat a balanced diet, but not all of us can or do. The hectic pace of real life often interferes. If you do not eat a balanced diet, including eight to ten servings of fruits and vegetables each day, and even if you do, you can get all the vitamin and mineral nutrition you need by taking a multivitamin twice daily, in addition to the other supplements recommended in this chapter.

Difficulty rating: Quick fix

■ Besides folate, B_6, B_{12}, vitamin D, calcium, magnesium, potassium, selenium, and vitamins C and E (if you aren't taking a statin), what should you be getting in your diet? This chapter discusses some of the latest nutrient, herb, and supplement treatments. What are the

possible benefits or side effects of such micronutrients as chromium picolinate, alpha lipoic acid, and L-carnitine, and such herbal remedies as echinacea, glucosamine and chondroitin sulfate, coenzyme Q10, and ginseng? Some might be taken regularly. For example, glucosamine and chondriotin sulfate decrease joint pain, decrease cartilage and joint space loss, help increase cartilage buildup in patients with osteoarthritis. Should all of us be taking this combination to prevent the ubiquitous osteoarthritis from disabling us? The data are not good enough to say that yet, but I know at the first sign of such in my own body, I will. Avoiding inappropriate supplements and fads and taking appropriate ones will make you one to four years younger.
Difficulty rating: Quick fix

A RealAge Makeover Success Story: G.G.

Dear Dr. Mike,

I was a 47-year-old woman who didn't want to be older but, by the tables in your book, my RealAge was 7.5 years older. But your book was so positive that I could get younger, that I had to try. You write in a great tone, so I believed you and I tried, and you helped me succeed. My Doc had told me I had premature osteopenia, low bone density, on my way to osteoporosis and bone fractures, and that my knee pain was probably due to that. He put me on Tums, 8 of them, so I'd get 1,600 mg of calcium a day. But my bone density test got worse over the first 14 months, so he wanted to start a medication to put calcium into my bones. About that time a friend gave me your book. I learned that I couldn't absorb all that calcium at once; that I had to take at most 600 mg of calcium in any 8-hour period, to take it with 200 mg of magnesium, and that if I took it with 600 IU of vitamin D, I would absorb the calcium better. And to take it with a prune every day to avoid constipation, if that began to bother me. I also learned that I should add vitamin C, 500 mg three times a day, to decrease the risk of osteoporosis—so my renewed bone would form correctly—and to do 12 lunges twice three times a week. You also said it was okay to take an aspirin two hours before I tried the lunges. I couldn't do two lunges very well, let alone 12, when I read your book. But I started vitamins D and C and split the Tums tablets so I took 3 at a time three times a day. Now 18 months later, my bone density test says I'm better; my knees no longer hurt; I do a full set of resistance exercises, lunges, back rows, the full thing, three times a week; and I am 4 years younger on your test. My Doc wants to know what I'm doing to make my bones so much better, and doesn't feel the need to talk me into the new medicine anymore. I gave him a copy of your book, with the vitamin chapter noted with Post-its. Thank you, thank you, thank you!

G.G., Des Moines, Iowa, via e-mail

Yes, it is possible to start your RealAge Makeover by taking the right vitamins and avoiding the wrong ones, just as the member of H.M.'s club and G.G. did. But do you really know which vitamins, and how much of them, you should be taking?

It's easy to find the choices overwhelming. If you walk into a health-food store, or down the vitamin aisle at your local drugstore, you will see shelves overflowing with vitamins of all sorts, not to mention minerals and a panoply of supplements. There are multivitamins, individual vitamins, "cocktails," stress vitamins, energy vitamins, herbs, minerals, pills, capsules, liquid vitamins, and drops, the same vitamins in different dosages and different formulations—and no clear instructions about what you should take, how much, or how often. You can even get vitamin boosts at your neighborhood coffee or juice chain.

Our thinking about vitamins changed in the 1960s when the Nobel Prize-winning chemist Linus Pauling asserted that taking high doses of vitamin C prevented the common cold. His claims became a folk remedy, and people readily began to take vitamin pills. Now, a quarter of all adults in the United States gulp down vitamin supplements regularly, and half take them occasionally.

I Was a Skeptic

In medical school, I had exactly two hours of education on nutrition out of more than 4,800 hours of lectures. First we were taught what symptoms and diseases each vitamin deficiency or excess caused. Then we were taught that if you ate a balanced diet, you would get enough of everything you needed, including vitamins and minerals. But this is not what actually happens. Of the more than five million people who have taken the nutrition portion of the RealAge program on our website, most don't eat a complete enough diet to get the RealAge Optimum of vitamins and minerals necessary for preventing aging and age-related disease.

Almost all of us on the RealAge scientific team started taking vitamins when we realized how powerful and consistent the data were about their importance. That was after reviewing the first 1,000 or so articles on vitamins and minerals in diet and supplements. Everyone else on the team started after we reviewed about 1,500 articles on this subject. We were further surprised to find that most multivitamins sold by the large companies are not formulated for optimal health. (At least, the companies don't make the vitamins to fit what the data indicate.) The RealAge scientific team learned that specific vitamins and minerals in specific amounts could actually help prevent age-related disease. Granted, the subject was complex. We had to spend much time sorting through all the data to find what would be an optimal vitamin combination and how we—and you— should take it. However, the data were so compelling that those of us who came in as skeptics went out as believers and began to take specific vitamins and minerals for our health.

Exactly how confusing and consuming the issue could be was made clear to me one day when a new patient, Frank T., walked into my office, opened up a bag, and began pulling out bottles. Brown bottles, blue bottles, small bottles, big bottles. (I always ask each patient to bring all the medicines and supplements they are taking.) When Frank was done, he had thirty-five containers of vitamins, minerals, and supplements lined up on my desk.

Incredulous, I asked, "You take all of these every day?"

"Absolutely," he replied. "Some I take twice a day." In all, he took about fifty tablets daily. Clearly, he was an organized man, and this was a full-time job. At fifty-four, Frank was in good shape. He exercised vigorously and often, was trim, happily married, and at the peak of his career. Recently he'd had a prostate scare, and that made him worry. He began reading up on his health and asking people at the health-food store for recommendations. The results of his research—all thirty-five bottles' worth—were spread out in front of me like a Thanksgiving feast. Now he wanted to know what I thought.

"Fifty pills a day is too much," I told him. "Some of them are doubtless good for you, but some of them could be bad for you." Then I gave Frank some basic guidelines for taking vitamins and outlined a specific plan that could do exactly what he wanted: keep him young.

What Should My Multivitamin Contain to Reach the RealAge Optimum?

Here's what you should be doing to make your nutritional supplements the most effective tool for your RealAge Makeover. When you shop for a multivitamin, first read the label. The multivitamin should have the usual RDAs of vitamins and minerals. You need to supplement those amounts so that you obtain the RAOs for each vitamin and mineral listed. Then you have to remember five minerals (sorry, there's no mnemonic). Just photocopy this list and take it with you when you go to buy your multi.

Table 10.1	**RealAge Optimum Amounts of Vitamins, Minerals, and Nutrients**

VITAMINS	REALAGE OPTIMUM (RAO)
A	No more than 2,500 IU
B_6	4 mg a day
B_{12}	800 μg a day (25 μg, in a supplement. B_{12} in a supplement is absorbed much better than the B_{12} found in food)
C	400 mg a day three times a day (remember it's water-soluble, so you need several doses over the day). Reduce this to 100 mg a day from supplements if you're taking a statin drug (for example, Zocor, Lipitor, Pravachol, or Crestor)
D	400 IU a day if under age 60; 600 IU a day if 60 or over
E	400 to 800 IU a day (400 to 800 IU of mixed tocopherols is the form I favor). Reduce this to less than 100 IU a day from supplements if you're taking a statin drug
F (folate)	800 μg a day (folic acid, folate, or folicin, sometimes listed as vitamin B_9)
Thiamin	25 mg
Riboflavin	25 mg
Niacin	At least 30 mg a day, preferably more if you're taking a statin drug (check with your doctor)
Biotin	300 μg
Pantothenic acid	10 mg
MINERALS	
Calcium	600 mg twice a day (1,600 mg total a day for women)
Magnesium	400 mg a day
Selenium	200 μg a day
Zinc	15 mg
Potassium	Four fruits plus a normal diet should do it.
ADDITIONAL VITAMIN-LIKE SUBSTANCES THAT MIGHT BE TAKEN DAILY	
Lycopene	Ten tablespoons of tomato sauce a week (400 μg) should do it
Lutein	A leafy green vegetable a day (40 μg) should do it
Alpha lipoic acid	Not indicated by data yet
Acetyl-L-carnitine	Not indicated by data yet, but if you want it, 1,500 mg a day

Add 200 mg of Coenzyme Q10 if you're taking a statin drug. Make sure your multivitamin contains less than 2,500 IU (less than 1.6 mg) of vitamin A, because too much vitamin A or beta-carotene ages you.
IU is the abbreviation for international units;
μg is the abbreviation for micrograms;
mg is the abbreviation for milligrams.

General Rules About Vitamins

Perhaps next to questions about food, the questions about vitamins and minerals on our website are the most common: "I take a drug called Zocor for my cholesterol problem," wrote one website user. "Is it okay for me to take the same vitamin preparation as everyone else?"

Other website users had different questions. "Is there any benefit to coral calcium over regular calcium?" "How about ester-bound vitamin C preparations: are they better than the usual?" "Are liquid vitamins better than chewable or regular vitamin pills?" and "Should I take vitamins on an empty stomach first thing in the morning?" Another asked, "I take an aspirin a day like you recommended. But I recently read that vitamin E can cause bleeding if I take it with an aspirin. Should I take vitamin E at a different time or should I not take vitamin E at all, or should I not take aspirin at all?"

Perhaps most confusing for many of my patients is that what they read in the newspapers may be completely different from what they're told at the health-food store. And to say that there's a difference between the advice of medical doctors and of practitioners of alternative medicine would be a vast understatement. The value of nutritional supplements is clearly a controversial issue.

For doctors, one of the most frustrating aspects of the large array of vitamins and supplements available is not that they don't work, but that we don't have any proof they actually do work. With the exception of a few basic vitamins (C, D, E, B, B_6, B_{12}, folate, niacin, and A) and a few minerals (calcium, magnesium, selenium, potassium, and iron), we have limited scientific information about the role and optimal dosages of most of the supplements on the market. For many minerals and vitamins, we know the minimum amounts of essential nutrients needed for survival—the recommended daily allowances (RDAs) or the daily values (DVs). We know much less about the optimal doses for health and the prevention, retarding, or reversal of age-related disease or aging in general. Most of what you learn in health-food stores has not yet been proven. It may prove right, it may prove wrong—we just don't know.

Few or no scientific studies have investigated the change in outcome from the vast majority of supplements on sale at any local health-food store. Most are sold without any description of what they are, why they are good for us, or how we should take them. Many of them are unnecessary, and some are even harmful.

Many people swear by herbal medicines, and I believe that in many cases they do so for good reason. Some herbal supplements do indeed have an ingredient that is beneficial. However, that does not mean you should just go ahead and take any herbal supplement you want. First, it is necessary to examine the supplement, find out exactly what that beneficial ingredient is, and in what doses it should be taken.

For example, aspirin is an herbal remedy, as it comes from the bark of a tree. However, if we still gave aspirin as an herb, we probably wouldn't get the dose right, and we would have many more side effects for the same therapeutic benefit. Aspirin is now purified and formulated; it costs less than a penny a pill but has enormous value. The same can be true for ginseng and, I believe, most other herbs: given properly and in the right dosage, they can have value. In order to deliver that value to you, we need to isolate the active ingredients and to purify and formulate them as we do drugs, and as we purified and formulated aspirin from tree bark. Unfortunately, for most herbs, minerals, and other food supplements, the necessary research has just not yet been done.

Because nutritional supplements are classified as food products and not medicines, they aren't regulated by the strict standards governing the sale of prescription and over-the-counter drugs, and manufacturers can sell them in any quantity or combination they want. Different brands of the same supplement might contain very different elements. Not uncommonly, some bottles contain ingredients and even contaminants not listed on the label. In addition, the law does not require that the manufacturers perform scientific studies to back up their claims of health effects, as needed for any new medicinal drug.

The law that allows herbs and supplements to be sold in the United States is called the Dietary Supplement Health and Education Act (DSHEA). If aspirin were formulated under such a law, we might have brands of aspirin that contain no active ingredient at all, and others that contained 250 to 500 percent of the amount claimed on the label. Imagine if aspirin were marketed as, for example, "cinchona bark." You would have to guess how much aspirin was in the bottle and if there was even any at all), and how many contaminants it contained, because the U.S. Food and Drug Administration (FDA) would not have controlled the purity of its manufacture as strictly. (The FDA would have been able to control the purity by removing the supplement only after a problem developed.)

That's how many of our herbal medicines are currently marketed. We do not know the dose, and we do not know how many contaminants are included. The DSHEA law makes it much tougher for the general public and physicians to find the kernel of truth in the remedy.

What to Do

If you do buy supplements, purchase from a large and reputable manufacturer. In addition, do not take any supplement without getting a recommendation from a reputable source. When I am going to buy an herb for myself or want to recommend it to a patient, I look it up on *www.consumerlab.com*, a subscription service. This website tests herbal preparations to ascertain the actual (versus claimed) amount of ingredients in the product, and contaminants. For example, of the thirteen preparations of glucosamine and chondroitin sulfate *www .consumerlab.com* tested one year, seven had little or no active ingredient of one or the other compound at all, and another had two and a half times as much of one ingredient as listed on the label.

I also advise against taking any supplement "cocktail" sold at a health-food store, from a vitamin aisle at a store, or from a catalog (many are sent from Canada where the laws are even more lax than in the U.S.). These mixtures of herbs, vitamins, and minerals often don't even list what they contain, or how much of any one ingredient is included, as the companies that sell them aren't required by law to do so. You could be taking all kinds of things you don't want. Most of these wonder pills are probably harmless, but we cannot say for sure. For example, all the data I have seen concerning the human growth hormone (HGH) preparations sold as over-the-counter supplements (not the injections in a physician's office) indicate that such preparations are ineffective. Your body sees no increase in your normal HGH level, in HGH-like compounds, or in any other substance that might produce the same effect. However, the good news is that most of these supplements aren't toxic, either. So as far as HGH supplements go, you're probably just out a little money, but at least you're not hurting your health. Even so, why take a chance? If you are trying to be smart about Age Reduction, don't take a pill or supplement cocktail just because a store clerk or infomercial tells you to do so. If you don't know what it is, don't take it.

What do we actually know about vitamins, minerals, and other supplements? Which ones should we take? Which ones should we definitely not take? In general, if you eat a balanced and healthy diet, with four servings of fruits, five servings of vegetables, and plenty of grains, you should get all the nutrients you need through your food. However, most of us have busy lives and hectic schedules, which means that it's not always easy to eat a balanced and nutrient-rich diet. In fact, of the more than 5 million people who have reported their diets on the RealAge website, fewer than 50,000—less than 1 percent—get the right amount of vitamins D, B_6, B_{12}, and folate and the minerals calcium and magnesium from food alone. To make up for the lack, I recommend taking a multivitamin every day, in case you have missed out on a little bit of one mineral or the other. Choose a multivitamin without added iron, and one that has less than 2,500 IU of vitamin A and beta-carotene, combined.

In fact, you should really take your vitamins (or your multivitamin) twice a day: several vitamins are water soluble and you will urinate them out so quickly that you need them twice a day just to have a minimally acceptable level in your blood at all times (especially if you do not eat a lot of fruit and vegetables). Further, for some such as calcium, you cannot absorb more than 600 mg at a time, so you need that twice a day; and if you take more than 500 mg at once of others such as vitamin C, you increase the risk of toxicity. So to keep a steady level, absorb the optimal level, and minimize the risk of toxicity from too much at once, you want a twice-a-day multivitamin. Although many may be unwilling to take their vitamins twice a day, that is the optimal way for health.

If you are worried about whether you are eating a balanced diet rich in vitamins and nutrients, talk to your doctor or see a clinical nutritionist to review your eating habits and develop food guidelines specific to you. You can also take the nutrient profile from your RealAge Age-Reduction planning session, available at *www.RealAge.com*, with you to facilitate the process. Vegetarians and others on special or restricted diets should be vigilant about getting the basics, especially B$_{12}$ and all essential amino acids, as these are not readily obtained in vegetarian diets. Quinoa is a grain that has all the essential amino acids you need, and it tastes great. Give it a try.

What other nutrients and vitamins should you be getting? What do vitamins do for you? What shouldn't you take? Let's explore your options.

Oxidants and Antioxidants: Rustproofing Your Body

Although oxidants and antioxidants were considered among the most crucial elements of vitamins in the past, new research indicates that oxidation may not be the main cause of arterial aging. It may be that anti-inflammatory properties are more important factors in producing the primary antiaging benefits of vitamins; we do not yet know for sure that antioxidation alone is responsible for the primary benefit.

Even if antioxidants aren't the magic bullet we first believed, they still have great value, because they purportedly can help prevent the damage from oxidation that has been linked to cancers and other types of aging. Taking the right amounts of antioxidant vitamins C and E, for example, can make your RealAge as much as one year younger. However, many people wrongly believe that if a little bit of antioxidant is good, a lot is better. Too many antioxidants, especially the wrong type, can actually cause oxidation and its subsequent damage. My recommendation is to use antioxidation in moderation.

To understand antioxidants, let's first think about the oxygen. Oxygen is necessary for our bodies to function at all. Breathing is fundamental to living. When we breathe, oxygen enters the bloodstream and is transported to our cells. Once it enters your cells, oxygen forms the basis of many of the cells' most fundamental processes. This same oxygen, however, in the form of unstable molecules or ions called oxygen radicals (or free radicals), can oxidize tissues—that is, cause those tissues to "rust." As a result, oxygen waste products, called lipofuscins, build up in organs such as the heart and brain, leaving brown discoloration on the tissues. Do these waste products cause or contribute to aging or age-related disease, or are they just innocent by-products?

Oxidation itself may not be the basic problem. There may be a more fundamental problem such as inflammation, or something else that causes immune dysfunction. Whatever the cause, these brown spots are signs of aging. The older you get, the more prevalent they become.

Imagine apples. If you slice an apple and leave it out in the air, it will soon turn brown. Exposed to air, the surface of the apple oxidizes (combines with oxygen). This process is similar to what happens when oxygen radicals build up in your body. If you were to take that same apple and sprinkle lemon juice on the slices, they would stay white. The apple does not turn brown because lemon juice is full of vitamin C, which works as an antioxidant. Lemon juice stops the oxidation process and keeps the apple from "rusting." In your body, antioxidants such as vitamins C and E do the same thing.

Think of your body as an exclusive club. Free radicals are the visitors who crash the scene without an invitation. They are so pesky, the body can't get rid of them without some help. Antioxidants function as a kind of security system, the bouncers. They seek out the roving oxygen radicals and bind to them—a kind of chemical handcuff. Bound together, the free radical and the antioxidant form an entity that the body can then flush out through the kidneys. As long as you have enough bouncers, free radicals and lipofuscins won't build up in the body. And your body literally has an army of antioxidants built in to protect you. Vitamins C and E seem to augment this army's work.

How does this rusting affect us? Mainly, oxidation ages your arteries. As you get older, your arteries are more likely to become clogged with fat deposits. These clogs contain high levels of oxidized lipids: fats that have been chemically altered through interaction with high levels of free radicals. Therefore, oxidation plays a significant role in the aging of our arteries.

Oxidation affects us in other ways, too. Oxygen free radicals are an unstable form of oxygen that causes genetic damage. Each cell in your body contains DNA (deoxyribonucleic acid) that instructs that cell what to do and when to do it. Every time your cells divide, DNA is copied into the new cell. Oxidation interferes with this process, causing DNA damage. This oxidation is thought to lead to cancer as well as the premature aging of solid tissues. However, we don't have great data that oxidation itself is the fundamental problem. Oxidation can also damage the immune system, the body's backup security system to ensure that cancer cells don't spread (see Chapter 5). Finally, oxidation ages our eyes. It can damage the lenses, promoting cataracts, and the retina. The gradual loss of sight is one of the very first things that can make us feel old.

There are still many gaps in what we know about oxidation, and a lot of what we do know is based on circumstantial evidence. We do know that people with extensive buildup of oxidized fats in their bodies have much higher rates of heart disease, and that their bodies appear to age more quickly in other ways, too.

In summary, the hypothesis is that aging and oxidation are connected, although we have a hunch this may not be the total story. Something else, such as inflammation, may cause oxidation that in turn causes damage through free radicals. Oxidation may be the result instead of the cause.

Regardless of the exact reasons why oxidation seems to age us, we know that people who consume the antioxidants vitamin C and vitamin E together (the studies of one or the other alone show no RealAge benefit) at specific levels have substantially lower rates of coronary disease, cancer, cataracts, and other forms of aging.

Twice Daily Basics: Vitamins C and E, but *Not* Vitamin A

Taken together, vitamins C and E help keep your cardiovascular system healthy by reducing the amount of harmful buildup (plaque) on the walls of your arteries. In addition, vitamin C strengthens the immune system, improves both eye and lung function, and helps the body heal. Vitamins C and E, taken in combination, help keep the arteries relaxed and elastic. You can make your RealAge one year younger by taking between 600 and 2,000 mg of vitamin C a day as supplements, in divided doses of no more than 500 mg in any six hours and 400 IU of vitamin E a day, in addition to eating a balanced diet with lots of fresh fruits and vegetables.

Table 10.2	The RealAge Benefits of Vitamins C and E

FOR MEN:

Daily Intake* Of Vitamin C (mg) and Vitamin E† (IU) Taken in Split Doses

Vitamin C (mg) Vitamin E (IU)	Less than 60 Less than 15	60 to 699 15 to 119	700 to 1199 120 to 399	1,200 or more 400 or more
CALENDAR AGE		REALAGE		
35	35.6	35.0	34.7	34.4
55	55.8	55.0	54.2	54.0
70	71.3	70.0	69.0	68.6

FOR WOMEN:

Daily Intake* of Vitamin C (mg) and Vitamin E† (IU) Taken in Split Doses

Vitamin C (mg) Vitamin E (IU)	Less than 60 Less than 15	60 to 699 15 to 119	700 to 1199 120 to 399	1200 or more 400 or more
CALENDAR AGE		REALAGE		
35	35.4	35.0	34.8	34.7
55	55.7	55.0	54.7	54.4
70	71.2	70.0	69.5	69.0

*The RealAge Optimum, the dose recommended for the greatest Age Reduction.
†Vitamin E is fat-soluble and thus does not need to be taken in split doses or twice a day.
IU is the abbreviation for international units;
mg is the abbreviation for milligrams;
If you are taking a statin drug for cholesterol or other arterial aging management, you should take much lower doses of vitamins C and E (100 mg of C and 50 IU of E twice a day), as very good data indicate these two vitamins inhibit the functioning of the statins in making your arteries younger.

Vitamin C and vitamin E complement one another. Vitamin C is water-soluble, whereas vitamin E is fat-soluble. What does that mean? Cells are made up of two components: the cell membrane and the cell interior. The cell membrane, the outer casing of the cell, consists of lipids, or fats. It is the cell membrane that has the buildup of lipofuscins, those brown spots. Because vitamin E dissolves in fat, it helps prevent oxidant-induced aging in the membrane. In contrast, the inside of the cell consists mostly of water. Because vitamin C dissolves in water, it can enter the center of the cell and collect the free-radical oxidants lurking there. Together, these two vitamins keep oxidants from damaging your cells both inside and out (see Table 10.2). Remember, however, that some effect other than antioxidation may be producing the majority of benefit associated with vitamins C and E.

Vitamin C: An Immune-Strengthening Antiager

Have you ever noticed that the minute you get a cold, everyone from the checkout clerk at the grocery store to your mother starts telling you take vitamin C? That is the legacy of Nobel laureate Linus Pauling. All of us know that vitamin C is good for us, but most of us probably couldn't say why.

What exactly does vitamin C do? Like vitamin E, vitamin C helps keep the arteries clear by inhibiting oxidation of fat in the walls of your blood vessels. It converts cholesterol to a form that can be washed out of the body easily, inhibiting lipid buildup. Because vitamin C is water-soluble, it enters the cells that make up the wall of the vessels, and binds to free radicals lurking inside the cells, precisely in the place where those free radicals are likely to cause DNA damage. Because of its healing capabilities, vitamin C helps maintain a healthy matrix (intracellular substance) in the blood vessels, repairing the vessel walls when they become damaged.

Vitamin C needs to be taken with vitamin E to obtain the antiaging benefit. In studies in which vitamin C was administered alone, there was no reduction in vascular disease. Thus, many of the review articles (and the United States Preventive Service Task Force study) report no benefit from vitamin C or from vitamin E with regard to arterial aging. They are absolutely right: when taken alone, no benefit occurs. Important arterial antiaging benefits have only been seen in epidemiologic studies of people who take these two vitamins together (see Table 10.2).

Vitamin C helps reduce high blood pressure, prevents cataracts, and promotes wound healing. It improves lung function, preventing aging of the respiratory system. Also, vitamin C really does keep your immune system young. We now know it decreases the likelihood of the one ager we all want to avoid: cancer. Vitamin C helps prevent infections from the bacterium that causes both stomach and duodenal ulcers and stomach cancer, *Helicobacter pylori*. Recent data from analysis of the National Health and Nutrition Examination Survey (NHANES) indicate that those who had the highest vitamin C levels in their blood were more than 70 percent less likely to be infected by this disease-causing bacterium than those with the lowest levels. The authors of that 2003 study speculate that this resistance to dangerous bacteria which promote cancer is caused by the ability of vitamin C to make the stomach more acidic, and thus less favorable for the bacteria. Whatever the cause, it is an additional RealAge benefit of vitamin C.

Because vitamin C is water-soluble, it washes out of your body when you urinate. Therefore, it is important to take several doses of vitamin C a day. I recommend taking at least two, usually three, doses daily. I do this by combining food and supplements. In the morning, I take a multivitamin containing 500 mg of vitamin C (that also has 200 IU of vitamin E) have an orange or grapefruit at lunch, and again take the same multivitamin with dinner, just to make sure I'm getting enough. I also get vitamin C, in smaller amounts from other things I eat, such as tomatoes and salads. The RAO for vitamin C is approximately 1,200 mg a day from food and supplements, taken in smaller amounts spread throughout the day. The RDA is only 60 mg, way short of the antiaging optimum. Vitamin C tends to leech out of packaged or cut vegetables, and cooking reduces vitamin C levels even more. That's another reason to eat plenty of fresh fruits and vegetables every day. Also, eat some fruit or take some of your vitamin C one to two hours before any vigorous exercise. Vigorous physical activity causes oxidant buildup, and vitamin C's antioxidant power may be one of the ways that it works to keep you younger.

It doesn't matter whether you take natural or synthetic vitamin C. Your body can't tell the difference. Personally, I stay away from "chewables," because the acid is hard on the teeth. Although it costs a little more, I prefer taking vitamin C that contains calcium ascorbate, which helps prevent the stomachaches that straight ascorbic acid (vitamin C) can cause. If you have a sensitive stomach, take the calcium ascorbate form of vitamin C.

One more comment on vitamin C: a recent headline said that vitamin C caused cancer by causing breaks in DNA. What the headline didn't say was that at the 500-mg level, vitamin C appears to repair ten times as many breaks as it causes. Also, if you take 500-mg pills, take them no more frequently than one every six hours not to get too much at once.

Finally, does vitamin C prevent colds? Unfortunately, no. But it does lessen their effect. When you begin to show signs of a cold, increase your vitamin C to as much as 4 grams (4,000 mg) a day, taken with plenty of water—eight glasses for 4 grams. Although this won't cure colds—Pauling wasn't exactly right—it will lessen the severity of the symptoms. For example, when you have a cold and take your C, you may find that you can keep exercising. If you are taking a statin, just increase your intake of chicken soup (not vitamin C). Chicken soup, zinc lozenges, and vitamin C seem to have the identical effect in lessening the severity of symptoms. (To my knowledge no one has studied these together to see if they have addictive effects.)

Vitamin E

Because vitamin E is fat-soluble, it is an especially vigorous antioxidant. In two studies, when taken by patients who had adequate levels of vitamin C, or along with vitamin C, vitamin E reduced the risk of heart attack in women by 35 to 40 percent. One study found that if a person already has arterial disease but not fibrotic, calcified, or permanently hardened arteries, vitamin E can decrease the risk of heart attack by as much as 75 percent. That's an outstanding impact! (However, in most of the other studies done on this subject, vitamin E has been given alone, without vitamin C. This may be a defect in these other studies. In all those studies in which vitamin C was not given with vitamin E, there was no reduction in arterial aging from vitamin E.) Like aspirin, vitamin E thins your blood, making clots less likely to form; quinone (a chemical part of vitamin E) has powerful anticlotting powers. Several studies have noticed an increase in bleeding when vitamin E and aspirin are used in combination, a condition implicated in both ulcers and strokes. It is rare, but discuss this possibility with your physician, especially if you have a history of ulcers or other blood-clotting problems.

Recent evidence indicates vitamin E is associated with a decreased risk of lung and prostate cancer, and perhaps other cancers as well. In two recently completed randomized studies, vitamin E decreased the progression of Alzheimer's disease and the development of Parkinson's disease. We do not know if these effects are due to its antioxidant properties or to other mechanisms. Further studies still need to be done, but the evidence appears promising. Vitamin E may also help the body build muscle strength. In addition, vitamin E has been shown to help prevent cataracts, and preliminary studies suggest it might help prevent progression of macular degeneration, a kind of blindness that can occur with aging.

You should be aware of several things before taking vitamin E. This vitamin therapy reduces the size of fatty buildup only before the arteries have become fibrotic (permanently hardened)—that is, when there is fatty buildup but no irreversible changes. Vitamin E seems to help reduce the size of small or medium-size lesions in the arteries, but not severe ones. That is why you want to start taking these vitamins as soon as possible, to foil aging before it begins.

How much vitamin E should you take? Vitamin E is found in fatty vegetables such as avocados, and in some vegetable oils. It is also found in nuts, leafy green vegetables, and some grains. But it is virtually impossible to get the necessary antiaging dose of vitamin E from food alone. The RDA is only 12 to 15 IU a day. This is the amount you need to survive without showing signs of deficiency disease. However, the RAO (RealAge Optimum) is 400 IU. Most multivitamins follow RDA recommendations and contain only 15 to 30 IU; the level of vitamin E in most multivitamins is often 370 IU short of the optimum for antiaging.

How often do you need to take vitamin E? Since it's fat-soluble, it stays in your body for quite a while. One dose a day is just the right dose. There is little risk of a vitamin E overdose unless you ingest more than 1,200 IU a day, and vitamin E is probably safe up to 3,000 IU a day. If you have high blood pressure, some physicians believe you should get the high blood pressure treated before you slowly start with vitamin E. They advocate you start with 200 IU of vitamin E a day. After a week or so, increase the dose to 400 IU.

The following bears repeating: if you are taking a statin drug for cholesterol management, you should take much lower doses of vitamins C and E (100 mg of C and 50 IU of E twice a day), as very good data indicate these two vitamins inhibit the functioning of the statins in making your arteries younger.

Now, let's consider another big antioxidant vitamin, vitamin A. What is it about vitamin A that makes it an aging vitamin and not an antiaging vitamin?

Vitamin A and Its Precursor, Beta-Carotene

Vitamin A is essential for sight and for normal development. What then could be bad about it? We still don't know the full story on vitamin A and its precursor, beta-carotene, but we do know that they can be an example of too much of a good thing. In the late 1980s, a study came out showing that people who ate foods with lots of vitamin A tended to have lower rates of cancer. People interpreted this to mean they should be taking vitamin A supplements, not eating more fruits and vegetables. Sales of vitamin A and beta-carotene, a substance the body breaks down into vitamin A, went through the roof. In 1988, Americans spent less than eight million dollars on vitamin A supplements, but by 1999, they spent eighty million dollars on vitamin A, often in the form of beta-carotene. What we didn't know at the time was that we were doing ourselves more harm than good.

Studies since then show that we jumped the gun. First, the correlation between vitamin A and the prevention of cancer has been disproved in randomized controlled trials of vitamin A and beta-carotene. Second, we've learned that too much vitamin A can actually be harmful. Although it is important to get sufficient vitamin A, you should do this by eating well, not by taking supplements. You should especially avoid megadosing (taking very large doses). In fact, taking more than 2,500 IU a day increases your risk of cancer and appears to increase your risk of bone fractures. Do not take more than 2,500 IU a day, which is below the standard dosage in many vitamin supplements.

While the body will not convert beta-carotene into vitamin A if it has no need for it, both substances in excess can increase your risk of cancer.

Why can megadosing be dangerous? Because vitamin A is a nutrient that is "level-sensitive." When vitamin A levels in the body are moderate, it works as an antioxidant and is important to the functioning of your body. However, when you megadose, the surplus vitamin A does the opposite. Rather than functioning as an antioxidant, high doses of vitamin A oxidize tissues, cause DNA damage, and deplete your bones of calcium. So taking too much vitamin A makes you age faster.

A 1993 study in Finland showed that people taking vitamin A had a higher risk of lung cancer, atherosclerosis, and, for smokers, stroke. Several other studies have confirmed these findings. Also, excessive amounts of vitamin A may cause liver damage. Smokers need to be especially careful about taking any kind of vitamin A, even the beta-carotene form of vitamin A; when combined with smoke, vitamin A and beta-carotene can be toxic and can increase rates of cancer. These two substances also increase rates of bone reabsorption or decrease rates of new bone formation, and can lead to an increased risk of hip and other bone fractures.

Although some health-food stores still push vitamin A and beta-carotene, remember that you probably get enough in your daily diet. For basic antioxidation, if you believe it's important, rely on vitamins C and E, plus carotenoids (found in foods such as cranberries, blueberries, green beans, broccoli, and tomatoes) and flavonoids (found in wine, onions, garlic, real chocolate, grapes, tea, and apples) which also seem to have antiaging power, decreasing aging of the arterial and immune system (see Chapter 8).

As good as vitamin C is, remember when it comes to vitamins, be careful with antioxidants, as they are a double-edged sword. Avoid excessive C and E if you are taking a statin drug. Also, take a total of no more than 2,500 IU of vitamin A and beta-carotene combined.

Anti-inflammatory Vitamins: Is Preventing Inflammation a Key to Making Your RealAge Young?

Many people think that the main benefit of vitamins in food comes from their antioxidant properties. Although it has been a logical theory for a long time, it is an unproven theory. The data are compelling that something other than—or in addition to—a purely antioxidant property is key to the benefit of vitamins. What now appears crucial is the ability of a vitamin, mineral, or other substance to confer an anti-inflammatory effect. Some of these anti-inflammatory properties may also be antioxidant properties. The anti-inflammatory properties seem to prevent stimulation of inappropriate immune responses that can cause autoimmune disease or aging of the arteries. In addition, these anti-inflammatory properties allow appropriate immune responses that can help defend your body against infections and cancer.

The Risk of Homocysteine, and the Folate Counterattack

A RealAge Makeover Success Story: Kevin D.

My patient Kevin D. was similar to the twenty-six-year-old man in the e-mail at the start of this chapter. Kevin D. had a family history of coronary artery disease. On the other hand, he had normal blood cholesterol levels, a relatively high HDL cholesterol level, and normal blood pressure. He didn't smoke, nor did any of his family members who had died of disease, premature stroke, or premature coronary artery disease. Thus, the classic teaching went, he and his family just had "bad genes," or else they wouldn't have had serious vascular disease. And this was correct, except that he and his family didn't realize that they could actually influence the bad genes by what they did.

When he came to see me at age forty-four, Kevin had the beginning of premature vascular disease. His lower legs ached when he ran; the aching stopped two or three minutes after he stopped running. He would then resume running and go longer before his legs started aching again. Despite this condition, he was able to perform all three forms of physical activity. Claudication (aching legs with exercise) was his first sign of arterial aging. He did not have overt heart disease or any symptom of chest pain. But he knew what happened to his family members and was desperate for preventative measures.

He said, "Doc, I do all the right things. I exercise, I don't eat much saturated fat, my HDL is high, and I have low blood pressure. Why else can I do?" After looking through his records and asking some questions, I ascertained that he wasn't taking folate or any of the B vitamins or a multivitamin, nor had he ever had his homocysteine level measured. Measurement of his homocysteine level showed it was 36, dangerously high.

Homocysteine is an amino acid by-product of the metabolism of protein and can build up in the blood. As you age, your homocysteine levels increase. No one is exactly sure how homocysteine ages your arteries other than by causing inflammation, but it is well established that people with high homocysteine levels have considerably higher levels of inflammatory arterial disease and much greater damage from plaque deposits on the arteries than those who don't have high levels of homocysteine.

Elevated homocysteine levels (18 micromoles per liter of blood—μmol/l—and higher) double the risk of heart attack, stroke, peripheral vascular disease, and impotence. More than 42 percent of people with cerebral vascular disease, 30 percent of those with cardiovascular disease, and 28 percent of those with peripheral vascular disease have homocysteine levels that are too high. And even levels above 12 seem to increase inflammation in your blood vessels. Taking 800 μg of folate a day in supplements, or 1,400 μg through your diet, can reduce homocysteine levels dramatically, essentially removing any excess homocysteine from your bloodstream and stopping its aging effects. It's a quick, easy, and painless way to make your arteries younger.

No one knows for sure why, but high levels of homocysteine seem to disturb the endothelium, the inner lining of the artery. Some scientists believe that homocysteine causes small openings between the endothelial cells that make up the inner lining of your arteries, leading to deterioration of the arterial wall, buildup of plaque, and inflammation. Other theories on how homocysteine ages your arteries suggest that homocysteine may decrease the production of relaxing factors which allow the blood vessels to dilate. It may also stimulate blood clots by changing the shape or form of cells that make up the epithelium. In addition, homocysteine might oxidize low-density lipoproteins (LDL cholesterol), promoting plaque buildup along the walls of arteries. Although we don't know all the reasons, an established link exists between high homocysteine levels and arterial aging.

By consistently taking 800 μg (micrograms) of folate a day, you can make your RealAge 1.2 years younger in just three months, and probably 3.7 years younger in three years. (Although most individuals need 400 to 800 μg for its antiaging effect in the arteries, you need 800 μg for its full anticancer effect, so I have simplified the RAO by just using 800 μg throughout. We know of no toxicity at any dose of folate, so taking 800 μg appears to be very safe.) If you already have elevated levels of homocysteine, you can make your RealAge three or more years younger in just three months. (Other names for folate are folicin, folic acid, and vitamin B$_9$.)

As homocysteine levels increase, folate levels decrease, and vice versa. The two compounds are part of a complex chemical reaction involving many steps, but the end result is that the more of one, the less of the other. The more folate you take, the lower your homocysteine levels.

There is a clearly established correlation between high folate levels and arterial health. One study estimated that if everyone had proper levels of folate, the number of heart attacks in the U.S. could be reduced by 40,000 to 150,000 a year. In fact, these numbers may actually be too conservative! Statistics from risk-factor studies predict that a more realistic estimate would be a reduction of one-third in the rate of heart attacks and strokes in the U.S. every year. In other words, perhaps as many as 450,000 heart attacks and 170,000 strokes occur because we don't get enough folate.

Naturally occurring folate or folic acid is part of the B-complex family of vitamins. Folic acid is often prescribed for pregnant women, because it is essential for the normal development of the brain and spinal cord of the fetus. Thus, we tend to think of folate as being essential only while we are *in utero*, but we also need it as adults.

As you age, the concentration of folate in your body drops; the most common vitamin deficiency among older people is folate. This deficiency not only causes vascular disease but can also lead to cancer as well. In four studies, colon cancer rates decreased 20 to 50 percent with folate supplementation. However, more than 50 percent of all Americans don't even get the RDA of folate. More than 90 percent do not get the amount necessary to decrease the risk of colon cancer (800 μg). In 1998, on average American men consumed 281 μg of folate a day in diet, and American women consumed 270 μg a day. Older people consume even less. Although we have supplemented bread and cereal with folate, the amount we consume still averages less than 400 μg a day.

Lots of foods contain folate. But folate from food is absorbed less well than folic acid from supplements. An eight-ounce glass of orange juice has 43 μg. To get enough folate, you would have to drink about twenty-five eight-ounce glasses of orange juice a day. A slice of white bread has only 6 μg of folate and green salad just 2 μg. Since the average intake of folate is 275 to 375 μg from diet, a 525 μg supplement is what you should take to get the RealAge Optimum of 800 μg a day. If you are trying to get all the folate from diet, you will have to consume even more—upward of 1,400 μg—because the body will absorb only about half of the folate in food. And remember: if you eat a lot of protein, you need even more folate because protein becomes metabolized by the body to homocysteine.

As for Kevin D., I quickly advised him to add 800 μg of folate, 4 mg of B_6, and 25 μg of B_{12} (you need 800 μg of B_{12} from food but only 25 μg in supplements) in a twice-a-day supplement. Within three weeks his homocysteine level was down to 8 μmol/l (micromoles per liter). His risk of subsequent premature vascular disease—aging of his arteries—was reduced by the equivalent of twelve years. Kevin continued working hard to reverse his existing disease, and he no longer has claudication (leg pain with walking).

On one subsequent visit, Kevin asked me why none of his other doctors had spotted this homocysteine problem. Many good physicians have missed the fact that homocysteine can be, and often is, more important than cholesterol. Luckily, we now understand its importance, which can help reduce your RealAge radically. I look at LDL cholesterol as petty crime, and homocysteine as grand larceny.

Folate supplementation may also help prevent cancer. Dr. Bruce Ames (the creator of the Ames Test for Cancer, the test most often used for predicting the potential of chemicals to produce cancer) believes that more that 50 percent of all congenital defects—not just spina bifida—and 50 percent of cancers might be caused by a shortage of folate. In DNA replication, if we don't have adequate levels of folate, B_6 and B_{12}, our bodies naturally substitute uracil for thymidine in the repair processes. Uracil is unnatural for your DNA. That substitution results in genetic mutations and cancer—all from want of adequate folate, B_6 and B_{12}. So there may be an extra bonus from taking these three B vitamins.

If a person has severe vascular disease or arterial aging disease, such as stroke, heart attack, peripheral vascular disease, or impotence; a strong family history of no known risk factors for arterial aging; and he or she is taking the right amount of folate, his or her homocysteine level should be tested at least once. Unless the person has a high level of homocysteine while he or she is taking the right amount of folate, B_6, and B_{12}, repeated measurements are probably not necessary. If the homocysteine level is above normal, then I would recommend repeated measurements. If B_6, B_{12}, and folate don't reduce the homocysteine levels into the normal range, then the person is one of a very rare group of people who may need another therapy. In that case, the repeated measurement of homocysteine levels would be important.

If your kidneys are not working properly, you should not only take folic acid supplements but also eat a low-protein diet. This will help you control homocysteine levels, which normally increase with a high-protein diet.

I believe all of us need to take folate, B_6 and B_{12} consistently for all our lives. Make sure you get adequate B_{12} (in supplements, 25 μg) and B_6 (4 mg) every day. Both of these vitamins lower homocysteine levels. The highest amounts of B_6 are found in beef, parsley, many fish (cod, catfish, crab, halibut, herring, mackerel, salmon, sardines, tuna), bananas, avocados, some fortified cereals, whole grains, eggs, chestnuts, peanuts, sunflower seeds, beans (garbanzos, limas, green beans, pinto beans, lentils), soybeans, spinach, potatoes, and green peppers. Most of us get the recommended amount of B_6 and B_{12} from diet and multivitamins; vegetarians may need to take supplements. As we age, we often have more difficulty absorbing B_{12} from food. Absorption of B_{12} in food requires a substance from our stomachs called intrinsic factor, the production of which decreases with age. However, the B_{12} in multivitamins does not need intrinsic factor for absorption.

Table 10.3	The RealAge Effect of Folate

FOR MEN:

Daily Intake of Folate (μg)

CALENDAR AGE	Less than 280	281 to 400	401 to 699	700 to 799	More than 800
			REALAGE		
35	35.7	35.1	35.0	34.3	34.2
55	56.0	55.2	55.0	54.2	54.1
70	72.2	70.2	70.0	69.1	69.0

FOR WOMEN:

Daily Intake of Folate (μg)

CALENDAR AGE	Less than 280	281 to 400	401 to 699	700 to 799	More than 800
			REALAGE		
35	36.2	35.0	35.0	34.6	34.5
55	56.0	55.1	55.0	54.5	54.3
70	72.2	70.2	70.0	69.0	68.9

μg is the abbreviation for micrograms

Tables 10.3, 10.4, and 10.5 show the effect of various levels of folate, vitamin B_6 and vitamin B_{12} intake, respectively, on your RealAge.

Another Wonderful Combination: Vitamin D and Calcium

We often forget that our bones are living tissues that need proper care. They undergo constant remaking and remodeling. Just as we can make our arterial and immune systems younger, we can make our bones younger as well: Doing so protects us for the long term, reducing our overall RealAge. How do we make our bones younger? By making them stronger.

Just imagine your skeleton as the structure of a house. Your bones are the wooden beams that buttress your body. In a house, you have to worry about

| Table 10.4 | The RealAge Effect of Vitamin B_6 | | | | |

FOR MEN:

Daily Intake of Vitamin B_6 (mg)

	Less than 1.2	1.2 to 1.5	1.51 to 2.2	2.21 to 3.7	More than 3.7
CALENDAR AGE			REALAGE		
35	35.3	35.1	35.0	34.9	34.9
55	55.6	55.2	55.0	54.9	54.9
70	70.7	70.2	70.0	69.9	69.8

FOR WOMEN:

Daily Intake of Vitamin B_6 (mg)

	Less than 1.2	1.2 to 1.5	1.51 to 2.2	2.21 to 3.7	More than 3.7
CALENDAR AGE			REALAGE		
35	35.3	35.0	35.0	34.9	34.9
55	55.6	55.1	55.0	54.9	54.9
70	70.8	70.2	70.0	69.9	69.8

mg is the abbreviation for milligrams

termites: they hollow out beams from within until the beams become so weak they collapse. As your body depletes the calcium stored in your bones, they also become weaker and weaker, until finally, like termite-eaten beams, they are almost hollow. Then you fall or move in a way that stresses the bone, and *snap*. They break. And a broken bone, especially a broken hip, is one of the things that can age you the fastest. Just six months of immobility can reverse all of your RealAge progress by a third or more. Every day you go without activity, you get older.

Bone weakening (osteopenia) and its more severe form, osteoporosis, affect more than 25 million Americans. It is the major underlying cause of hip fractures and bone breaks in the elderly. Approximately 1.35 million bone fractures, including 300,000 hip fractures and 700,000 fractures of the vertebrae of the spine are caused annually by osteoporosis-weakened bones coupled with a fall or movement that stresses the weakened bone. Although osteoporosis

Table 10.5	The RealAge Effect of Vitamin B$_{12}$				

FOR MEN:

Daily Dietary Intake of Vitamin B$_{12}$ (μg)*

	Less than 280	281 to 400	401 to 699	700 to 799	More than 800
CALENDAR AGE			REALAGE		
35	35.3	35.0	35.0	34.9	34.8
55	55.5	55.1	55.0	54.8	54.7
70	70.7	70.1	70.0	69.7	69.6

FOR WOMEN:

Daily Dietary Intake of Vitamin B$_{12}$ (μg)*

	Less than 280	281 to 400	401 to 699	700 to 799	More than 800
CALENDAR AGE			REALAGE		
35	35.3	35.0	35.0	34.9	34.8
55	55.5	55.1	55.0	54.8	54.7
70	70.8	70.2	70.0	69.7	69.6

μg is the abbreviation for micrograms
*See text for nondietary (supplement) requirements for B$_{12}$.

affects women disproportionately, especially small-boned women of northern European or Asian descent, we are all at risk.

Hip fractures are astoundingly common. Thirty to 40 percent of women over age sixty-five have fractured their spine or vertebrae, and 25 percent of these women will suffer a fractured hip. Doing what you can to prevent a fracture is one of your best protections against aging. Remember, it's not just women who are at risk, either. Men traditionally have been much less susceptible to bone fractures than women. Just 15 to 20 percent of men over age sixty-five have these kinds of debilitating fractures. Because historically, men have not lived as long as women, we know less about bone strength in men as they age. It appears that men also suffer bone loss as they get older, although they start out with higher bone density than women. As we see more men living longer, bone loss and severe fractures have become an increasing problem for them, too.

Why is breaking a hip so bad? It's not the fracture itself that ages a person, but rather the complications that stem from such an injury. A hip fracture may be the beginning of a downward spiral, triggering a chain of aging events. When a person is bedridden, the immune system becomes more vulnerable, and the body weakens, becoming susceptible to pneumonia and other infections that can often be fatal or leave severe lung or kidney problems that disrupt your quality of life. With less exercise and movement, arteries start showing signs of aging, becoming less elastic and more prone to disease or failure. For older people, the mortality rate from hip fractures is as high as 40 percent (12 to 20 percent of older women and 40 percent of elderly men who have had hip fractures die within six months). Furthermore, 40 percent of those who survive that initial six months will require long-term nursing care. More than half will never regain their former quality of life.

Victor P. used to be a vigorous sixty-eight-year-old man who avoided the sun. He didn't do any weight-lifting exercise, but he did play tennis periodically. He should have taken calcium and vitamin D, but didn't. He had tried taking calcium and vitamin D, but that had made him constipated. Then, one day, he fell while stretching for a volley at the tennis net. He couldn't get up because of the pain in his hip. He was taken by ambulance to the local orthopedist. Victor received a hip replacement.

Within three weeks, the site of the hip replacement had become infected, and he was admitted to the hospital again. After three weeks of high-dose antibiotics and all the immobilization and discomfort that ruined the quality of his life, he had to have his hip replacement removed and the hip joint irrigated with antibiotics for two weeks. The antibiotic caused kidney insufficiency and then kidney failure. Eventually his renal function improved to the point where he could come off dialysis and undergo another hip replacement. However, he never regained his enjoyment of life or his prowess on the tennis court, to the same degree. All because he didn't take calcium and vitamins and didn't lift weights. Pretty severe penalty for just avoiding constipation, a side effect that could have been taken care of with a little magnesium and a little prune juice.

Calcium

Your body stores excess calcium until you reach your early thirties, when you reach your peak level of bone density. After that, your body stops storing extra calcium. You must then get all the calcium you need from your daily diet, or you will begin to deplete the calcium stores in your bones. As you age, your bones lose calcium, becoming progressively weaker.

If you're working to make yourself younger, you should make sure that your bones stay young, too. For the best RealAge advantage, men and women should make sure to get enough calcium: 1,000 to 1,200 mg a day for men and 1,200 mg for most women over thirty (pregnancy and other conditions may change requirements slightly). Take 500 or 600 mg twice a day. (This refers to the amount of actual calcium, not calcium in combination as citrate or carbonate. If the label reads 1,000 mg of calcium citrate, read on to find the amount of calcium by itself.) Any kind of calcium supplement, even over-the-counter antacid tablets, should fit the bill, just as long as you are getting the right number of milligrams.

What about coral calcium? What about calcium carbonate versus calcium citrate? Some people favor coral calcium, because a study showed that calcium absorption was 17.5 percent better with coral calcium than with calcium carbonate. But why pay three times as much for just this small difference in absorption? Why not just take 200 mg more a day? You'll get the same amount in your body. That extra 200 mg may cost you perhaps a dime more, whereas the coral calcium would cost you something like a dollar extra a day.

I advise against taking calcium supplements that contain bone meal, dolomite, and/or oyster shells, as these can contain lead or other heavy metals that may be toxic. Calcium carbonate is best absorbed when taken with food. Calcium citrate may be taken at any time (by itself or with food). Both forms can cause constipation. If this occurs, eat more fruits, whole grain cereals, and vegetables, or rely on that old standby, a prune a day. I recommend taking about 400 mg of magnesium in conjunction with calcium (see the section on magnesium later in this chapter).

Although calcium is plentiful in dairy foods (milk, cheese, and yogurt), most people do not eat enough of them to get adequate amounts of calcium from diet alone. Also, while most dairy products have added vitamin D, they do not contain the magnesium that you need. (Each glass of milk contains 25 to 30 milligrams of magnesium, so you would need to drink ten to twelve glasses of milk a day to obtain enough magnesium.)

Eat dairy foods for extra calcium, but do not rely on them as your only source of calcium unless you eat and drink a lot of dairy products (and, of course, remember to eat low-fat versions). If you consistently drink three or four glasses of milk a day, you can modify the amount you take in supplemental form accordingly. However, most adults do not drink anywhere near that amount. Of the five million or so people who have taken the full nutrition program on the RealAge website, fewer than fifty thousand (1 percent) drink four glasses of milk a day or get enough calcium and vitamin D from their diet alone.

You must be very careful to make the 1,000- or 1,200-milligram marker daily. Here's a reminder to anyone under thirty, or even thirty-five: you need lots of calcium to build bone strength for the future, because the calcium the body stores in bone until about the mid-thirties then becomes the surplus stores for the rest of your life.

Not only does calcium help your bones, it may also help to lower blood pressure. Three recent studies show that men taking 1,000 milligrams or more of calcium a day had a 12 percent or greater reduction in blood pressure. This evidence remains controversial, as some studies have reported no such decrease in blood pressure; however, they were less well controlled. Although the data are still not complete on this topic, blood pressure reduction may be just one added benefit of taking calcium, which you should be doing anyway. Another side note for people with high blood pressure: a common treatment for high blood pressure is the administration of calcium channel–blocking drugs. But these drugs have nothing to do with calcium supplements, so don't be concerned. Go ahead and take calcium supplements.

Vitamin D

Sometimes you can't imagine one without the other. Bonnie and Clyde, Abbott and Costello, Charlie Brown and Snoopy. The same is true for calcium and its vital partner, vitamin D.

Vitamin D is essential for proper absorption of calcium. Vitamin D helps strengthen bones and prevents the joint deterioration that accompanies arthritis. Vitamin D and its metabolites also appear beneficial in reducing certain kinds of breast, colon, prostate, and lung cancers.

Production of vitamin D is a three-stage process. In the first stage, the body takes in food that contains a kind of cholesterol which is a precursor to vitamin D. Our bodies cannot use this form of the vitamin without converting it to another form. (Only a few foods, such as cod liver oil and certain fatty fishes—tuna, salmon, sardines, oysters, mackerel, and herring—naturally contain vitamin D in the form that can be used by the body.)

For the second stage of the conversion, we need sun. The energy of the sun's radiation is necessary to create the right chemical reaction that turns the precursor cholesterols into the form of vitamin D the body can use.

In the final stage of the process, the liver and kidneys convert that vitamin D into yet another form of the vitamin: vitamin D_3, the active form of the vitamin that our bodies can use. As mentioned in the section on sun exposure (see Chapter 5), you need just 10 to 20 minutes of sunlight a day to ensure that your body is producing enough vitamin D. Most of us do not get enough sun, especially in northern climates. In Boston, Chicago, and Seattle, for example, it is almost impossible for the body to produce the necessary levels of vitamin D from sunlight alone during the months of October through March, because the energy of the sun is not sufficient.

After we reach our seventies, the precursor to vitamin D generally found in skin diminishes three- or four-fold, making it increasingly difficult for us to produce vitamin D naturally, with sun exposure. The second and less risky way of getting enough vitamin D is through food and supplements. Some foods, mainly fish and shellfish, contain vitamin D naturally. Such foods as milk (the major source of vitamin D in food) and most breakfast cereals contain vitamin D as an additive. These additions, which help prevent rickets (a vitamin D deficiency disease), are synthetic.

Vitamin D appears to work to decrease immune aging and cancer by strengthening the functioning of your proofreader gene. Whether or not this works the ways the theories propose, the ability of vitamin D to decrease the risk of cancer is consistent in both epidemiologic and test-tube studies. The first theory is that the D_3 form of the vitamin kills cell mutations. Somehow, vitamin D is directly toxic to potentially cancerous cells. The second theory, supported by more data, is that adequate levels of vitamin D are necessary for proofreader genes to spot cancerous cells and cause them to die.

As noted in Chapter 5, the proofreader gene recognizes mutated DNA and cells. Vitamin D_3 is an essential component used in this attempt by the body to rid itself of the cells. Vitamin D_3 helps make protein for the functioning of the P53 gene, which is one of the body's main proofreader genes and cancer watchdogs. This gene helps prevent cancer by regulating protein production of specific oncogenes—genes that, when mutated, can cause cancers. Indeed, vitamin D not only helps in the proper functioning of the gene, but also appears to actually help safeguard the P53 gene itself from damage. Although studies still need to be done to confirm the link between vitamin D and cancer prevention, it is very possible that vitamin D does double duty by helping prevent aging of both the musculoskeletal and immune systems. When I think of vitamin D, I think of "defense." Vitamin D helps your body defend itself.

Vitamin D may also help protect the body from the onset and aging effects of arthritis, although the data on this are still somewhat speculative. Osteoarthritis is a disease that afflicts more than 10 percent of people sixty-five and older, and 95 percent of people eighty-five and older. It is painful, disabling, and aging. Recent studies have shown that taking calcium, vitamin C, and particularly vitamin D can retard the progression of arthritis, and perhaps even prevent its progression. These studies found that people who had high levels of vitamin D in their bodies had less joint deterioration and fewer of the painful bone spurs and growths that can accompany arthritis as it worsens. Arthritis patients with low levels of calcium and vitamins C and D were reported to be three times more likely to undergo rapid progression of the disease than those who had high levels of these nutrients. Arthritis caused them to age faster.

Most American adults do not get enough vitamin D. Estimates are that 30 to 40 percent of adults are deficient in vitamin D. In three studies of elderly people who live north of Raleigh–Durham, North Carolina, by the end of April as many as 65, 87, and 89 percent were deficient in vitamin D. Thus, their proofreader genes could not function appropriately, putting them at risk of cancer. To repeat an important point: You get vitamin D from three and only three sources: the sun, food, and supplements.

How much vitamin D do you need to get the maximum antiaging protection? The RDA of 55 IU only prevents the deficiency disease, rickets. I recommend at least 400 IU a day in a supplement if you are seventy or younger, and 600 IU a day if you are older than sixty, unless you are absolutely sure you are getting enough from your diet. This is what I consider the RAO. For 400 IU that means four glasses of nonfat milk a day. Vitamin D overdoses are exceedingly rare among adults. To develop toxic levels in your blood, you would have to consume more than 2,000 IU a day for more than six months. In one study, elderly patients were given 100,000 IU as one injection every four months, the equivalent of 800 IU a day. These individuals did not develop kidney stones or other scientific evidence of toxicity, and did have adequate levels of vitamin D for the entire four-month period.

In addition to a supplement, I recommend getting some sunlight. Ten to twenty minutes a day outside without sunscreen should provide sufficient vitamin D protection, although the farther north you live, the less likely you can produce all the D you need this way. If you are going to be in the sun for more than twenty minutes, put on a sunscreen. Note that an SPF 8 sunscreen reduces your vitamin D production by 95 percent, and SPF 30 cuts it to zero. The risk of skin cancer from a little bit of sunlight is probably less than the benefit you gain from having healthy vitamin D levels, especially the older you are. Finally, if you are worried about vitamin D deficiency, you can ask your doctor to test your blood levels. A test will quickly determine whether you are getting enough vitamin D.

Table 10.6 shows the effects of various levels of vitamin D intake on your RealAge.

Table 10.6	The RealAge Effect of Vitamin D

FOR MEN:

Daily Intake of Vitamin D (IU)

| Under age 60 | Less than 55 | 55 to 150 | 151 to 299 | 300 to 400 | More than 400 |
| Age 60 and older | Less than 55 | 55 to 250 | 251 to 399 | 400 to 600 | More than 600 |

CALENDAR AGE		REALAGE			
35	35.6	35.0	35.0	34.8	34.7
55	55.7	55.2	55.0	54.7	54.5
70	71.1	70.2	70.0	69.3	69.2

FOR WOMEN:

Daily Intake of Vitamin D (IU)

| Under age 60 | Less than 55 | 55 to 150 | 151 to 299 | 300 to 400 | More than 400 |
| Age 60 and older | Less than 55 | 55 to 250 | 251 to 399 | 400 to 600 | More than 600 |

CALENDAR AGE		REALAGE			
35	35.7	35.1	35.0	34.8	34.6
55	55.8	55.2	55.0	54.6	54.4
70	71.2	70.2	70.0	69.1	68.7

IU is the abbreviation for international units

Beyond the Basics: Minerals, Eye Vitamins, Herbs, and Miscellaneous Supplements

We have reviewed the four basic vitamins—E, C, D, and folate—and one mineral—calcium—that I recommend you get each day to retard aging. What about the panoply of others? What else do you need? First let us review the other minerals your body needs to function. Then we'll consider a few of the more popular herbal remedies.

Minerals

Besides calcium, a number of other minerals are found in our bodies, all of which are necessary for basic metabolic function. Like calcium, magnesium, potassium, sodium, chloride, sulfur, and phosphorus are needed in relatively large quantities. Usually our food provides sufficient quantities of all these minerals. In the case of sodium, we may get far more than we need; people with salt-sensitive high blood pressure, arterial disease, and excess weight gain often need to reduce their sodium intake. Minerals we need in trace amounts include chromium, copper, cobalt, iodine, iron, fluoride, manganese, molybdenum, selenium, and zinc. Our bodies demand these in much smaller amounts, and we generally get them from our diet. Although silicon, vanadium, nickel, lithium, cadmium, and boron are other trace minerals we seem to need, science knows much less about these. If you are eating a well-balanced diet, you can make sure you're getting enough of all of these minerals by taking a multivitamin at least once a week. (I really believe everyone should take a multivitamin of appropriate makeup twice a day, but in no case (unless your doctor tells you not to) should you take one less than at least once a week.) Do not take extra mineral supplements.

Why not? Minerals are insoluble elements (they don't dissolve) that come from the earth's crust. Many of them are heavy metals (dense metals), which can be toxic in excess amounts. With minerals, we want to make sure to get enough without overloading. Extra minerals can build up in the body. Iron is a perfect example.

IRON

Unless you have been diagnosed as having an iron deficiency, you're almost certain to be getting enough iron. Iron deficiency is a condition seen almost exclusively in premenopausal women, growing children, people who have ulcers or cancers that cause bleeding into their gastrointestinal tract and subsequent tarry black stool, trauma victims, postsurgical patients, and occasionally vegetarians. Men and postmenopausal women are at the lowest risk of iron deficiency, and most of us—no matter who we are—get plenty of iron from meats, fortified breakfast cereals, breads, and pastas. In fact, the United States has been criticized for adding too much iron to such foods as breakfast cereals. The critics aren't all wrong: the consequences of taking too much iron can be grave. Iron overload can be life-threatening and, not surprisingly, may make your RealAge older.

Perhaps this news sounds surprising. After all, most of us were raised with cartoon images of Popeye gulping down spinach to revitalize his strength. We all thought we needed our iron. Don't get me wrong, spinach is good. However, needless iron in supplements ages us. Avoid iron unless it is prescribed for you by a physician. And when you do take iron, take it separately from your calcium and your vitamin C as iron decreases the absorption of these, and vice versa.

When Jason P., a twenty-four-year-old body builder, came to see me he should have been at the peak of health. Instead, he was near death. A few months earlier he had looked like a twenty-four-year-old Arnold Schwarzenegger. Now he felt and acted like he was over eighty. He had congestive heart failure, which is unusual for someone so young. A few more months of decline and he would have needed a heart transplant. He had once been able to bench press three hundred fifty pounds, but by the time I saw him he could barely get out of a chair. His progression from a young man to an old one in just a few months was a mystery. Luckily, the histories of other patients had convinced me of the need to ask all of my patients about their use of vitamins and supplements. I learned that Jason was taking 10 grams of iron a day. He thought it would build muscle, but it was killing him. Fortunately, the treatment to remove the excess iron that had built up in his body worked, and he recovered completely, his heart intact.

Although this extreme degree of iron overload is relatively rare, Jason's story proves an important point. Iron stays in the body for a long time and, when present in large amounts, can be toxic. The body rids itself of iron primarily through bleeding, which is why menstruating women sometimes suffer from anemia, or iron deficiency. Early symptoms of iron overload include abdominal pain, fatigue, and loss of sex drive. Later symptoms include enlargement of the liver, diabetes, arthritis, and shrinking of the testicles. In severe cases such as Jason's, abnormal heart beat and even heart failure can occur. (Since I wrote about this in the first book, no patients have called or seen me about possible iron overload. Since patients come to see me or e-mail me about every other subject discussed in this book, iron overload may be less common than the medical literature would have us believe.)

Hemochromatosis (chronic iron overload) is thought to be a fairly common affliction, and as many as one in two hundred fifty people has a genetic predisposition to this condition, making hemochromatosis one of the most frequently occurring inherited genetic disorders. Even people who don't carry the gene can develop the disorder, which damages key organs such as the liver and heart, and causes needless aging.

Even slightly excessive levels of iron in the body can be damaging. Studies link elevated iron levels with increased rates of cardiovascular disease and cancers. Although in both cases the evidence is somewhat preliminary, and we still need to do more studies to prove the links, taking extra iron is not worth the risk. In RealAge terms, it can increase your aging.

There are two possible ways that even low levels of iron toxicity can age us. First, iron appears to contribute to arterial aging. No one knows exactly how, but the theory is that because iron is an oxidant, it increases the oxidation of LDL cholesterol. When LDL cholesterol is oxidized, it is more likely to be incorporated into plaque, causing atherosclerosis. Some scientists have speculated that one of the reasons menstruating women have lower rates of cardiovascular disease is that they have lower levels of iron in their blood. One Finnish study showed that the rate of heart attacks doubled when the concentration of iron in the blood exceeded 220 mg/dl (milligrams per deciliter of blood). This risk was four times higher for patients who had both high iron levels and an LDL cholesterol reading of 190 mg/dl or higher. Other studies have been unable to confirm this link, and the connection has been strongly contested.

Elevated iron levels have also been linked to cancers. The data remain preliminary, and we still don't completely understand the relationship, but two major theories suggest why this may be the case. First, as noted above, iron is an oxidant. In contrast to antioxidants such as vitamins C and E that remove free radicals from the body, iron enhances the production of free radicals, which in turn seems to be linked to increased levels of cancer. Second, cancer cells appear to demand more iron than other cells. When cancers do develop, the increased iron in the body may fuel them to grow at a faster rate. Although neither theory has been proved, studies in the United States and Finland have shown an increased risk of cancer for people with elevated levels of iron.

If you are not iron-deficient, make sure your multivitamin does not contain iron. Eat normally. Only take iron if anemia is a chronic problem and you are specifically directed to do so by a doctor. If you are a vegetarian, be sure to have your red blood cell count checked annually to ensure that you are not iron-deficient. If you are a vegetarian and are eating a balanced diet, you are probably getting enough iron from other sources. If you are a woman and still menstruating, have your iron levels checked before you decide to take iron.

CHROMIUM

Chromium, a mineral involved in glucose metabolism, is important for the synthesis of cholesterol, fats, and protein. Health-food gurus advocate chromium, usually in the form of chromium picolinate, for everything from weight loss, to cholesterol reduction, to alleviation of depression, to treatment of hypoglycemia and diabetes. Chromium has also been said to prevent osteoporosis, to build muscle, and to promote longevity. In light of these claims, should you take chromium as a supplement?

Chromium is certainly a necessary mineral, but we generally get enough from our diet to provide for our needs. Chromium is found in many whole grains, meats, dairy products, and even beer! Clearly, having proper levels of chromium in your body is necessary to metabolize blood sugar, and most of the benefits associated with chromium are tied to proper glucose metabolism. Doctors sometimes advise people with type II diabetes to take chromium to boost insulin tolerance. However, even if you have diabetes, you should not take chromium or any drug without first consulting your doctor.

Most of the longevity claims for chromium come from animal studies, and are tied to the fact that a low body mass index increases life span. Several studies in the 1980s glorified chromium as a wonder nutrient, but the results have largely been disproved. It is still unclear whether chromium supplementation promotes safe weight loss, and some studies indicate that it may even cause weight gain. Indeed, one study links the intake of chromium picolinate with weight gain among already-overweight women. As for other claims, studies show little evidence that chromium adds muscle mass. Because I believe in that germ of truth in all folk wisdom, I think there is probably something valuable about chromium. We just have to find out what it is.

We don't know exactly how much chromium a person can take without a negative effect. Too much chromium can cause heart palpitations, high blood pressure, and even psychosis. Animal studies have shown that chromium can cause chromosomal damage and so may pose a risk of cancer as well. I recommend eating a balanced diet and taking a multivitamin as a backup, that should provide all the chromium you need.

SELENIUM

Selenium is one of the trace minerals needed by our bodies. We get selenium largely from plant foods such as garlic, that absorb selenium from the soil they grow in. The soil in different regions of the country varies considerably in selenium content.

A 1998 study published in the *Journal of the American Medical Association* reported a 50 percent reduction in cancer deaths among cancer patients who took 100 μg of selenium twice a day. Other research suggests selenium may have an immune effect as well, boosting resistance to certain viruses. These findings are still very preliminary and have been much criticized by some cancer researchers. But shortly after 1999, the National Institutes of Health started funding at least five studies on this potential benefit of selenium. We expected to know considerably more by now. Unfortunately, those studies haven't been completed. Of the five primary medical advisors on the RealAge team, three thought the data sufficiently convincing to start taking selenium themselves. The other two are waiting for more information.

Although we may find that selenium has important antiaging properties, it is a trace mineral that is not easily excreted by the body. It can build up to toxic levels, causing needless aging. The current recommended daily allowances for selenium are 70 μg a day for men and 55 μg a day for women. I recommend that you get at most 200 μg a day as a supplement. That way, you probably won't overdo it. Most Americans eating a balanced diet should not worry about a deficiency, as selenium is plentiful in many foods: garlic, whole grains, cereals, meats, and some seafood. Because garlic in particular has been well documented as providing numerous health benefits, I recommend getting selenium by loading your meals with lots of garlic.

POTASSIUM

Strokes are the major cause of cognitive aging (aging of the brain). Thankfully, strokes can largely be prevented. One easy thing you can do is increase your intake of potassium. Four major studies have shown that increased potassium intake is linked to a decrease in the incidence of strokes and other kinds of arterial aging as well. (Three studies have also shown decreased rates of heart attacks and peripheral vascular disease.) It's pretty clear that potassium prevents aging of the arteries.

If you already eat a diet rich in fruits and vegetables, adding the potassium equivalent of three bananas a day to that diet can make your Real Age as much as 0.6 year younger in just three years (see Table 10.7).

What makes potassium so important? Potassium is an electrolyte: an electrically charged particle needed by the body for proper cellular functioning. Every time a nerve impulse is conducted or a muscle is contracted, potassium— because it carries an electrical charge—has made that reflex possible. Potassium, in conjunction with other minerals, regulates blood pressure and allows the heart and kidneys to function properly.

In human clinical trials, the Rancho Bernardo study found that people who ate comparatively little potassium had 2.6 to 4.8 times the risk of stroke as those who ate considerably more. Of the 287 people who had high potassium intake, no one had a stroke during the study. Among the 572 people with lower potassium intake, 24 had strokes. Possible explanations? Three studies found that increased dietary potassium intake decreased blood pressure, thus decreasing the rate of arterial aging, which can cause both heart attacks and strokes. That, however, could not have been the whole story, as the decrease in blood pressure

Table 10.7	The RealAge Effect of Potassium

FOR MEN:

Daily Intake of Potassium (mg)

CALENDAR AGE	Less than 1,600	1,600 to 1,800	1,801 to 2,400	2,401 to 3,000	More than 3,000
			REALAGE		
35	35.2	35.1	35.0	34.9	34.8
55	55.6	55.1	55.0	54.8	54.4
70	70.8	70.2	70.0	69.7	69.2

FOR WOMEN:

Daily Intake of Potassium (mg)

CALENDAR AGE	Less than 1,600	1,600 to 1,800	1,801 to 2,400	2,401 to 3,000	More than 3,000
			REALAGE		
35	35.1	35.0	35.0	34.9	34.9
55	55.5	55.1	55.0	54.8	54.5
70	70.7	70.2	70.0	69.7	69.3

mg is the abbreviation for milligrams

does not account for the entire RealAge benefit. Other biological mechanisms that may account for the RealAge effect include stabilization of arterial plaques, decreased oxidation of lipids, and stabilization of nerve cells when they get inadequate oxygen.

There is no RDA standard for potassium, but nutritionists recommend you consume about 3,000 mg a day. If you eat a balanced diet, you will probably get a little more than half of that in normal consumption. Bananas and avocados are, ounce for ounce, the richest sources of potassium. One banana contains about 467 mg of potassium, and both Florida and California avocados contain over 1,000 mg of potassium. Although avocados are highly caloric because of their high fat content, they are rich in monounsaturated fat, the kind of fat that's good for you (see Chapter 8). Potatoes, citrus fruits, tomatoes, spinach, celery, cantaloupes, and honeydew melons are also excellent sources of potassium, having

400 to 500 mg a serving. Even though they are relatively high in calories, dried apricots and peaches provide over 1,500 mg of potassium per cup. Dairy products, lean meats, and fish (tuna, mackerel, and halibut) contain over 500 mg per serving. Sardines are extremely rich in potassium, with over 1,000 mg per serving. Skim milk and low-fat yogurt are excellent sources of potassium (400 mg per serving). To get the RealAge benefit of potassium, try to eat plenty of fruits and vegetables rich in potassium. By doing so, your total intake would be about 3,000 mg a day.

Under no circumstances should you take potassium supplements, unless advised to do so by your doctor, as overdosing (taking much more than 3,000 milligrams a day) can be a problem. Although most of us do not consume the optimal amount of potassium, actual potassium deficiencies are truly rare, except in people with very specific medical conditions. Because certain medications may deplete potassium supplies, supplements may be advised, but they should be taken only under strict medical supervision. Remember, too, that increasing potassium intake can actually cause aging in people who have kidney disease or are taking certain medications. So talk to your doctor before increasing your potassium intake. For most, however, increasing potassium intake through diet is a quick, easy way to make your RealAge 0.6 year younger and to decrease your risk of stroke and the associated cognitive aging it can cause.

SODIUM

Although sodium is vital for the proper functioning of your body, you don't need to worry about getting enough sodium. In fact, most Americans consume far more than they need. The minimum needed for good health is 116 mg a day, and the average American gets more than 4,000 mg a day.

When we hear "sodium," we think of table salt (sodium chloride). Actually, table salt is only 40 percent sodium. Sodium comes in many other forms. Approximately 75 percent of the sodium you consume comes from processed foods, not the salt shaker.

Numerous studies have found that high consumption of sodium is associated with higher blood pressure in some, and perhaps all, people. The most famous was the INTERSALT study, which evaluated sodium consumption in more than 10,000 people in fifty-two study centers in thirty-two countries. Sodium intake correlated with an increase in blood pressure, and, correspondingly, high blood pressure correlated with an accelerated rate of arterial aging. Indeed, the first correlation between sodium intake and high blood pressure was made by Ambard and Beaujard in 1904. As a result, early in the last century, and for many years, low-sodium diets were frequently prescribed as a way to successfully lower blood pressure. However, the development of blood pressure medications encouraged many doctors to move away from prescribing low-sodium diets, except for the rare patient who was sodium-sensitive.

Newer data suggest that perhaps all of us age faster when salt consumption is excessive. Even so, the theory of sodium-sensitivity is problematic. A chief drawback is that no one knows who is sodium-sensitive until after high blood pressure develops, and by then significant aging has already begun. Many people's sensitivity to sodium changes with age, as their metabolism undergoes other changes as well. The best action is to cut back on sodium intake. Salt restriction, exercise, and weight control form the triad of behavioral changes that can best help you reduce the likelihood of high blood pressure and subsequent arterial aging.

Although the average American consumes about 4,000 mg of sodium a day, most reputable medical associations, including the U.S. Surgeon General's Office, the National Institutes of Health, the National Academy of Science's Research Council, and countless experts in the field, suggest that sodium intake should not exceed 2,400 mg (about a teaspoon of salt) a day. I go further and suggest that for the maximum Age-Reduction benefit, you try to keep sodium consumption to less than 1,600 mg a day. A fifty-five-year-old man who has consistently consumed only 1,600 mg of sodium a day is as much as 2.8 years younger than his counterpart who has put no limit on sodium intake.

How can you reduce sodium intake? The easiest way is to decrease consumption of processed and prepackaged foods, as a lot of sodium is used to preserve these products. Most fast foods are also high in sodium. By contrast, fresh fruits and vegetables and fresh meats and poultry contain very little sodium. If these foods make up most of your diet, you will already have significantly reduced your sodium consumption. When you do buy packaged or canned foods, read the labels. Foods you would never describe as salty can have an astounding amount of sodium. Processed cheese, preserved meats, many condiments, and some shellfish are very high in sodium, so beware. Often similar products will have surprisingly different sodium levels; many companies now offer "no-sodium" and "low-sodium" variants of their products. Even though you should also cut back on table salt, remember, it is the hidden salt in processed foods that accounts for most of your sodium consumption.

Although sodium deficiencies are virtually unheard of, strenuous exercise on a hot day can lower salt concentrations in the body, a condition that can trigger other complications that age the body. When exercising, drink plenty of water to keep yourself properly hydrated.

MAGNESIUM

Magnesium is a mineral essential for energy metabolism. Muscle contractions, nerve impulses, and even the most basic processes of cellular energy storage require magnesium.

It has been known for some time that heart attacks are less common in areas where the water supplies are rich in magnesium. Magnesium is also known to lower blood pressure, dilate the arteries, and when given after a heart attack, restore normal heart rhythms. Magnesium is especially important in the regulation of calcium. Because we do know that taking calcium helps reduce RealAge, it is also vital to get enough magnesium to allow for the proper absorption of calcium.

A ten-year study on four hundred individuals at high risk of coronary disease found that those who ate a magnesium-rich diet had less than half as many complications from cardiovascular-related problems as those who ate only about one-third of the recommended amount of magnesium. Overall mortality rates for people who ate a magnesium-rich diet were lower as well. Although this ten-year investigation is the first in-depth study on magnesium, the results have been buttressed by several smaller studies. That means that eating a magnesium-rich diet makes your RealAge as much 0.9 year younger (see Table 10.8).

The suggested intake of magnesium is about one-third the intake of calcium, which means that women should get at least 400 mg of magnesium a day, and that men should get at least 333 mg a day. Current studies show that the average intake of Americans is less than 300 mg. People who need to be extra careful to get the right amounts of magnesium include women who are pregnant or lactating, people with kidney disease, diabetics, those on low-calorie diets, and those taking digitalis preparations and diuretics. All of these people should consult their physician before beginning any new regimen.

Magnesium is found largely in whole grain breads and cereals. Breads made with refined flours unfortunately have very little magnesium, as most of the mineral is lost during the refining process. Most fortified and whole grain cereals contain 100 to 200 mg per bowl. Soybeans and lima beans contain 100 mg per serving, and most nuts contain 100 to 300 mg per one-ounce serving. Fruits and vegetables such as avocados, bananas, beets, raisins, and dates are also good sources of magnesium.

Unfortunately, magnesium deficiency is increasingly common. Experts estimate that 40 percent of Americans are getting less than 70 percent of the RDA for magnesium. Life in the modern world seems to be especially hard on our magnesium levels: stress, sugar, alcohol, and the phosphates commonly found

Table 10.8	The RealAge Effect of Magnesium

FOR MEN:

Daily Intake of Magnesium (mg)			
Less than 161	161 to 266	267 to 333	More than 333

CALENDAR AGE	REALAGE			
35	35.7	35.1	35.0	34.3
55	56.0	55.2	55.0	54.1
70	71.1	70.2	70.0	69.0

FOR WOMEN:

Daily Intake of Magnesium (mg)			
Less than 171	171 to 293	293 to 400	More than 400

CALENDAR AGE	REALAGE			
35	35.6	35.1	35.0	34.4
55	55.9	55.2	55.0	54.2
70	71.1	70.2	70.0	69.0

mg is the abbreviation for milligrams

in soft drinks and processed foods all deplete our stores of magnesium. Even exercise, one of the most important factors in preventing aging, can cause magnesium deficiency, because we lose magnesium when we sweat. Moreover, magnesium deficiency often provides no symptoms. The first sign that something is wrong can be a heart attack caused by an abnormal heart rhythm.

When you choose your daily vitamin supplements, obtain an amount of magnesium that is about one-third the milligram amount of calcium you take. If you worry that you are not getting enough magnesium, consider supplementing your diet with 250 to 300 mg daily. As with all Age-Reduction behaviors or plans you adopt, check with your physician first, as those who have kidney problems can accumulate too much magnesium and have serious side effects.

ZINC

Zinc is linked to antioxidant activity and immune system response. Zinc is also vital to the synthesis of DNA and RNA (ribonucleic acid), and is therefore important for cell division. Several zinc trials in infertile couples have improved deficient sperm count and sperm function. In fact, increasing zinc levels to a normal level increased the pregnancy rate in those studies. Zinc is most commonly found in animal products but is also found in nuts, legumes, and fortified cereals. Shellfish contain high quantities of zinc. Unless you are a vegetarian or are on a restricted diet, you probably get enough zinc from food.

Zinc deficiencies are rare. As with most trace minerals, I do not recommend you take supplements beyond your multivitamin, and then make sure yours does not have more than 15 mg. Although zinc deficiencies may cause various problems, boosting zinc beyond basic levels appears to do no good and may even cause harm. For example, too much zinc may interfere with the workings of another needed trace mineral, copper. As with most minerals, high intake may prove toxic, and too much zinc can damage the immune system. Take no more than 30 mg daily. (If you take 6 of the zinc cough drops—the recommended maximum per day—that's 80 mg, so you see why I believe in chicken soup, which has an equivalent effect for my patients.) The RDA is just 15 mg for men and just 12 mg for women; the 2003 nutrition panel of the FDA recommended that the daily recommended value of zinc be decreased to 6 mg. More than that can be harmful. For example, taking just 50 to 75 mg a day can actually reduce your healthy (HDL) cholesterol, which is something you want to avoid.

Recently, zinc has received a lot of attention for its role in fighting colds. Two studies found that zinc lozenges may help ease cold symptoms; another two showed it did not. The effect is about the same as having a bowl of chicken soup every day, and the soup seems less risky to me.

Herbs and Miscellaneous Supplements

I have talked about vitamins and minerals, but what about all those other bottles you see on the shelves of any health-food store? As little as we know about minerals, we know even less about most herbal remedies and food supplements. Drawn from various folk treatments, as well as from traditional Eastern medicine, herbs no doubt can provide some benefits. As you will read in the story about ginseng below, I strongly believe there is a germ of truth in folk wisdom, such as "Chicken soup reduces colds." In fact, the trials involving chicken soup show that chicken soup does reduce the severity and duration of colds to the

Eye Vitamins: Preventing Loss of Sight

I recently received an e-mail from a woman who was interested in preventing macular degeneration and glaucoma for herself; her husband already had glaucoma. She wanted to know if I could recommend any vitamin or mineral products.

I told her the following: a number of epidemiologic studies have indicated that high doses of vitamin C, vitamin E, beta-carotene, zinc, and copper were associated with less progression and less age-related degeneration of the macula (the central part of the retina). These findings were and are important, as four to ten million Americans have some form of age-related macular degeneration (AMD). Several large randomized trials have been started, and one in particular has generated some very important and interesting results. The Age-Related Eye Disease Study (AREDS) is sponsored by the National Eye Institute of the National Institutes of Health. In this study, 3,640 patients with AMD were studied for an average of 6.3 years. (This very large, important, and well-designed study is still in progress.)

Most people with AMD have the nonvascular ("dry") form, meaning there's no new, excess growth of blood vessels. Many of these patients keep most of their vision. Some AMD progresses to the neovascular ("wet") form, which is caused by uncontrollable growth of tiny blood vessels that leak fluid and can scar the macula. Ninety percent of people who suffer severe sight loss from AMD have this form of the disease. The AREDS study found that certain vitamins and minerals taken together provided a major benefit for preventing vision loss in patients with active disease (active AMD lesions). Those who had active AMD had a more than 25 percent reduction in the risk of vision loss if they took 500 mg of vitamin C, 400 IU of vitamin E, 15 mg of beta-carotene, 80 mg of zinc, and 2 mg of copper a day. Fifty percent also took an RDA multivitamin daily.

This benefit did not prevent AMD from starting, nor did it prevent cataracts. However, some of the pigment compounds (two of the carotenoids—lutein and zeaxanthin) in green vegetables (spinach and broccoli) and vitamin E by itself have been shown to reduce the risk of cataracts by 20 percent or more.

One benefit of the AREDS study was confirmation of the safety and lack of side effects of long-term use of these vitamins and minerals in nonsmokers (In other studies, zinc at this high a dose has some significant side effects, as does beta-carotene in smokers: namely, an increased risk of lung cancer.)

What do I recommend to the person who fears AMD but does not yet have it? Eat three green vegetables a day. If you can't, take lutein (40 μg) and zeaxanthin (400 μg) supplements every day. I would also take a twice-a-day multivitamin with vitamin

C (500 mg) and vitamin E (400 to 800 IU) a day, and with a low level of zinc (12 mg) and beta-carotene (about 3 mg). If I had AMD or a patient who had AMD at any stage, I would recommend all the vitamins as defined by the AREDS study but would be afraid of the zinc, copper, and beta-carotene in those larger doses taken for a long period of time.

same degree as increased vitamin C or zinc lozenges do. And, as you'll see in the story of ginseng, the DSHEA might have done us a disservice by not forcing an evaluation of what the germ of truth is in each of the herbal remedies, so that all of us could have remedies sooner.

More scientific studies are being done on such remedies each year. Most of the herbs do not cause harm, but some cause needless aging. For example, never take anything that contains comfrey. This herb is known to cause liver damage. Also, sassafras, chaparral, germander, and pokeroot have been linked to severe and even lethal effects. Since St. John's Wort alters the metabolism and effectiveness of over 50 medications, while useful for minor depressions, it should not be taken by anyone taking any other medication without checking with his or her doctor first. A large study of patients who had to be hospitalized due to such drug interactions with St. John's Wort has been published. In fact, several European countries have made St. John's Wort a prescription drug.

If you want to try some remedy that sounds interesting, find out about it first. Do not simply ask the clerk at the health-food store or rely on a book there. Do research at the local library or on the Internet. If you don't have access to the resources, ask your doctor or local librarian to find out more information for you. With the right search, you can find out about popular claims as well as the status of that herb in the scientific literature. Remember you can log on to *www. consumerlab.com* (for a fee) and find out how much of the actual ingredients on the label are in the product. Sometimes you may decide that you want to try an herb even though its claimed effects remain unproven. As long as your remedy causes no harm, go ahead. It might or might not prevent you from aging, but you want to make sure that it does not cause aging.

Here's my review of some of the more popular herbal remedies and food supplements. The list is almost endless, and is everchanging.

COENZYME Q10

Coenzyme Q10 has gained popularity recently for allegedly preventing cardiovascular aging. I believe that it does that, in specific situations. Found naturally in the body's organs, coenzyme Q10 helps stimulate energy pathways at a cellular level, notably in the muscle tissue of the heart and, in fact, all muscles. Coenzyme Q10 has gained some popularity for therapy of critically ill patients awaiting heart transplants, and several clinical studies lend support to those claims. Our bodies naturally produce Q10 when they are not lacking vitamin C or any of the B-complex vitamins. In studies of diabetes, Parkinson's disease, and hypertension, high doses of coenzyme Q10 ranging from 300 to 1,200 mg a day seem to improve glucose control in diabetes, decrease symptoms of Parkinson's disease, and decrease high blood pressure. In my own practice, patients who were already doing a set treadmill routine and were then started on a statin drug found the treadmill routine more difficult to complete within two weeks of starting the statin drug. I found that initiating a daily 100-mg dose of coenzyme Q10 at the same time that I prescribed the statin drug eliminated this problem. According to one study, this large group of potential patients would receive a definite benefit from taking coenzyme Q10: those who use statins (for example, Zocor, Pravachol, Lipitor, or Crestor)—that's more than fifteen million people in the United States alone—will benefit. Those with severe and life-threatening heart failure, Parkinson's symptoms, diabetes, and hypertension would also benefit. These eighty-million-plus individuals should only take a supplement including coenzyme Q10 or medication under the strict supervision of their physician. However, I cannot recommend taking coenzyme Q10 as an antiaging supplement for everyone, as no scientific data suggest it has antiaging benefits if no disease or defect is present.

ALPHA LIPOIC ACID

This substance is an important part of the process by which our bodies produce energy. Animal studies and one human study have shown that alpha lipoic acid reduces aging of nonnuclear cellular DNA and the "power plants" of our cells: the mitochondria, which use glucose and oxygen to generate the cell's power requirements. Although the data are not yet extensive enough for us to give alpha lipoic acid a RealAge effect, two of the five members of the RealAge scientific team are now considering taking alpha lipoic acid themselves. Stay tuned: we will discuss any new studies in the RealAge "Tips of the Day," and when more evidence occurs, we will post it prominently on *www.realage.com*.

L-CARNITINE

This amino acid (a building block of protein) is found in our mitochondria (the cell's power plant) and is important in the transfer of energy within our cells. L-carnitine definitely improves some conditions in specific patients, such as low function of thyroid (hypothyroidism), heart failure, specific childhood liver dysfunction requiring kidney dialysis, and vascular disease. In animal studies, supplementation with its precursor, acetyl-L-carnitine, decreased aging of the arteries, improved memory, and decreased defects in the nonnuclear DNA of cells and in the energy-producing system of cells. I am beginning to think the data will be well enough developed by early 2005 or 2006 to determine if acetyl-L-carnitine has a RealAge benefit. Two of the five primary RealAge scientific advisors now take 1,500 mg of L-carnitine a day. I believe that L-carnitine should be considered by physicians for all patients who are over sixty years of age; or have arterial aging, or hypothroidism, or heart failure; or need dialysis.

ECHINACEA

Come cold and flu season, I always see individuals taking echinacea, an herbal powder derived from the leaves and stems of the coneflower. A popular folk remedy, echinacea is said to boost the body's natural immunity. Unfortunately, the very few studies on echinacea in both Germany and the United States have produced mixed results. Some found an immune response, others found no effect. At this stage, we really don't have any proof as to whether it works or not. It may have gotten a bad rap in some studies because a contaminant that was found in some of the preparations of echinacea did cause liver disease. People with allergies to plants in the sunflower family should steer clear of echinacea, and those with autoimmune diseases will want to talk to their doctors before taking this herb. In general, echinacea appears harmless. Do not take echinacea for long periods; even fans of the herb recommend taking it for only a few weeks at a time, when cold or flu symptoms set in.

GINKGO BILOBA

Ginkgo biloba is an herb that comes from the leaves and seeds Chinese ginkgo tree. It is reputed to have antioxidant properties and is best known for its supposed enhancement of mental clarity. Ginkgo is also reputed to lower blood pressure and to have other antiaging properties. Are these claims valid? No one knows. Ginkgo biloba does contain flavonoids and other compounds that are known to scavenge free radicals. Although several early European studies indicate possible benefits for people with Alzheimer's disease, these studies were not performed using a proper clinical trial design, and therefore their results cannot be viewed as reliable.

However, several scientifically credible clinical trials on ginkgo biloba have been conducted since 1998. One indicated that the herb may help improve cognitive functioning in people who have Alzheimer's disease or other forms of dementia. As reported in the *Journal of the American Medical Association*, the study found a cognitive improvement in 37 percent of those given the extract, as opposed to 23 percent of those given a placebo containing no ginkgo. The data offered by the study were preliminary, merely a first-round screening of the supplement. The study relied largely on subjective social indicators, such as whether caregivers noticed any change in behavior when patients with dementia took the drug, rather than on concrete physiological or psychological tests. Other large studies using both subjective and objective measures have not found any benefit. More research needs to be done on ginkgo biloba before we know if it really has any substantial effect.

Ginkgo biloba appears to be another of many possible antioxidants found in fruits and vegetables. A known side effect of ginkgo biloba is an antiplatelet effect (it inhibits the ability of platelets to clump together and cause blood clotting), which does not appear to be significant for most patients. It is unclear if ginkgo biloba has any unique properties not found in any other antioxidants. Thus, at this time, ginkgo biloba cannot be recommended for its memory-preserving or antiaging benefits.

GINSENG

Ginseng is a root that has been used for a long time in Eastern medicine to increase energy. Recently, medical reports claim that ginseng can boost the immune response and white blood cell count. As with most herbs, ginseng has undergone very few rigorous studies, so most of our information comes from personal testimonials and word-of-mouth. One study linked ginseng to a reduced incidence of the common cold and flu, but another showed that mice fed ginseng actually had damage to the immune system. The ginseng mice had more illness and aged more rapidly than they would have normally. Some claim that the American variety of ginseng has more active properties than the Asian variety. Some reports indicated ginseng should not be used for more than approximately two weeks at a time.

At the University of Chicago, I helped start an herbal study unit called the Tang Center for Herbal Studies. One of the first scientists we recruited was Chun-Su Yuan; early on, he sought to study ginseng. Ginseng had been reported to improve glucose control in diabetes. When Dr. Yuan looked at this issue in animal models of diabetes, only one of six or more preparations of ginseng had a beneficial effect on glucose control. Why did this one preparation consistently show a benefit while none of the others did? Dr. Yuan then discovered that a contaminant in the ginseng herbal preparation was responsible for the benefit. It seems that some of the ginseng berries were mixed with the herb in this one company's preparation. Those ginseng berries—not the root—contained a substance that normalized glucose levels.

Dr. Yuan went farther and found there were eleven ginsenocides (the active ingredients in ginseng) in the berry, of which two had beneficial effects, one of them eleven times more powerful than the other. Dr. Yuan has purified and patented these compounds, and preparations are now being tested for Food and Drug Administration approved studies in humans. So far, no major side effects have occurred. So the germ of truth that I believe present in almost every herbal remedy seems to be not that ginseng was not effective, but that the contaminant was. It is hoped that Dr. Yuan's pursuit of this topic will produce a purified form of a therapeutic agent that will have benefits that exceed the risks, and that can be controlled because it is prepared in a pharmaceutical formulation.

GLUCOSAMINE AND CHONDROITIN SULFATE

A number of studies stimulated and were stimulated by the 1997 book *The Arthritis Cure* by Jason Theodosakis, Brenda Adderly, and Barry Fox. These studies found that the herb combination of glucosamine and chondroitin sulfate decreases symptoms and repairs joint destruction in osteoarthritis. This herb combination decreases the severity of arthritis pain through an anti-inflammatory effect, and might decrease the basic inflammation and cause of osteoarthritis. Again, it may be an anti-inflammatory effect that helps preserve cartilage. Dr. Theodosakis believes it is more, that something in glucosamine prevents degradation, and something in chondroitin stimulates regrowth of the cartilage. Interested readers are encouraged to log on to *www.drtheo.com* to learn the current preparations of glucosamine and chondroitin sulfate that contain the active ingredient as specified on the label, and *www.consumerlab.com* to learn the current preparations that do not meet standards. Over 50 percent of the products sold as this combination are either devoid of the active ingredients, or contain less than 25 percent of the amounts claimed on the label.

But the data are clear: preparations that contain glucosamine and chondriotin sulfate decrease joint pain, decrease cartilage and joint space loss, and help increase cartilage buildup in patients with osteoarthritis. Should we all be taking this combination to prevent the ubiquitous osteoarthritis from disabling us? The data are not good enough to say that yet, but I know at the first sign of such in my own body, I will log on to *drtheo.com* to find the best preparation, and start taking it. You might ask, if 95 percent of us will have osteoarthritis by age 85, why do you not advise preventing it with glucosamine and chondriotin sulfate? I would if we knew for sure it works and works for the 25 year period it will take me to hit that calendar age. But such data do not yet exist. So for now I advise taking it if you have symptoms, and after you check with your doctor.

THYMUS EXTRACT

Because of its alleged antiaging benefits, there has recently been a stir about thymus extract. Should you take it? No. Why not? The thymus is a gland that is active during childhood and adolescence. It helps control and modulate the immune system. By age twenty, the thymus begins to dry up, and by age fifty it has virtually disappeared. The theory behind taking thymus-extract as a supplement is that the extract will help stimulate immune functioning and protect you from cancers, arthritis, and other ailments that age you. Because the thymus is active during youth, it is wrongfully assumed to be able to keep us young. No studies and absolutely no data indicate that thymus extract helps in any way. Furthermore, taking the extract poses a potential hazard. Thymus extract that is introduced into the body is different from that produced by your own body. Because supplemental thymus extract is a foreign protein, it may trigger an immune reaction, which in turn may cause your body to develop antibodies against itself.

OTHER SUPPLEMENTS

Many other miscellaneous supplements and herbs could be discussed here. However, except for a few supplements that treat specific conditions—for example, saw palmetto for benign prostatic hypertrophy (noncancerous enlargement of the prostate gland); creatine building rapid response muscles; and SAM-e, which has been useful in some studies for preventing and treating depression—there are no data on the antiaging effects of many of these other supplements. St John's Wort has so many interactions with other medications and supplements that I do not advise taking it unless you are under a doctor's care who prescribes it. So even though it is more expensive, SAM-e is the one I advise for those patients of mine who want a herbal antidepressant.

Eat a Nutrient-Rich Diet, Take Your Get-Younger Pills, and Avoid the Get-Older Ills

Now, instead of feeling confusion when faced with the wide variety of supplements available, you can feel confident and use vitamins as an effective part of your RealAge Makeover. If you're worried about arterial aging, make sure you get the anti-inflammatory/antioxidant vitamins E and C, the homocysteine-lowering vitamins folate, B_6, and B_{12}, and lutein and lycopene. If you're concerned about osteoporosis, arthritis, or immune aging, pay careful attention to your intake of calcium, magnesium, selenium, lycopene, and vitamins B_6, B_{12}, C, and D. Before you go shopping at your local pharmacy or health-food store, evaluate what you already have at home. Check expiration dates. Throw away the vitamins that contain more than you need in one day. And always ask your physician before you take any vitamin or mineral.

As for my patient Frank T.—the one with the thirty-five bottles of vitamins, supplements, and minerals—I told him that I thought keeping them straight must be a full-time job. My recommendation was that Frank take a twice-a-day multivitamin that contained 400 µg of folate, 2 mg of B_6, 15 µg of B_{12}, 500 mg of vitamin C, 200 IU of vitamin D, 600 mg of calcium, 200 mg of magnesium, and 200 IU of vitamin E as mixed tocopherols (each time he took it so the dose per day would be twice as much). I encouraged him to get at least two servings of vitamin C from fruit in the middle of the day. He was also told to make sure that the multivitamin contained no iron and 2,500 IU or less of vitamin A and beta-carotene combined. He learned to reduce his sodium intake to 1,600 mg a day and to boost his potassium intake to 4,000 mg a day with good food choices and without pills. Other than that, he was instructed to continue to eat his four fruit and five vegetable servings a day, and to keep his diet high in nutrients and low in calories (see Chapter 8).

"Mike," he said, "Are you sure I'm getting what I need?"

"Yes, and more important," I told him as I looked into my wastebasket filled to the brim with bottles, "I'm even more sure you're not getting what could be harmful to you. Those will stay here in the trash, where they belong."

He laughed as he walked out, carrying a much lighter load.

Daily Dose of Goodness

Five Habits That Can Give You More Energy

A RealAge Makeover Success Story: Joan D.

Joan D. had gained twenty-eight pounds slowly over the last nine years. Her bank account was full enough to support three closet renovations, she told me when we first met in 2001, and had to: she had now begun to purchase all her clothes in three sizes at once: 8, 10, and 12. As the first of her three children left home, she took over his room—which adjoined her bedroom—and made it into a large closet. She said she was desperate, feeling some twinges of what she thought might be heart pain, only to be reassured by her prior physician that it was indigestion. But she had lingering doubts. And she felt desperate as none of the diets she had tried—Atkins, Sugar Busters, Sommers—had worked for long. Oh, all had worked she said, but she would yo-yo from a size 8 to 12 to 8 to 12 to 8 and back again as she went from diet to diet, with only brief stops at size 10. Her last child had now left home, so she felt she had to take care of herself and her husband; she wanted to be around to advise her daughters and to enjoy the life she and her husband had saved for. But her blood pressure had also gone up, and she wanted to become thinner now for her own health as well as to please her husband. She asked a friend who was my patient, whom she had seen become a fraction of her former self, and decided if I was able to help her friend, I'd be able to help her.

Weekdays she arose at 7 a.m., made coffee for her husband, and then started working at home. I learned she was a successful author, writing and publishing about two mystery books a year. She worked in a home office while her lawyer husband often worked long hours as a successful corporate litigator. She skipped all food save for black coffee until about 2 p.m. daily to avoid the calories and then, famished, would snack on Oreos or Triscuits while waiting for her lunch soup to boil. She'd have an afternoon snack of nuts and fruit (her friend taught her that one), which would end her writing day. She then read the newspapers and watched TV, often snacking on Triscuits, Oreos, and decaffeinated coffee until her husband came home sometime between 6 and 10 p.m. They would have a big dinner, often prepared for them by one of a number of local restaurants (she cooked only once a week or so, even when the kids were at home), watch some TV together, then go to bed after the 10 o'clock news. On weekends she followed a similar routine since her kids left home, but often went to benefits on Friday and Saturday nights. She used to do StairMaster, never did resistence exercises, and occasionally walked thirty minutes with her husband on weekends. I asked her how many packs of Oreos and boxes of Triscuits she bought a week; four and four was the answer.

There were three problems we could fix immediately if she wanted to: she could benefit from eating cereal and fruit for breakfast, start walking every day with a goal of being able to walk 30 minutes every day, no excuses, and change her snacks. I told her the last one would be easy if she started eating breakfast. After a discussion explaining these three ideas, she committed to them. I heard from her by phone and e-mail daily for the first three months. One month into the program she worked with a trainer and learned the fourteen resistance exercises (see Chapter 9). By the end of three months, she had lost fourteen pounds, her blood pressure came back to 120/76 from 140/85 she loved her new energy, and had decided to buy a treadmill to place in front of a TV in the basement. A month later she said she needed to call only once a month. I last saw her two years after we first met, for her yearly progress report. She was a size six, happy, and committed to a breakfast of cereal, fruit (or egg white omelet on weekends), and coffee. She was deliriously happy with her RealAge Makeover, which started with eating breakfast daily.

Occasionally, our RealAge Makeover requires a big, one-time decision, such as the need for surgery to correct a medical problem. But much more commonly, what influences your health are small, daily issues that add up with a cumulative effect. Much of what you do is decided by sheer force of habit. Just becoming aware of the choices you're making, and being conscious of how they contribute to your RealAge Makeover, is the first step toward ensuring that your normal, daily routines are making you younger. Whether it's getting enough sleep, eating breakfast, drinking alcohol in moderation, enjoying coffee, or walking the dog, some daily routines and overall life strategies can help you live longer, healthier, and younger lives. Learn how to incorporate these habits into your daily life.

- Often it's the simple things that matter most in Age Reduction. You don't have time to sleep seven or eight hours a night? You don't have time *not* to. Your body needs time to rest and regenerate, and getting enough ZZZZs will give you more energy and make your waking hours more productive and enjoyable. Regularly sleeping just two hours less than normal impairs your judgments and reaction time to the same extent as a blood alcohol level of 0.12. This level is 50 percent higher than the level most states say drivers are inebriated. And you need your sleep to prevent aging of your immune system. So enjoy a full night's sleep every night. It can make your RealAge at least three years younger.
Difficulty rating: Moderately easy to very difficult

- Once you've slept the whole night through, don't forget to start the day off right. Eating a high-nutrient, high-fiber breakfast with some healthy fat gives a power-start to the day and helps keep you three years younger than those who never eat breakfast.
Difficulty rating: Moderately easy

- Do you love coffee and caffeinated beverages as much as I do? If so, you're in luck. A cup of joe or can of diet soda can make you younger. (Granted, of course, that you don't have any of the negative side effects such as migraine headaches, abnormal heartbeats, or gastrointestinal upset.) Studies consistently show that coffee and caffeine reduce the risk of Parkinson's disease and Alzheimer's. So go ahead and have that diet soda, or espresso, or latte. Six cups a day will make you more than a third of a year younger. This seems like an awful lot, but that is the amount supported by the data. Just be sure to filter the coffee, use skim milk, don't add sugar, and take a little extra calcium and B vitamins.
Difficulty rating: Moderately easy

- Do you like a drink now and then? Well, if you're not at risk of alcohol or drug abuse, moderate drinking—one half to one drink a day for women and one or two drinks a day for men—may help you stay younger longer. A little alcohol can help your heart and arteries keep their spring. It's the alcohol in wine, spirits, or beer that provides the benefit. Red wine may produce an extra benefit, and I'll show you how to get that benefit, even if you don't like red wine. Moderate drinkers may gain as much as 1.9 years in RealAge. However, drinking too much and too often can be dangerous, even life-threatening. The Real-Age of heavy drinkers can be three years older than that of nondrinkers.
Difficulty rating: Moderately easy (moderate alcohol consumption) to most difficult (cutting back on excessive alcohol consumption)

■ Dog owners, rejoice. People who own pooches actually gain energy and stay younger longer. Think of your furry friend as an exercise-promoting stress-reducer. Sorry, cat owners: the greatest RealAge benefit of pet ownership has gone to the dogs—one year younger. **Difficulty rating: Moderate**

As human beings, we're creatures of habit. The trick is to make this fact work for you by developing a habit of making healthy choices—so that you make them without even thinking. Until you do, it's far too easy to live on autopilot, unconsciously making bad health choices. Pressed for time, you may skimp on sleep. Feeling guilty about last night's bowl of double chocolate fudge ice cream, you skip breakfast. However, you can learn habits that make you younger, too, even some that you will come to look forward to. Drinking alcohol in moderation—one half to one drink a day for women and one or two drinks a day for men—can help prevent arterial aging. ("One drink" is 12 ounces of beer, 4 ounces of wine, or 1.5 ounces of 80-proof liquor) One of the best habits is walking the dog. Why? It's exercise. As the twentieth-century physician William Osler said, "Walk your dog. Even if you don't have one." Being rested can be a key to maintaining a positive attitude, keeping your energy level high, and being able to handle the rest of the day in a nonstressful, youth-promoting way. Maintaining the quality of your life affects the quantity of your life: the better you take care of yourself, the younger you stay.

How many times have you heard, "Do everything in moderation" and "Achieve balance in life"? Until recently, those sayings were more folk wisdom than science. When it comes to aging, research has confirmed that these commonsense ideas are actually correct. Let's now consider a few changes that are easy to make, simple to integrate into your life, and don't necessarily require the resolve that getting in shape or changing your diet does.

Beauty Rest:
It's Not Just the Eye Bags and Wrinkles

In years past, when it came to the bad habit of buying extra time by skipping sleep, I myself was a guilty culprit. Of course, I was also not the only one—not by a long shot. When I was training to become a doctor, interns and residents were expected to survive without sleep. Luckily, times have changed. Most residents and interns now work less than eighty hours a week and must have eight hours off after every twenty-four-hour shift. Still, most of us in academic medicine want to accomplish more as we become successful in our patient care and research careers. For example, when I was invited to speak somewhere on a weekend, I was afraid that saying no would mean I wouldn't be asked again, so I always accepted, even if it cost me several hours of sleep. I was guilty of even worse behavior, though. To continue my career and have a family life, I just kept cutting down on sleep, relying on only five hours a night. I didn't realize I was making my RealAge older. Chronic fatigue was robbing me of energy and making all my waking hours less productive and less fun. And more aging.

The fact that sleeping seven to eight hours a night protects against needless aging has been shown in reports from around the world. The best known study on sleep patterns, the famous Alameda County, California study, found that men who slept seven to eight hours a night and women who slept six to seven hours a night were significantly less likely to die than those who did not sleep that amount. In RealAge terms, regular sleep patterns can make more than a three-year difference (see Table 11.1). Even so, this benefit doesn't do justice to the true value of sleep, because insufficient sleep causes a ripple effect, in which you can start to slide in other areas of your daily routine. For example, if you're feeling tired and less energetic, you might skip your daily walk. You're more likely to say, "I don't have the energy to cook a wholesome meal. I'll just grab some fast food." Recent studies indicate that chronic reduction in sleep to a level that seems acceptable—to four or five hours a night—makes everyday stress more aging. And lack of sleep decreases immune responses; lack of a good night's sleep before immunization against flu decreases the success rate or protection you receive from that immunization. So sleep, just like attitude and stress, is one of the key areas that has a greater overall effect than their direct effect on RealAge.

At the same time, as with many other RealAge choices, it is possible to get too much of a good thing, and oversleeping will make you older. Sleeping more than nine hours on a regular basis is too much for most of us, and is often a sign of an underlying health problem. If you find yourself consistently sleeping this much, see your doctor.

In today's modern world, with a 24/7 lifestyle where we can grocery shop or get gas at 4 a.m. if we want to, we can virtually ignore the cycles of night and day. But our bodies really aren't designed to live this way. Our bodies evolved over thousands of years to adapt to the natural cycle of the day. Our natural rhythms follow the schedule of sunup and sundown, assisted by hormones such as melatonin, serotonin, and cortisol that are secreted at different times of the day to push us through our sleep-to-wake cycle. For example, as it begins to get dark, your body begins to secrete melatonin, a hormone that increases drowsiness. As the sun starts to rise, your adrenal gland begins producing cortisol, a hormone that gets you up and going. A hundred and twenty years ago, before the invention of the light bulb, our lifestyles were in synch with these natural

Table 11.1   The RealAge Effect of Sleep

FOR MEN:

	Regular Sleep (Hours Per Night)			
	Less than 6	6 to 7.5	7.6 to 9	More than 9
CALENDAR AGE	REALAGE			
35	38.6	34.5	33.2	35.4
50	53.9	49.4	48.1	55.6
70	74.3	69.3	67.8	70.9

FOR WOMEN:

	Regular Sleep (Hours Per Night)			
	Less than 6	6 to 7.5	7.6 to 9	More than 9
CALENDAR AGE	REALAGE			
35	36.0	32.9	34.5	39.2
50	51.9	47.5	49.5	59.6
70	72.8	67.5	69.3	74.8

rhythms. But today they are not. You might be up working half the night under an electric light, or set an alarm to be up extra early. And this has an adverse effect on your biological system. Your internal clock becomes confused, your hormones become irregular in their on and off times, you become fatigued, and you undergo unnecessary aging.

On the whole, as a nation, we aren't getting enough sleep. More than 20 percent of American adults find themselves dozing off at inappropriate moments or during quiet and sedentary activities, which is a sign of sleep deprivation. And I should know. One of the most—if not *the* most—embarrassing moments of my life was caused by sleep deprivation. When I was an intern, I woke up after the dessert course of a dinner party at my professor's house with pie on my face. After a night on call, I had fallen asleep into the dessert. Try to gracefully sweep cream pie off your face. In front of a date, two peers, your boss, the president of the hospital, and a dean of a medical school.

In two studies, sleep deprivation exaggerated the hormone responses to normal, irritating stresses. That overreaction probably contributes to aging. Sleep deprivation reduces task performance in almost all mock and real worksites where tested. Two hours of sleep deprivation can also make you irritable, disagreeable to be around, and less focused mentally.

Sleepy people are at greater risk of accidents, and not just auto accidents. For auto accidents, the greatest risk occurs during periods of maximum sleepiness, such as the late afternoon or after midnight. As your body gets increasingly tired, your *sleep latency window*—the time it takes to go from being bored to dead asleep—decreases from as much as three minutes to as little as thirty seconds.

Most of us require at least six hours of sleep a night, and usually seven to eight hours. When we are younger, we need more sleep, and the quality of our sleep is better. As we age, the quality of our sleep decreases. Our periods of slow-wave sleep (the kind of sleep needed to ensure mental alertness and motor coordination) decrease from one hundred fifty minutes a day to just twenty-five. These periods of slow-wave sleep are vitally important but don't occur until an hour and a half or more of continual sleep. Thus, if you are frequently awakened by some physical condition—for example, the need to urinate because of an enlarged prostate, or sleep apnea—you will not get the restorative sleep you need. (Sleep apnea, as discussed in Chapter 9, is caused by an obstruction in the airway. It's a key reason why people who are older or overweight don't feel rested in the daytime.)

Naps don't make up for loss of restorative sleep time because they are usually shorter than the time you need to reach slow-wave sleep. You need both rapid-eye-movement sleep and slow-wave sleep to feel refreshed, and both of these kinds of sleep require a period of continuous sleep before they start. I don't know why our systems were made this way, but we can't get right into slow-wave sleep or rapid-eye-movement sleep without a period of regular sleep first. (Although naps can give you more short-term energy, they don't restore your energy long-term, nor do they reverse the aging that lack of sleep causes.)

Making up sleep on weekends is a tradition of high school and college students, and of the many people who work two jobs or care for infants. The Real-Age effect of such sleep debt and makeup sleep periods has not been well studied. The little data I have on such weekend catch-up patterns indicate that one can restore slow-wave and rapid-eye-movement sleep debt and hormone cycles by making up for lost sleep in this way. However, it does not easily repair the lost friendships due to your grouchiness from sleep debt earlier in the week.

The more sleep-deprived you are, the more likely you are to doze off at the wheel or to put yourself and others in a life-threatening situation. Remember, driving while sleep-deprived is the same as driving with a blood alcohol level well into the inebriated range: your judgment is impaired and your reflex time for corrective action is diminished, even if you do not actually doze off. So driving while exhausted is another way, in addition to reducing your ability to manage stress, that sleep deprivation can quickly make your RealAge substantially older.

If giving yourself a RealAge Makeover means learning new habits, what kind of habits can we learn to ensure a good night's sleep? Sleeping in a cool, dark room is one. If you find it hard to get to sleep, do something relaxing before going to bed—reading or watching TV—to calm yourself down. You can also drink a glass of milk (skim!) or eat a banana or some other food that contains melatonin (oats, sweet corn, rice, barley, tomatoes) or serotonin (complex carbohydrate-rich foods such as whole-grain pasta and vegetables) to help make you sleepy. If you need to rise early in the morning, skip late-night activities. The best sleep schedule is a regular schedule, and one that is in sync with the natural rhythms of the day. If you need to, sleep late on weekends to repay sleep debts. Sleeping late on weekends is at least a good way to get your restorative sleep and reset your stress hormone patterns.

Because bad sleep patterns are so disruptive to daily life and a general feeling of well-being, you probably already know if you have sleep problems. Often, sleeping too little or too much is an indicator of an underlying problem, such as illness or stress. For example, two common signs of clinical depression are waking up too early in the morning and sleeping an endless numbers of hours. Other diseases can disturb your sleep cycle, causing chronic sleepiness or fatigue. If you notice changes in your sleep cycle, talk to your doctor about possible causes. If you are under a lot of stress, try to find new ways of relaxing. Exercise may help. One study found that exercising in the early evening more than two hours prior to your normal sleep time—walking, lifting weights, or any kind of workout—improved both the quantity and quality of sleep. However, too much exercise close to sleep time will make it difficult to fall asleep because it increases your metabolic rate too much.

Many people try to conquer sleep problems by taking sleeping pills or drinking alcohol at bedtime. While these quick fixes might produce short-term sleep benefits, in the long run they disrupt sleep. Regular use of these substances can confuse your circadian rhythm (internal clock), which means that you may then need the drug if you are to sleep at all. Occasional use is usually not a problem. (For example, you can take melatonin supplements to help avoid jet lag during international flights. However, for some people, this increases asthma symptoms.) If you feel you need sleeping pills, talk to your doctor. Sleeping pills can be physically and psychologically addictive and may have long-term aging effects. In fact, a recent study found that people who used sleeping pills more than fourteen days a month were 1.9 years older, and that those who took twenty-nine or more a month were 2.8 years older. It is a good idea to use sleeping pills for only a limited time or to abstain from them altogether.

Remember, giving yourself a RealAge Makeover is all about treating yourself well and enjoying the best life has to offer. And there's little that can beat the pleasure of a good night's sleep that leaves you refreshed, restored, and ready to face the challenges of the day. And like most RealAge Makeover habits, you'll look better when refreshed by a good night's sleep, once again a makeover from the inside out. So when time constraints make you think of skimping on shut-eye, make self-care a priority instead. Because rest is one of the healthy habits that keeps you young. Sleep helps strengthen your immune system, boosts your attention span, and dissipates excess stress that can damage your arteries, stomach, and, once again, immune system. Also, normal sleep prior to driving and other activities helps prevent accidents that can make your RealAge older, a lot older, real fast.

Don't Skip Breakfast: Starting the Day Off Right

A RealAge Makeover Success Story, Karen L.

Karen L. was a patient who came to me complaining that she was not losing weight despite her best attempts. We discussed her eating patterns carefully; she was very proud of the fact that she saved calories by skipping breakfast every morning. Like Joan D., the patient at the start of this chapter, she thought she would keep her weight down and thereby make her RealAge younger. She was wrong on both counts. Skipping breakfast makes your RealAge as much as three years older, and causes a slowing of metabolic rate that we think increases fat gain when you do eat. Besides, she didn't realize how hungry it was making her later in the day. Like most people, she greatly underestimated how much she actually ate. When we went over her diet carefully, it was clear she made up for her missing breakfasts like Joan D., by eating an incredible volume of high-calorie snacks. She changed that one habit and lost 18 pounds the next year.

Studies consistently show that people who eat meals at regular intervals, and particularly those who eat breakfast, stay younger longer. Indeed, non-breakfast-eaters have a mortality rate that is 1.3 to 1.5 times higher per year than those who eat breakfast regularly.

Breakfast is the first part of a day-long eating plan. Eating breakfast helps our bodies metabolize food more efficiently, and cuts down on the urge to snack between meals. Unhealthy snacking for more than three days a week can increase your RealAge. Eating regularly helps break up long periods of fasting, meaning that your body doesn't have to gear up to digest a big meal after doing nothing for hours, which is not an efficient process. In addition, some researchers have hypothesized that we burn more fat during our waking hours, since we are more active. This means that we might burn off our breakfast calories more effectively than we would an overly large late-night dinner. However, this is still speculation.

A perhaps surprising health effect of eating breakfast is that it also makes your cardiovascular and immune systems younger. We don't know exactly why, but several theories exist. First, many cereals contain lots of soluble fiber, which prevents lipid buildup and thus helps prevent arterial aging. Fiber also helps decrease the risk of cancer. The average American eats 12 grams of fiber a day, but increasing your fiber intake to 25 grams a day can reduce arterial aging and make your RealAge as much as two years younger. Fiber is one of the fifteen food choices (see Chapter 8) that has definitely been shown to make a difference in how long and how well you live. Second, cereals are usually fortified with extra vitamins, minerals, and micronutrients. During breakfast, we get many of the essential nutrients that we may not get during the rest of the day. This is even more important if you don't eat lots of fruits and vegetables during the day, or if you don't take vitamin and mineral supplements regularly. Other typical breakfast foods (fortified fruit juices, yogurt, and whole fruit) contain essential nutrients such as vitamins C and D, calcium, and magnesium.

If we want to eat a breakfast that will benefit our RealAge Makeover the most, what exactly should we eat? Lots of cereals, fruits, and juices and low-fat dairy products such as fat-free yogurt or skim milk. Choose a whole grain cereal with no saturated or trans fats or sugars that just add empty calories. As usual, start with healthy fat. Become a label reader and watch out for "healthy" breakfast foods, including many brands of granola, that actually contain a lot of calories and unhealthy (aging) fat. Use skim milk instead of whole milk on your cereal and in your tea or coffee. Drink plenty of juices—pure juice or fortified pure juice, not juice cocktails or blends. (Juice blends or cocktails often contain a lot of added sugar and less real juice.) Whole fruits are even better than juice, as they contain lots of fiber. Both are good sources of vitamin C and potassium.

Eat whole grain or multigrain toast; again, read the labels, because many commercially manufactured breads contain added sugars, salt, and other ingredients that you may want to avoid. Instead of a pastry or croissant, which is high in unhealthy fats, choose an English muffin or bagel. The average breakfast croissant contains more than one and one-half days' worth of aging fat (more than 30 grams) and over 400 calories. (By comparison, the average 3-ounce piece of top sirloin steak only has 3 or 4 grams of aging fat.) Another staple of the American breakfast—the donut—is an absolutely empty breakfast, with lots of calories and artery-aging trans fat, but no nutrition. Try peanut butter (the healthy kind, made with peanuts only), avocado spread, nut spread, or olive oil instead of high-fat cream cheese, butter, or margarine. Nut spreads are a good substitute for high-sugar, calorie-laden jams and jellies.

Unfortunately, many staples of the classic American breakfast, such as bacon and sausage, are full of four-legged or saturated fats, and should be avoided. What about another classic staple: the egg? Luckily, only the yolk of the egg is high in fat and cholesterol, so an egg-white-and-vegetable omelet with salsa—no cheese—is a delicious, low-cholesterol, low-fat breakfast choice. (The average omelet made with three egg whites in a little canola oil has less than 2 grams of healthy fat and only 75 to 125 calories.) Or, if you can't bear to go completely yolk-free, one yolk included with three whites makes a scramble or omelet look and taste almost like a regular one. If you crave pancakes or waffles for breakfast, cook them in a nonstick pan or one coated with low-fat vegetable oil spray. Top with chopped fruit and a sprinkle of powdered sugar instead of mounds of butter and syrup.

Instead of eating the same thing every morning, use breakfast time to stimulate your imagination: try unconventional breakfast foods, such as chopped vegetables with a handful of low-fat whole grain crackers, or a corn tortilla loaded with beans, lettuce, and tomato. If you own a juicer, you can make carrot or tomato juice mixed with celery, spinach, and other vegetables. It's a time-saving, nutrient-rich, and fat-free way to begin the day.

Like Joan D. and Karen L., many people mistakenly believe they're making a good dieting choice by skipping breakfast. Others think that they don't have time. They can barely bolt a cup of coffee before it's time to leave for work. If this is the case with you, try "blender blasters" or smoothies, which you can make very quickly. These are delicious and usually contain fruit and other healthy ingredients. For example, try the "Double Strawberry Blender Blast" (*Cooking the RealAge® Way*, page 192): take 3 cups of fresh or frozen strawberries, 1 cup of fat-free milk or light soy milk, 1 cup of strawberry sorbet, blend together, and in minutes you've got a delicious blast of nutrition, big enough for four servings. Or try the "Frothy Raspberry–Orange Smoothie" (page 195): 2 cups

Table 11.2	The RealAge Effect of Eating Breakfast		

FOR MEN:

		Breakfast	
	Rarely/Occasionally	2 to 5 Times/Week	Almost every day
CALENDAR AGE		REALAGE	
35	37.0	34.8	34.5
50	52.2	49.7	49.2
70	72.0	69.8	69.5

FOR WOMEN:

		Breakfast	
	Rarely/Occasionally	2 to 5 Times/Week	Almost every day
CALENDAR AGE		REALAGE	
35	36.2	35.0	34.8
50	51.2	50.0	49.8
70	71.3	70.0	69.8

of fat-free milk or 1 percent vanilla soy milk, 2 ripe medium bananas, 2 cups of frozen raspberries, and 2 tablespoons of frozen orange juice concentrate. Again, simply blend and enjoy. Or "Linda D's Orange Fruit Smoothie" (page 197). Take 2 cups of cut-up honeydew melon, 2 cups of frozen or fresh strawberries, 2 cups of frozen raspberries or other berries, 2 tablespoons of frozen orange juice concentrate, 4 ice cubes, and 1 large tablespoon of quick oats. Blend together for a delicious treat. These blasters all take less than five minutes to prepare from start to finish.

There are other ways to work breakfast into a hectic schedule. Anything you can eat on the go—in line at the bus stop, or in your car (but not while you're driving!)—can make breakfast possible even for the busiest person. As we discussed in Chapter 8, you'll usually want to eat in only a couple of special places. However, in this case, the antiaging benefits of breakfast justify eating elsewhere. Carry a small bag of cereal with you to munch on in your car. Or pack a low-fat yogurt. Buy small boxes of real juice, not juice drinks or juice cocktails and carry them in your purse or briefcase. Keep plenty of fruit around, to start the day and to munch on between meals. Becoming a breakfast-eater can make your RealAge as much as three years younger (see Table 11.2). That's not even counting the RealAge benefits from all the vitamins, minerals, and other nutrients such as carotenoids, flavonoids, and fiber you get from eating nutritious food.

Finally, remember that mealtimes are a RealAge double-dip when they are fun social events, and breakfast is no exception. For many families, the weekend is a time for everyone to get together and talk about what happened during the week. Saturday and Sunday morning brunches are a good time to see friends and strengthen the social ties that keep us younger.

Coffee and Caffeine Make You Younger

At work, I was always teased about my caffeine intake. Whenever I went on a TV show or did a personal appearance, I would keep a Diet Pepsi, Diet Coke, or Diet Dr Pepper near me. When people would see me drink four to six cups of coffee during a four-hour meeting, they would ask, "Doesn't coffee make you older?"

I would tell them we didn't have any data one way or another. But I wanted to know, so the rest of the RealAge scientific team explored the issue. (I was kept out of the research because of my possible bias.) Before 1999, the scientific team found no data that showed coffee made you either older or younger. In addition, diet soft drinks that had not been exposed to heat (which turns the aspartame to formaldehyde) seemed to have no effect on aging, unless you consumed more than one hundred 12-ounce cans a day. (In contrast, regular soft drinks are full of simple sugars, so they of course do cause your blood vessels to age.)

However, in late 1999, the data started coming out and haven't stopped yet. The headlines said, "Coffee Decreases Parkinson's Disease," "Coffee Decreases the Risk of Alzheimer's Disease," and "Coffee Decreases the Risk of Type II Diabetes." These results initially came from risk-factor epidemiologic studies, observational studies that can establish relationships between factors but not cause and effect. Three of the studies used questions to track the lifestyle and health of 120,000 nurses, 50,000 health professionals, and 15,000 physicians. Enough studies have now been performed that we can say with confidence that drinking six or more 4-ounce cups of coffee a day decreases your risk of Parkinson's disease by approximately 40 percent and your risk of Alzheimer's disease by approximately 20 percent. Are these intervention studies—that is, controlled trials, which are the gold standard of scientific research? No, but even when you

| Table 11.3 | The RealAge Effect of Coffee Consumption | | |

FOR MEN:

Coffee Consumption*

	Rarely/Occasionally	2 to 5 Cups/Day	6 or More cups a day
CALENDAR AGE		REALAGE	
35	35.1	34.9	34.8
50	50.2	49.8	49.7
70	71.0	69.7	69.6

FOR WOMEN:

Coffee Consumption*

	Rarely/Occasionally	2 to 5 Cups/Day	6 or More cups a day
CALENDAR AGE		REALAGE	
35	35.1	35.0	34.8
50	50.2	50.0	49.8
70	71.3	70.0	69.4

*A cup is a 4-ounce cup of coffee or 12-ounce can of caffeinated soft drink such as Diet Coke, Diet Dr Pepper, or Diet Pepsi.

take into account every other factor we know that is associated with arterial aging, immune aging, or accidents, caffeine seems to decrease your risk of these severe, incapacitating, neurologic diseases.

What are the hazards of coffee? For a few people, too much caffeine will increase abnormal heartbeats; if you already have a tendency to have abnormal heartbeats, caffeine may make them worse. Furthermore, if you develop benign prostatic hypertrophy (enlargement of the prostate gland that often makes older men awaken to urinate several times during the night, disrupting sleep), caffeine may make it worse by causing a spasm of the urethra. So if you have an enlarged prostate, caffeine may make it more difficult to urinate. In addition, for a few people, caffeine will cause migraine headaches, and too much caffeine will cause gastrointestinal upset.

Remember to make adjustments for caffeine: take 20 additional milligrams of calcium and 3 percent more of each of the water-soluble B vitamins, including folate, a day for every 4-ounce cup of coffee or 12-ounce can of caffeinated soft drinks you consume a day. And only drink coffee that has been filtered through paper; the paper filter removes oils that increase fat uptake into arterial plagues.

Assuming you don't have any bad reaction to caffeine and are not "stressed by it," coffee can make your RealAge younger. How much younger? The data indicates that six 4-ounce cups of caffeinated coffee, six 12-ounce sugarless soft drinks, or combinations of the two make your RealAge three to six months younger.

By the way, the agent most used prior to about 1994 to decaffinate coffee caused cancer. This substance is no longer used to decaffinate coffee in the United States. But it is the caffeine that apparently has the Age-Reduction effect, so decaffeinated coffee affords no RealAge effect.

Mixed Drinks: The Pros and Cons of Alcohol Consumption

In 1996 the U.S. government—the same institution that brought us Prohibition—declared that a moderate intake of alcohol appeared to be beneficial to human health. The announcement was astounding. After years of fighting alcohol consumption, the government was actually encouraging it. However, the government was careful to emphasize "moderate." That means one half to one drink a day for women and one to two drinks a day for men—nothing more.

Alcohol is a complicated issue, and one that requires careful thought, because alcohol can either help you or harm you. Regular consumption of alcohol in small amounts helps prevent arterial aging and heart attacks. Too much alcohol consumption can lead to alcoholism, liver disease, increased cancer rates, and increased risk of death due to accidents during intoxication. Approximately 5 percent of all deaths can be attributed to excessive consumption of alcohol, and the medical and social consequences can be severe. Approximately 100,000 Americans die every year of alcohol-related disease, and 20 million have problems related to alcohol addiction.

So how can you know if alcohol can play a role in your RealAge Makeover? Should you have a glass of wine in the evening? Or are you someone who can't drink in moderation and probably shouldn't drink at all?

First of all, the RealAge Age-Reduction effect of alcohol consumption begins only when a person reaches the age at which the risk of cardiovascular disease increases: after menopause for women, and about age thirty-five for men. Second, the antiaging benefits of alcohol apply only to some people. Therefore, you would need to weigh your risks and decide whether or not alcohol consumption should be part of your Age-Reduction plan. You would also need to determine if you could consume alcohol in moderate amounts, considering your own genetic and social risks of developing alcoholism, liver disease, or cancers.

The Pros

The connection between alcohol and reduced arterial aging—the so-called "red wine factor"—was first observed in France. The southern French, with their traditional diet heavy in fatty cheeses, butter, and red meats, had rates of cardiovascular disease that were, surprisingly, lower than anyone would have predicted. The hypothesis was that all the red wine the French used to accompany their saturated-fat-laden food was helping to protect their arteries from fatty plaque buildup. The hypothesis has now been modified, as suggested in Chapter 8. The French do not consume more saturated and trans fats than Americans, because the French use nine-inch plates, and, more important, eat small servings. Americans use eleven- or thirteen-inch plates, and our portions are almost twice the size of French portions. And that's only our first serving: we may have two or three. Also, Americans eat a lot of trans fats which, until the last few years, were rare in France.

No one knows exactly how alcohol retards or reverses arterial aging. It appears to prevent clotting by decreasing the rate of platelet aggregation, meaning that the platelets don't stick together as fast as they normally would. Also, alcohol appears to prevent the oxidation of fat that leads to accumulation of fatty plaques along the walls of the arteries. Alcohol promotes health of the endothelium, the layer of cells that lines the arteries, and helps promote proper blood flow. In test-tube studies, alcohol decreased inflammation in the endothelial cells of arteries. Although some may be better than others, all types of alcoholic beverages help reduce the level of atherosclerosis. All alcohol causes an increase in healthy (HDL) cholesterol levels.

Red wine does provide an extra benefit. It contains resveratrol, a flavonoid that seems to decrease aging of the DNA in the mitochondria, the cell's energy plant. Red wine has this benefit because the skin of the grape contains resveratrol, and red wine has been in contact with that skin for a longer period of time than white wine (hence its red color). Red wine, presumably because of the presence of flavonoids in grape skins may have other antioxidant benefits as well (see Chapter 8). The flavonoids act as an antioxidant and free-radical scavenger, resulting in reduced arterial and immune system aging. A fun way to incorporate moderate drinking into your life—and one that is less likely to lead to over-consumption of alcohol—is to become a wine lover. By learning about vintages and types of wine, you can have even more fun making your RealAge younger.

Would you like to get the benefit of red wine from white wine? Take three grapes of any color, freeze them, and put them in the bottom of your wine glass. Then pour the white wine over the grapes. Whether the grapes are green, red, or purple, their skins contain resveratrol. Pouring white wine over frozen grapes also makes the wine taste better, as the taste of white wine is brought out when it's served at a cooler temperature. Eating the grapes after you've drunk the wine gives you the benefit of the resveratrol. By the way, the resveratrol content of grapes is thought to be highest when the grapes have been grown in damp, northern climates, such as the New York State Finger Lakes region. In the studies I've seen, that was not actually correct. The reservatrol content of grapes varies greatly, and it's unclear to me how the resveratrol content of a grape can be predicted by its origin: some of the highest resveratrol content occurred in table grapes from California. The effect of resveratrol slows or reverses aging of your immune system and your arteries to a small degree, but it is the alcohol that works to reverse aging of your arteries.

Mounting evidence now suggests that not just red wine but any alcoholic beverage helps protect us from arterial aging. When it comes to Age Reduction, all alcoholic beverages seem to have the same effect: 4 ounces of wine is the same as one 12-ounce can of beer, which is the same as 1.5 ounces of 80-proof liquor. Moderate and regular consumption of alcohol reduces the risk of heart attack by as much as 30 percent, making your RealAge 1.9 years younger (see Table 11.4).

The benefit you receive from alcohol is at its maximum with one or two drinks a day if you're a man and with one half to one drink a day if you're a woman. If you drink more or less than that, the benefit decreases. Therefore, to realize the maximum benefit from alcohol—that is, the least aging—you must drink in moderation. The curve representing the RealAge benefit from alcohol is U-shaped: the least aging occurs with moderate intake of alcohol, and the greatest aging occurs at either end of the curve, with either no alcohol consumption or more than moderate consumption.

What is the evidence that alcohol reduces arterial aging and thus the incidence of heart disease? An analysis of the health habits of almost ninety thousand female nurses found that those who drank three or more drinks a week (the equivalent of one half to one drink a day) had a 40 percent lower rate of nonfatal heart attacks and arterial disease than those who did not. A study on mostly male health professionals and two other corresponding studies on men found similar

Table 11.4	The RealAge Effect of Alcohol Consumption

FOR MEN:

Alcoholic Drinks Per Day

	Rarely/Never	1 to 2	2+ to 3	3+ to 5	More than 5
CALENDAR AGE			REALAGE		
35	35.5	34.1	34.8	35.3	36.4
50	50.7	48.3	49.6	51.5	55.0
70	70.9	67.7	69.5	73.2	77.6

FOR WOMEN:

Alcoholic Drinks Per Day

	Rarely/Never	½ to 1	1+ to 3	3+ to 5	More than 5
CALENDAR AGE			REALAGE		
35	35.0	34.8	35.1	35.7	36.4
50	50.4	49.2	50.3	52.3	55.0
70	70.6	67.8	70.4	73.8	77.6

results. These studies also indicated there was an ideal range of alcohol consumption. Women who had one half to one drink a day and men who had one or two drinks a day were at lower risk of coronary and arterial aging, yet did not have a higher risk of aging from immune aging, liver disease or cancers, or accidents—the events that higher alcohol intake can contribute to. Individuals who drank less than the moderate drinkers were also at higher risk of cardiovascular diseases. Those in the low-to-moderate drinking range had the longest life expectancy, the fewest health problems, and the youngest RealAge at any calendar age.

By the way, kids at college who hear me talk about the health benefits of alcohol often ask, "Is seven drinks on a Friday night the same as one every night?" The answer, of course, is "No." Bingeing on alcohol is never good for your health, and in extreme cases can be fatal.

Why can women get the same antiaging effect from less alcohol? First, women tend to be smaller, which affects the overall amount of alcohol they can tolerate at any one time. Second, women have less alcohol dehydrogenase in the lining of their stomach. This enzyme breaks down alcohol before it enters the bloodstream. Women tend to absorb more alcohol into their bloodstream per drink. Third, when you drink a lot, the enzyme that breaks down alcohol (cytochrome CYPE2A) increases. Unfortunately, this enzyme also breaks down hormones, such as estrogen, that help protect women from heart disease (at least when normally secreted before menopause). Fortunately, this CYPE2A enzyme also breaks down some toxins, and in this way may benefit you.

The Cons

People at high risk of cardiovascular disease because of a family history of heart attacks or because of signs of developing atherosclerosis will get the most Age-Reduction benefit from a drink a day. Smokers and those with a family history of alcoholism, cirrhosis of the liver, hepatic cancer, or other alcohol-related illnesses are also strongly urged to avoid all alcohol consumption.

The liver is the principle site of metabolism of alcohol and as such remains at the highest risk of damage—and aging—from alcohol use. Liver scarring from use of alcohol (cirrhosis) or its precursor, alcoholic hepatitis, can cause considerable aging. In some urban areas, it's the fourth leading cause of death for individuals twenty-five to sixty-four years of age. Because cirrhosis of the liver causes irreversible structural damage, there are few treatment options for the disease once it reaches an advanced stage. Damage to the liver also appears related to a higher risk of cancer.

There are two theories of why excessive drinking causes cancer. The first and most widely held explanation is that use of alcohol induces or increases the production of an enzyme that breaks down the alcohol, CYPE2A. This enzyme breaks down not only alcohol but also other foreign substances, often creating carcinogenic compounds in the process. That is why smokers in particular need to avoid drinking alcohol. The combination is deadly: the same enzyme that breaks down alcohol (CYPE2A) and increases when you are drinking, also breaks down the nitrosamines in cigarette smoke into a carcinogenic form. By stimulating the production of this enzyme, alcohol increases the risk of cancer from smoking. The RealAge effect can make someone five to ten years older.

That's why the state legislature and especially State Senator Joseph Bruno did the citizens of New York such a huge favor by banning cigarettes from bars. By not allowing a mixture of smoke and alcohol, the extra toxicity and carcinogenic elements you would get by drinking alcohol and inhaling cigarette smoke were and will be diminished.

A second explanation for the higher incidence of cancer among heavy drinkers is that alcohol itself contains low levels of cancer-causing substances. The risk of throat and digestive tract cancers increases two to ten times among heavy drinkers, depending on the kind of cancer. Women in particular have to be careful: women who drink too much are at twice the risk of uterine and cervical cancers, and probably breast cancer, although the data are not definitive enough to assert a direct cause and effect.

Since alcohol has a high caloric content, heavy drinkers tend to carry around more paunch, which is another way that excessive drinking can age. And that fat doesn't just make you look older—it actually makes you older. It is, after all, fat around your waist that secretes substances that increase inflammation and damage to your arteries and immune system. The impurities that are stored in the fat also increase your risk of cancer to that of someone five to ten years older. Finally, heavy alcohol consumption impairs the absorption of crucial nutrients and vitamins, leading to nutrient deficiencies and even malnutrition. Heavy alcohol consumption is associated with a decreased intake of thiamine, folate, iron, zinc, vitamin E, and vitamin C.

And there's almost no other way to make yourself older faster than in alcohol-related accidents, in boats, automobiles, or other vehicles. Never, ever drink and drive. You put yourself and others at risk. If you are out with friends, make sure to choose a designated driver or take a cab home. Operating a boat, swimming, skiing, or putting yourself in other potentially risky situations while drinking can also cause rapid aging.

If you are wondering whether or not you have a drinking problem, the answer is that just the fact that you're wondering means that you probably do. Like any other health issue that ages you, this is a problem best confronted head-on. Talk to your doctor about possible medical risks, as well as strategies for quitting and getting younger. There are also many well-known clinics, and organizations such as Alcoholics Anonymous, that are extremely effective in helping break the addiction to alcohol. If you are a heavy drinker, the best RealAge plan for you is to quit drinking altogether.

As we stated during our discussion of cigarette smoking, kicking an addiction is no easy task. It was a real wake-up call for me when, as a medical student at San Francisco General Hospital, I went to an afternoon beer gathering for the medical students and residents. At the tavern, I was shocked to see some of the hospital patients who were being treated for complications of alcoholism, in their hospital gowns and with their IV poles, having drinks at the bar! That's how strong the desire for alcohol can be when you're addicted. That said, you *can* quit drinking. Start by talking to your doctor.

Walk Your Dog,
Even If You Don't Have One

One day I got a phone call from my friend Joy. Her husband George had been one of my patients before his death at age eighty-nine, and she often called me just to ask about health and other related issues. Now, however, she found herself in a quandary. Younger than George, and with newfound freedom, she wanted to travel and see the world. But her cocker spaniel Lucy kept her tied to home.

"Mike," she said, "I feel so torn. I adore Lucy, and she's one of my last ties to George. We picked her out together when she was a puppy, we named her, we housebroke her, and she nursed him right through to the end. The night he died, she lay curled on the bed right next to him, offering comfort. But now I want to travel, and I feel guilty about leaving her. Do you think that I should get rid of her?"

"Let's see if we can find a way for you to keep Lucy but have some relief from the full-time demands," I told Joy. Part of the reason I felt she should keep Lucy is that owning a dog is good for you. Pet owners, particularly dog owners, stay younger longer. Indeed, the RealAge benefit is as much as one year younger, and perhaps even more so during particularly stressful times.

Little research has been done on the effects of pets on health and aging, despite the fact that one third to one half of all households in the English-speaking world have pets. The problem is that it's difficult to perform randomized studies: can you imagine assigning a dog to one person, a cat to the next person, a hamster to the third person, and a rattlesnake to the fourth? Even if those people wanted a pet and were willing to care for one, those particular pets might not be their first choice. So most of the medical literature on pets deals only with the negative aspects of pet ownership, such as allergies or the increased risk of disease. These issues should not be of concern to most people. Even if you are vulnerable to allergies or immune diseases, you might still be able to have a pet if you really want one. Talk to your doctor about the possible solutions.

Unfortunately, most studies on the benefits of animal ownership have not been rigorously controlled, and the results are often skewed. Everyone involved in pet research seems to enjoy animals, and it is often difficult to be objective about the actual health benefits pets may provide. Also, one needs to consider whether people who own animals are different in other respects from those who do not. Perhaps they are more social and less stressed, which is why they wanted a pet in the first place. Finally, pet owners themselves are not all alike. Some clearly get enormous enjoyment out of their pets, whereas others see caring for them as just one more chore. To get a RealAge benefit from owning a pet, a person presumably should enjoy having the pet. What this means is that you shouldn't get a pet just because it can make you younger. Those of you who already own a pet can take comfort in knowing that your animal companion makes you younger.

A 1980 study on heart attack survivors found that the survival rate within one year of the heart attack was 94 percent for pet owners and only 72 percent for non-pet-owners. It didn't matter what kind of pet the person owned, either—dog, cat, bird, or iguana. Other confounding variables, such as differing life circumstances, could not account for the difference. In an expanded and more rigorous study, the results were similar. In fact, it showed that the survival rate for dog owners after a heart attack was even better. When translated into Real-Age terms, the heart attack sufferers who owned dogs were as much as 3.25 years younger during their recovery period than those who did not own dogs. Other studies have found that pet owners have lower blood pressure and lower lousy (LDL) cholesterol levels. Also, pet owners seem to suffer fewer headaches, cold sores, and other chronic infections, and seem to have a better overall sense of psychological well-being. It appears, too, that pet owners fare better during especially stressful times, suffering major life events less severely than those who don't own pets. Pet owners do not have as many bouts of depression, and maintain better self-esteem.

In particular, dog owners show the most substantial benefit. Cat owners often ask why this is the case. The real answer is that we don't know; the data on cat ownership do not lead us to a conclusive answer. And since I do not own a dog or a cat, I have no personal experience on which to base an opinion, either. However, the data concerning dogs and their effect on your RealAge are compelling. (By the way, if you want to calculate your dog's RealAge, try our sister website, *www.DogAge.com*.)

I assumed that all the walking that dog owners have to do might have something to do with the benefit, but the studies weren't clear about the reasons. William Osler, one of the preeminent clinicians of the nineteenth century, had observed that dog ownership boosted activity and exercise. After some ad hoc research of my own, I agree that the habits of dog ownership promote a healthier lifestyle. Speaking to some dog owners at a local park, I learned that dog ownership promotes other good choices in addition to extra physical activity. Having a dog often means keeping a more regular schedule, including a more regular sleep schedule, to accommodate the dog's need for regular walks. Also, I learned that dog owners who walk their dogs at the same park often form a social community, providing a support network for each other. All of these are factors that can keep their RealAge younger.

In order to advise Joy about her cocker spaniel, I took another look at the literature. The data were so compelling, it was easy to see that the health benefits the dog provided were worth the extra trouble to keep her. I called Joy and said, "It's true Lucy keeps you younger. I think you should keep her and find a dog sitter—someone you can count on to take care of her when you are away."

You should not get a dog just for the sake of your RealAge Makeover. Animals require time and care, every single day, and if you take on that workload unwillingly, you'll only end up feeling stressed, which will age you. It won't be fair to the dog, either. If you want to spend time with animals but aren't sure about the total commitment of pet ownership, consider volunteering at your local SPCA, which is always on the lookout for people to help with daily dog walking. After all, you'll get the same exercise benefits whether the dogs you walk are yours or just on loan, and the dogs will love you for it.

Of course, it's entirely possible that the benefits of spending time with dogs are more than physical. While Osler and others have attributed the advantages of pet ownership to physiologic benefits, countless pet owners believe otherwise. Many feel their pets give them an enormous psychological boost, something that in RealAge terms would make them much more than the one year younger attributed to dog walking. That may well be true. Most pet owners are extremely attached to their pets, and a high percentage of them find their relationship with their pet absolutely essential to their emotional well-being. Unfortunately, since no scientific data accurately measure this relationship, we cannot calculate a RealAge benefit for these emotional factors. The only scientifically reliable information is that pertaining to physiologic benefits. All we can say is that, for animal lovers, one more thing pets give you besides love and affection is added youth. And that's pretty hard gift to beat.

A Doctor's Note

How to Get the Best Medical Care

A RealAge Makeover Success Story: Sean

Sean's life had almost ground to a stop because of severe chest pain caused by arterial aging. He said, "I have hardly any energy, and I feel so old. You say I can actually reverse some of this and make myself better? That's the best news I've had in ages."

Susan, his wife, nodded in agreement. Things had taken a turn so fast. Just four months before, they had been touring the world, playing tennis and golf. However, the most active thing Sean had done in the last three months was walk from the living room to the kitchen.

Sean said, "You say that 75 percent of this could have been prevented. But we're beyond prevention now. The question I have is, how much of this can be reversed?"

I told him, "We know that at least 35 percent of plaque can be removed through diet and exercise and other changes you can make, and that 100 percent of inflammation can be stopped. That means that all symptoms and disability can be reversed and eliminated."

"I'm so tired all the time," Sean said again. "If I can reverse some of this and get my arteries to dilate again, how much will that increase my energy?"

I told him I didn't know and couldn't say for sure, but felt we should focus on the positive, and that much of the damage to his arteries could be undone through a RealAge Makeover. With proper changes in lifestyle, Sean could reverse his risk of subsequent heart attack, stroke, and impotence by 80 percent. Susan could get back the active husband she'd had just four months ago. I told Sean that it would be more difficult and would require more discipline to get younger now than if the situation had been prevented in the first place, but that it could and would happen, if he was motivated enough.

"Let's get started!" he said.

Sean did a great job on working to reverse the damage that had been done to his system. Even though it took three years for a complete RealAge Makeover, Sean felt much younger within ninety days. After three years, Susan said, "I've regained the active, vibrant husband I had ten years ago."

What did the three of us do together to help Sean regain his arterial youth and vigor? That's what you'll learn in this chapter, and much more: how to help yourself, no matter what chronic disease you are unfortunate enough to have.

The whole point of RealAge is to keep you out of the doctor's office. However, visiting the doctor for screening and preventative purposes can be a vital part of your makeover plan. Learning how to obtain the best possible care even before you get sick will keep your RealAge younger. Those who patrol their own health, learn how to manage chronic conditions, get regular checkups, keep vaccinations current, and demand quality care can have a RealAge as much as nine years younger than those who do not do these things. It's wise to evaluate your family medical history and your genetic risks, because knowing which diseases you might be predisposed to develop can help you counteract those conditions before they begin. If you do get a chronic medical condition, properly managing the illness can save you from much of the aging that it can cause. Being a savvy patient will help make you a younger patient.

- No one is in a better position—or is more motivated—to monitor your health than you. You know your own body better than your doctor ever will. You know if something aches, if something isn't working right, or if something has changed, even if it's just a subtle change. Persistence in pursuing your problem is key. So is taking it seriously when we don't feel good. One of the real reasons we may not feel good is that when we have illness we have an "acute phase" reaction. That acute phase reaction shuts down production of some hormones and increases production of others. Dehydroepiandrosterone (DHEA), one of the hormones that make us feel good, is shut down when we have acute illness. In the future, we may learn more about why we don't feel as good when we have an acute illness. Whatever the reason, not feeling well is a clear warning sign that you should take seriously, and that should get you to your doctor. Patrolling your health can make your RealAge as much as nine years younger.

  Difficulty rating: Moderately difficult

- You deserve the best medical care. How do you find the best doctor for your condition? You'll find out in this chapter. You may need to pay for tests that help you detect subclinical problems (before they give you symptoms) and prevent conditions before they affect your health, but it's worth it. It can make you more than 5 years younger. This chapter also tells you which tests you should obtain, and when.
Difficulty rating: Difficult

- How long did your parents live? How long did your grandparents live? Does the length of their life spans help predict the length of yours? What is the correlation between heredity and longevity? Learn how to evaluate and modify your inherited biological risks.
Difficulty rating: Moderate

- Only 40 percent of American adults keep their immunizations current, and just 47 percent of those who should be getting their yearly flu shots and their pneumococcal vaccination actually do so (even when the publicity about flu is as extensive as in 2003). By simply keeping immunizations current, you can give yourself quick and easy protection against unnecessary aging.
Difficulty rating: Quick fix

- Mixing and matching prescriptions, or taking medicines erratically or beyond the prescribed time course, can age you. Taking too many drugs can make you as much as 4.5 years older. But don't stop taking a medicine without consulting your doctor first; not taking necessary medicines can make you more than one year older.
Difficulty rating: Moderately easy

- The bad news is that the vast majority of us—eighty percent—will have a overt chronic illness such as diabetes, arthritis, heart disease, kidney disease, or asthma at some time in our lives. (Almost all of us will have test detectable disease; for example by age 85, more than 95 percent of us will have x-ray evidence of osteoarthritis). The good news is that in many cases we can manage a chronic disease and still be able to live healthily in spite of it. Getting a diagnosis of a chronic illness does not mean our lives are over—there are healthy behaviors that can help us to stay as young and vital as possible.
Difficulty rating: Moderately difficult

After giving yourself a RealAge Makeover and learning new lifestyle habits such as eating well and staying active, you'll find yourself healthier and needing to make fewer visits to the doctor's office for treatment. However, you shouldn't visit your doctor only when you're sick: your doctor is an essential part of your new RealAge plan. Over the next ten years, you will have to enlist your doctor's help more often if you want to stay as young as science will allow you to be. The science of disease prevention is advancing so fast that only your doctor will be able to give you the data and tests you need to make yourself younger. One example would be the test for high-sensitivity C-reactive protein, an indicator of inflammation in the body (explained in Chapter 4).

Keeping a clean bill of health helps us stay young, and detecting and managing new conditions in the early stages is the best way to prevent the aging they can cause. Learn to patrol your own health, looking for any early warning sign that something is amiss. Evaluate your family history, so you know the diseases you might be genetically predisposed to acquire. (Someday, a gene chip may be available and affordable, and you would be able to know what specific actions you can take to control your genetics and make your RealAge the youngest it can be.) By knowing your risks, you are in the best possible position to counteract them. Careful monitoring of any chronic conditions that do exist can save you years and years of unnecessary aging.

Patrolling Your Health:
How to Be a Member of the Age Police

A RealAge Makeover Success Story: Nathan R.

Nathan R. is a great example of how vigilant monitoring of your own health can keep a RealAge Makeover firmly on track. Nathan was fifty-five when he noticed his hearing wasn't quite right and his equilibrium was off. He was dizzy when he stood up abruptly. He kept having the sensation that he was going to faint, particularly whenever he expended any energy. He went to one doctor after another. The doctors ran him through all the tests they could think of, including an MRI (magnetic resonance imaging, a kind of three-dimensional x-ray) of Nathan's brain but couldn't find anything wrong.

Just because they couldn't find anything wrong didn't mean that something wasn't wrong. Nathan, who was feeling worse and worse, kept persisting. After going to several specialized clinics and seven different doctors, Nathan found a neurosurgeon who decided to repeat the MRI. The neurosurgeon also couldn't find anything wrong. However, Nathan was so insistent, that the doctor went over the images again, showing Nathan exactly what doctors look for when reading an MRI. Explaining how to read the images, pointing to the different lobes of the brain, the doctor began to study the images very carefully. Suddenly, he spotted it: a small telltale bump on a nerve, a tumor.

"It's so small that I can't believe I even saw it," the neurosurgeon told me when he called me to do the anesthesia for Nathan's surgery. Normally, brain tumors aren't detected until they are well over one centimeter. Nathan's was one third that size. However, the tumor was potentially deadly if allowed to grow too large.

"You're one heck of a lucky guy," I told Nathan in the recovery room after surgery. The tumor that was removed turned out to be a fast-growing cancer. It might well have killed Nathan in a matter of months had it not been discovered. However, I knew that Nathan wasn't just lucky: he was vigilant, persistent, and wise enough to listen to the messages his body was sending. He was saved not only by modern medicine but by his own persistence and savvy.

Because his tumor was discovered early, Nathan suffered virtually no consequences. After a few weeks of recovery, he went right back to life as usual. Since he already exercised, ate right, and took care of himself, his RealAge (around forty-five) was more than ten years younger than his calendar age. The only side effect of the surgery was some hearing loss in one ear. It's not much, considering the mortal danger he had barely escaped.

It's a great story, but it also raises some questions. If something small and vague began to affect you and lasted several weeks, would you see a doctor? If the doctor told you there was nothing wrong but you knew in your heart there was, would you persist in asking for more investigation? Or would you just hope that the problem would simply go away? Unfortunately, too many of us take that head-in-the-sand approach to our health.

The next story also illustrates the need for persistence in caring for yourself and may be more common than many of us had previously thought.

A RealAge Makeover Success Story: Ted D.

Ted D. was a long-term patient who in 1993 had experienced angina (chest pain) from severe coronary artery disease. As a result, he had undergone surgery for insertion of two stents. (Stents are metal springs that are placed in an artery after dilation of the artery, to keep the artery open.) When I first saw him in 1995, he was "chair-incapacitated": he moved from chair to chair, unable to walk or even to stand for any period of time.

We devised a plan to rehabilitate him totally through a complete RealAge Makeover. He began using a treadmill, starting at two minutes a day at 1.5 miles per hour (no incline), took statin drugs for cholesterol, lost weight, and controlled his blood pressure (with medications at first) and stress. By 2002, he was back to playing tennis, walking the golf course, and enjoying sex regularly. He had now lived ten years since his stent surgery, and ten years longer than his father, brother, or uncle had lived.

Then, on the tennis court, Ted noticed some vague discomfort, not in his chest but in his back left ribcage. We ran a series of extensive tests on his heart and arteries, but they all came back negative. However, like Nathan, Ted took the message his body was sending him—that something was wrong—seriously. He called me every day to tell me about his pain, and his daily phone calls led me to talk to his two cardiologists several times. What were the chances that all the tests we'd done were negative but that he still had heart disease?, I wondered. The answer was about 2.5 percent.

I debated whether or not to recommend coronary catheterization with one of his cardiologists. At first both of us had thought no, as we estimated that his chance of having a serious complication from the procedure (stroke, kidney damage, impotence, or even a heart attack) was also around 2.5 percent, meaning there was no clear benefit when we weighed the benefit against the odds of risks. However, when Ted awoke at night and called me, I decided it was time to recommend that he take the risk. He asked, "Are you just recommending that procedure so I don't wake you up at night?" But of course, that wasn't the reason. It was his persistence that led me and his cardiologists to suggest that he undergo catheterization, despite the risks.

I was gratified to see that the initial squirt of dye into his right coronary artery showed a narrowing of more than 95 percent near the beginning of the artery, as it meant we had advised him correctly. I was also gratified to see that the other coronary arteries looked better than they had in 1993 or 1998; the healthy behaviors of his RealAge Makeover had reversed his coronary artery disease except in the one localized area.

Coronary catheterization is a tricky procedure. The first attempt to move the catheter across the diseased area of the affected artery failed; the second attempt failed. I was getting tense and worried. On the third attempt, the cardiologist did it! He had succeeded in the tricky procedure and was able to dilate the artery. I was thrilled; Ted was going to be much better. He probably had a sizable risk, perhaps a 33 percent chance of sudden death with this narrowing, and yet it hadn't shown up in the two most common tests for detecting this condition. The tests may have been misleading, but the signals Ted's body was sending him were not. Ted's instinct to take them seriously, as well as his persistence in keeping us searching for the problem, undoubtedly saved his life.

How healthy do you believe you are? Comparing your health with that of others your age, would you rank yours as excellent, good, fair, or poor? If you say "excellent" or "good," your RealAge is probably a bit younger than calculated. If you say "poor," your RealAge is more than a bit older (see Table 12.1). Studies show that most people can assess the general state of their own health relatively accurately. That is, when something's not right with our bodies, most of us know it. One study found that those who ranked their overall health as poor were as much as twenty times more likely to die in the next year as those who ranked their health as good. This is not surprising. If you are sick, chances are you already know it. This statistic held true even for people who didn't know there was anything wrong with them; they just had a sense that their general health was not very good. Furthermore, at least seven studies, including the recent Baltimore Longitudinal Aging Study, have shown that the following fact is consistently true: Patients who suspect that something is wrong, even though their physicians have diagnosed them as being disease-free, are generally right. Something *is* wrong.

The sense that something is wrong may come from a decrease in your native hormones. When you have an acute disease or illness, your body shuts down production of some hormones. We know the mechanism of some of these. For others, we don't. One of the hormones that shuts down is dehydroepiandrosterone (DHEA), a steroid produced by the adrenal glands. In fact, we now know that if you are a smoker and have a low DHEA level, your chance of dying in the next year is more than one hundred fifty times higher than if you are a smoker and have a high DHEA level. That isn't because DHEA is so beneficial; it's because a low DHEA level is an indicator of acute illness in your system. Whatever the reason, you have a built-in warning system, one you should take seriously. If you sense that something is wrong, be persistent and do something about it.

It is difficult to quantify exactly how much patrolling your own health affects your RealAge. But there is no doubt that it markedly affects it for the better. For example, if you spot an early cancer and have it removed before it has a chance to metastasize (spread), you may save yourself ten, twenty, even thirty years of aging. For this reason, you should never skip routine testing: there are now many more beneficial tests available than even five years ago. The Cardiovascular Health Study examined three tests in 2,932 individuals over age 65; the investigators found that those without symptoms but with abnormalities on these three tests were the equivalent of 5 years older than if they had no abnormalities on these tests. Skipping routine maintenance on your body puts everything at stake—your memory, IQ, health, and enjoyment of life.

I do everything that I can for my patients to help them stay as healthy and to live as long as possible. I feel that is a physician's moral duty. But patients have a duty, too, when it comes to their health care. You are obliged, for the sake of your own health, to be as proactive as possible: you should take your medica-

Table 12.1	The RealAge Effect of Patrolling One's Health			

FOR MEN:

Compared with Others My Age, My Health Is:

	Excellent	Good	Fair	Poor
CALENDAR AGE		REALAGE		
35	33.8	35.1	37.7	40.7
55	51.8	53.5	58.7	60.8
70	68.4	69.6	71.9	72.6

FOR WOMEN:

Compared with Others My Age, My Health Is:

	Excellent	Good	Fair	Poor
CALENDAR AGE		REALAGE		
35	31.9	34.8	38.6	40.8
55	50.9	54.0	57.6	60.9
70	66.4	69.5	71.7	73.1

tions exactly as prescribed, explore your different treatment options, and research the people who are caring for you, to ensure your health is in the best hands possible. Not taking the extra trouble to do so can have devastating results, as illustrated by the following sad story.

A physician in the rehabilitation department at a nearby university had a seventy-four-year-old father. The father, who lived in rural Pennsylvania, had a very enlarged prostate. He went in for prostate surgery—not cancer care but routine surgery for noncancerous enlarged prostate. Should the patient have had drug therapy first? Probably. However, his urologist apparently believed he was a candidate for whom it was appropriate to do surgery right away. As the story is related to me, the patient did not investigate the local surgeon's background, nor did he explore his other, nonsurgical treatment options. He simply went in for surgery, as he was told to do. Sadly, the patient died right after surgery.

His son came to me to ask if his father had died because of the anesthetic that had been given. I looked at the chart; the answer was clearly no. The anesthetic was not the problem, but the surgery itself. His father had surgery for resection of the prostate for approximately two hours, a procedure that should not have lasted more than an hour.

I said to the physician, "I'm afraid your dad died of medical malpractice." I explained that when a prostate resection continues for more than an hour, there's a risk of transurethral prostate resection syndrome. This syndrome, known for more than the thirty years I've practiced medicine, can send a patient into congestive heart failure. The risk of this syndrome increases for every minute of resection that exceeds one hour. At the two-hour point, the rate of death or severe disability is over 10 percent. Although the surgeon should have been well aware of the risk of this syndrome, he apparently wasn't.

"How did you select the surgeon?" I asked.

The son looked down at his shoes and said, "I didn't. My dad went to him and wouldn't listen to me when I said I wanted to get him to a major medical center."

You, as a patient, deserve to select good physicians. Are all rural physicians no good? Of course not. But there are ways of getting the best care for yourself, no matter where you live. It's all a matter of being proactive, doing your research, and working in tandem with your physician so that you can both make the best decisions possible.

The changing nature of the insurance industry, and of the healthcare industry itself, means there is less chance that you will have just one doctor you see all the time. Many news reports lament the "sorry state of health care." But the news isn't all bad. We now have better facilities, better treatments, and better diagnostic tools. Which means that the best possible care is better than it's ever been. The trick is to get that care for yourself.

Here's a patient's e-mail that illustrates the power of persistence:

Dear Dr. Mike,
I've had migraines since age 5. As I grew older, they became more frequent and more intense. I went to a neurologist for years and tried many medications, including mega-narcotics. I even tried meds that cost $700 a month. I went to numerous pain clinics, but no one could find the source of my problem. At one point I was taking 180 Vicodin a month. I would miss a month of teaching because I could not move because of pain.
The older I got, the more time I spent in the ER. CAT scans consis-

tently showed that nothing was wrong, and I was told that my pain was psychological. But I knew the pain was real, and kept going back for help. One day my nurse practitioner saw me holding my neck and asked if I had ever had an MRI (which I had not). I had an MRI and within the day was told by my practitioner that I had a rare brain disorder called "Arnold Chiari Malformation II." The brain herniates through the base of the skull, cutting off spinal fluid. Since there is no room for the brain at the base of the skull, tremendous pressure builds up, causing unbearable, crushing pain.

I had brain surgery, was in intensive care for a week, and when I finally regained consciousness, I had NO HEADACHE. It was a miracle! It has been 3 years and I am still headache free. The surgery changed my life. I would like other migraine sufferers to know about this condition. I told two people who also had severe migraine headaches about it, and although the condition is rare, it turned out they had it, too.

I want to get the word out to others: don't let them tell you the pain is psychological. If something's really wrong, you know it. Keep asking for help.

D.Z.

How do you get the best possible care for yourself? It's more difficult than you or I think. The first thing to do, if you need to have a surgical procedure, is to be a proactive patient. It may seem embarrassing, but it is your body. You deserve to know. When you are about to have a procedure, be it catheterization of the heart or neurosurgery, ask about the number of times the doctor who will be doing it has performed the procedure. Always choose a doctor who has done it many times (more than twenty-five times a year is the rule) and can show you her or his results. Find out how many, if any, malpractice cases have been filed against him. It's easy. Go on the Internet. These are poor criteria, but you don't have the luxury of doing what I do.

What do I do? I call an anesthesiologist. Anesthesiologists are connoisseurs of surgical quality. They watch and observe the quality of surgery every day, and the quality of preoperative and postoperative judgments and care. I ask an anesthesiologist who the three best surgeons would be for this procedure at their hospital. (Do not wait to do this the morning of surgery, when you see the anesthesiologist for that day's procedure. At that time, he or she is trying to reassure you.) If it's such a small hospital that the anesthesiologist can name only one or two, personally, I would go to a bigger hospital. Other things you can do to obtain the best possible care for yourself include first finding a primary care doctor you like and trust. Choose someone who is competent, conscientious, and

Checklist of Tests for Men
(Yearly, Unless Otherwise Indicated)

At age fifteen, you should get the following:

- ☐ Blood pressure measurement (yearly, or more frequently)
- ☐ A dental exam yearly and teeth cleaning every six months or as indicated

At age twenty-five, you should also get the following:

- ☐ LDL level (you want it to be less than 100 mg/dl) every five years
- ☐ HDL cholesterol level (you want it to be higher than 45 mg/dl) every five years
- ☐ Fasting triglyceride level (you want it to be less than 100 mg/dl) every five years
- ☐ C-reactive protein (you want to test "normal") every five years
- ☐ A screen for diabetes (if you are overweight)

At age thirty, you should continue the tests above and in addition get the following:

- ☐ A screen for thyroid disease
- ☐ A test for diabetes and every five years thereafter

At age forty, you should continue the tests above and in addition get the following:

- ☐ A Hemoccult test for occult (hidden) blood in the feces
- ☐ An eye examination every three years until age 60, then yearly

At age fifty, you should continue the tests above and in addition get the following:

- ☐ A rectal examination for screening for rectal cancer and prostate cancer, and every year thereafter
- ☐ A colonoscopy (to rule out colon cancer), and every three to five years thereafter
- ☐ A PSA (a blood test for prostate cancer) and every year thereafter

At age sixty, you should continue the tests above and in addition get the following:

- ☐ A bone density test
- ☐ A screen for thyroid disease
- ☐ Tests for memory (like the one in Chart 2.1)

Checklist of Tests for Women
(Yearly, Unless Otherwise Indicated)

At age fifteen, you should get the following:

☐ Blood pressure measurement (yearly, or more frequently)

☐ A dental exam yearly and teeth cleaning every six months or as indicated

Starting when sexually active, you should get the following:

☐ PAP smear every one to three years

At age twenty-five, you should also get the following tested:

☐ LDL level (you want it to be less than 100 mg/dl) every five years

☐ HDL cholesterol level (you want it to be higher than 45 mg/dl) every five years

☐ Fasting triglyceride level (you want it to be less than 100 mg/dl) every five years

☐ C-reactive protein (you want to test "normal") every five years

☐ A screen for diabetes (if you are overweight)

At age thirty, you should continue the tests above and in addition get the following:

☐ A screen for thyroid disease

☐ A test for diabetes

At age forty, you should continue the tests above and in addition get the following:

☐ A mammogram

☐ A Hemoccult test for occult (hidden) blood in the feces (and yearly thereafter)

☐ An eye examination every three years until age 60, then yearly

At age fifty, you should continue the tests above and in addition get the following:

☐ A coloscopy (to rule out colon cancer), and every three to five years thereafter

☐ A bone density test

At age sixty, you should continue the tests above and in addition get the following:

☐ Tests for memory (like the one in Chart 2.1)

☐ A screen for thyroid disease

These tests will ensure that your RealAge Makeover stays on track. But, of course, the key is not just to obtain the tests but also to do whatever is necessary not to age should the test result be abnormal.

attentive to you and your problems. Your primary care physician should make you feel comfortable. If you don't feel comfortable, find someone else. Also, he or she should listen to you and be able to explain clearly what is going on with your body. Ask friends, neighbors, or pharmacists about the doctors they use, and consider such sources as "top physicians" guides. Also, you might want to find out where your doctor went to medical school and how well he or she did there. For example, membership in Alpha Omega Alpha indicates that your doctor graduated at the top of his or her class. Many HMOs or health service networks have services that provide information about their physicians. If a particular condition runs in your family, consider getting a specialist physician who is board-certified in that field.

Second, get regular checkups. You should see a doctor and a dentist at least once a year. Do not wait until you are sick to find a doctor, or you may not have the luxury of being able to see one you might want to see (few primary care doctors want to meet a patient for the first time in the middle of a night during an emergency); at such a time, you may be referred only to a primary care doctor who does not have enough patients to fill his schedule. And a clean bill of health is not a waste of money and time; it provides a baseline for how you are when everything is "normal." Then, if something does arise, you have a better framework for knowing what is wrong and when it started to go wrong. In addition, the more information your doctor has about you when you are healthy, the easier it will be for him or her to know when you are sick.

Remember the lesson learned from Nathan's story: if you sense that something is wrong but your doctor doesn't find anything, don't be afraid to keep pushing. Ask your doctor, "What does this test tell you?" or "What does this number mean?" And don't forget this one: "Is there anything else that it could be? Something we're not thinking about?" Part of your doctor's job is to explain to you exactly what is going on inside your body. If you don't understand what's ailing you, you won't be prepared to take the best care of yourself. Don't hesitate to get a second opinion. Or a third or fourth. If the second agrees with the first, you can relax and feel more comfortable about the diagnosis and treatment that you have selected or agreed to. Also, ask how to manage the condition. If the opinions differ, you will have a chance to compare them and reconsider your options.

Unfortunately, despite the great strides we've made in modern medicine, we still can't cure everything. Although we are discovering more about how our bodies work every day, many aspects of human biology remain elusive. It may take time for a condition to manifest itself in such a way that it can be diagnosed. However, the more aware of your body you are, the more likely you will be to catch a serious illness in its early stages.

Part of a RealAge Makeover is learning new habits, and you can learn to be a better patient when you visit the doctor by making it a habit to arrive prepared and informed. Write down your questions before you go so you won't forget any important points. If you've noticed a particular problem, write down your symptoms. Keep track of how often that problem bothers you. Make a copy to give your doctor. If you are going to see the doctor for a chronic condition, keep a log. If you have a pain that comes and goes, note when it comes and how long it lasts. Keep track of the foods you eat, the activities you perform, and anything else that might seem relevant. Write down all medicines including herbs, supplements, minerals, and vitamins you take, and the dosages you take. The more information your doctor has, the better he or she will be able to help you.

Even if a symptom seems too minor to be mentioned, err on the side of caution and tell your doctor anyway. Some conditions manifest in very odd ways. When something hasn't felt right for a while, it's probably not just in your head.

Get into the habit of doing research. Go to the library and look up a basic medical textbook, or use the Internet to find information on whatever ails you. A number of health information websites are run by major medical centers, and hundreds more are sponsored by organizations of credibility. For example, *Mayoclinic.com* and our own *Realage.com* are really excellent websites. At *Mayoclinic.com*, you can ask questions, as you can at the *Naturemade.com* website. Perhaps you will stumble across a description of exactly what you are experiencing but haven't been able to put into words.

On the other hand, don't be a gullible reader. Not everything you read is true, especially information that doesn't come from well-respected research institutions or hospitals. Some websites are not as reliable in providing accurate data for you. For herbal information, *www.consumerlab.com* is an objective information site, and if it does list a brand as substandard, you can be sure it is. Its report of a pass does not guarantee excellent status; if one of three batches passes its quality standard, that company's product is given approval as acceptable by *consumerlab.com*. So a failure means do not buy that company's product of that herb; a pass means only that at least one out of three times it will be acceptable. *Consumerlab.com* subscribers also have access to the Nature's Pharmacist site link that gives the benefits and risks of each herb and supplement, including all the situations in which you might avoid an herb. (For example, people taking warfarin need to adjust dosages if they take St. John's Wort.)

At the other end of the spectrum, I believe, in terms of critical review, is *www.supplementinfo.org*, a website on supplements provided by the supplement industry. I could find no mention of any toxicity or warning about vitamin A and smoking, or vitamin A and bone loss, or St. John's Wort and its effects on other drugs. That may be due to my inability to navigate the site (that is, the information may be there, but I cannot find it). Regardless, you need to understand that not all websites will be unbiased or provide you with information that gives the benefits and the risks. But as you learn more about your health, you will also learn how to distinguish what's likely to be true from what's likely to be rubbish. Remember to ask questions. What is it likely to be that I have? What could I have? What do I take these medicines for? What other things could it be? Do these medications interact with other things? All of these questions are important for you and your health.

Of course, the truth is that health care is expensive. People may hesitate to see the doctor because of the cost. And that sad fact is that in this country, not all of us can afford health insurance. This issue is clearly too complicated to discuss here. However, what we can say about healthcare with certainty is that, generally speaking, a few dollars saved in the short-term may mean many more lost later on. That is because the longer you wait to seek proper healthcare, the more likely the condition will worsen. Not only will it be more expensive to treat in the long run, but you will also be more likely to have experienced the aging and illness that the condition can cause. Prevention is always your cheapest healthcare option.

Is It All in the Genes?
The Impact of Family Heredity

We have already discussed the fact that more than 75 percent of aging (age-related disease and disability) can be linked to behavior and other environmental factors, meaning that you exert enormous power over how you will age, at least until age ninety or one hundred. But what about the other 25 percent? Exactly how should you view your genetic inheritance? How can you avoid the aging and age-related disease and disabilities associated with it?

The answers to those questions may change radically in the future. That is because the process of dealing with genetic inheritance will greatly change when a gene chip becomes available. Imagine if you knew everything about your genes, what would make them worse, and what would make them better. The U.S. Human Genome Project may make that dream a reality within five to ten years. I believe the gene chip will be ready by 2015. When that occurs, you will know much more about what to do to prevent *your* age-related diseases.

But we aren't there yet, and in the meantime our process isn't anywhere near as precise. One way to start is by looking at your family history, because the past may offer hints to what may happen in the future—although it's by no means a flawless predictor. (Note that we are discussing, for the most part, death related to disease. If a parent dies at age forty in a car accident, for example, that provides little information about how long the child will live, although alcohol-induced accidents are a possible exception.) Although many studies have looked at the family history of disease in relation to the onset of disease, only three major studies have correlated overall longevity trends between parents and their children. The Framingham Study, the "Termite" Study, and the Alameda County Study looked at the age of parental death to determine if it predicted longevity of the offspring. Did the two correlate? Yes, but minimally. Each study showed a minor effect. The Framingham Study, the most comprehensive of the three, found about a 6 percent correlation between life span of the parents and life span of their offspring, meaning that many other factors affect longevity as well. If both your parents lived past the age of seventy-five, the odds that you will live past seventy-five increase to some extent. But to what extent?

If you are a man and both of your parents died before the age of seventy-five, then your RealAge will be as much as 3.9 years older. If you are a woman, your RealAge will be as much as 3.4 years older. If both parents lived past the age of seventy-five, then your RealAge will be 3.8 years younger if you are a man, and 3.2 years younger if you are a woman (see Table 12.2). If no first-degree relative (parent, brother, sister) had breast, colon, or ovarian cancer diagnosed early, you are an additional 0.2 to eleven years younger than if your siblings or parents had those diagnoses.

Some genetic conditions, such as being a carrier of the BRCA-1 breast cancer gene, can make your RealAge as much as 17 years older (see Chapter 5). This is one of the instances where genetics can make a big difference. With BRCA-1, it's easy to say, "Yes, you must have bilateral mastectomies and bilateral oophorectomies (removal of breasts and both ovaries)." But, if you decide to go through that, and you have the BRCA-1 gene, you will make yourself seventeen years younger. I know that's easy for me to say: I'm not the one who will experience the physical trauma of surgery and the emotional trauma of losing the body parts that many women feel are at the essence of what makes them a woman. But I know the aging that severe breast cancer or ovarian cancer can cause. I have seen the disability that can result when people have gotten the BRCA-1 gene test and then ignored the results.

As I've said before, it's not that your genetic makeup has no effect at all on your health and quality of life, it's just that your lifestyle choices have a much bigger effect. Remember how the studies of twins showed that your choices make more than 70 percent of the difference in how well and how long you live? And that's even for twins who have just average risk of heart disease, stroke,

| Table 12.2 | The RealAge Effect of Parents' Life Span | | | |

FOR MEN:
Parents Living Past 75 Years of Age*

	Neither	Father	Mother	Both*
CALENDAR AGE		REALAGE		
35	38.3	36.0	34.0	32.0
55	58.6	56.1	53.7	51.5
70	73.9	71.2	68.6	66.2

FOR WOMEN:
Parents Living Past 75 Years of Age*

	Neither	Father	Mother	Both*
CALENDAR AGE		REALAGE		
35	38.0	35.9	34.1	32.3
55	58.2	56.0	53.9	52.0
70	73.4	71.0	68.9	66.8

*Make yourself 0.5 years younger at age 55 and 1.0 year younger at age 70 for every 5 years longer than age 75 the longest-lived parent lived.

or memory loss, or the normal age-related processes. With the genetic traits that cause severe disease, such as BRCA-1, your choices make even more of a difference than 70 to 75 percent.

When it comes to calculating the role of family history, many factors complicate the issue. Your parents not only influenced your genes, they influenced your environmental choices. We divide that into your genetic inheritance and your nongenetic inheritance. Until recently, for many people, if their father was a plumber, they were a plumber; if their mother was a schoolteacher, they were a schoolteacher. If your parents smoked, you smoked. If your family lived in Oshkosh, Wisconsin, you grew up and lived in Oshkosh, too.

We know that your genes account for only approximately 25 percent of how long and how well you live. Once you reach the late teen years, your choices determine more than 75 percent of the difference in how long and how well you live.

Remember, too, that just because there is a familial tendency for a certain kind of aging does not mean that that kind of aging is genetically inherited. For example, a family history of heart attacks may or may not be genetically coded. Smoking may be a habit that runs in the family: this is a nongenetic inheritance. Working in a steel factory where your Dad also works and where small bits of steel can go to your lungs is another nongenetic inheritance.

In general, you should review your family history for three factors:

1. a history of cardiovascular disease or any condition that increases the risk of genetic predisposition to vascular disease, such as too much LDL cholesterol, triglycerides, or homocysteine in the blood; high blood pressure; diabetes; or smoking;
2. a history of one particular type of cancer, such as breast cancer or colon cancer; and
3. a history of rare genetic illness such as Huntington's disease, Parkinson's disease, multiple sclerosis, or even Alzheimer's disease.

If more than one case of these diseases has occurred on one side of the family, you may have a genetic predisposition to that condition. The first step in determining if there is a family history of an illness is to count the number of occurrences of that condition. Then determine how these individuals are related to each other and to you. (Everyone must be related by blood, not marriage.)

A family history of a certain disease does not necessarily mean that you are genetically predisposed to develop that condition. It indicates a possibility, not a certainty. Even if a genetic illness does run in the family, there is currently no inexpensive way of knowing if you have inherited the disease gene or genes. In most instances, your odds of inheriting any condition are less than 50 percent. Even if you have inherited a predisposition for a specific biological condition that can cause aging, you may very well not adopt the behaviors and choices that trigger the onset of the disease.

Here's another example. You undoubtedly know a family with type II diabetes. There are certain people who have a predisposition to develop it. In fact, type II diabetes is thought to be a genetic disease with clinical manifestations at a rate dependent on many of your choices. That is, if you are a monozygotic twin (an "identical twin"), and your twin gets type II diabetes, you will get it 100 percent of the time. And it will age you. On the other hand, almost 90 percent of those who are diagnosed with the disease are also overweight. Many do not exercise and a large percentage smoke. When a person is genetically predisposed to type II diabetes, environmental factors such as weight gain, lack of exercise, and smoking can trigger the disease. A slim and fit person may well have the genetic predisposition but never know it, because the conditions that trigger the disease never occur. Indeed, taking care to protect your "youth" is the very best disease management. Living in a youthful manner can offset the genetic predisposition before a disease develops at all.

Another example is cardiovascular aging. As doctors have begun targeting high-risk patients (those who have a long family history of arterial disease and aging), they have seen the onset of premature aging diminish. By exercising and making Mediterranean (RealAge) food choices, anyone, no matter what his or her inherited risk, can reduce the rate of arterial aging. If a risk factor applies to you, you will want to do whatever you can to offset it. For example, if you are male and your father, grandfather, and great-grandfather died of heart attacks before the age of fifty, you will want to pay extra special attention to preventing arterial aging, not allowing the conditions to develop that would make you the next heart attack victim.

The genetic predisposition is not always negative, either. For example, in many instances we inherit a gene that can actually help us live longer. Some people have a gene that boosts healthy (HDL) cholesterol levels. This gene is a trump. All that HDL cholesterol helps prevent arterial aging to such an extent that the gene gives carriers a RealAge benefit of as much as ten years!

Immunizations: Staying Disease-Free

When we were kids, we all got immunizations. As adults, we can still benefit. Keeping our immunizations current is one of the easiest ways to prevent aging, although many people don't do so. Only 47 percent of American adults keep their vaccinations current, and just 60 percent of those who should receive yearly flu shots do so. Fewer than 50 percent of those who should get pneumonia vaccinations get them. Other vaccinations that adults should consider getting include hepatitis B, tetanus-diphtheria, and MMR (measles-mumps-rubella). Ask your doctor what you need. You can also visit the website for the Centers for Disease Control and Prevention, *www.cdc.gov*.

While you're hoping to take off years and years with your RealAge Makeover, keeping your vaccinations current makes a RealAge difference of only one hundred twenty-six days (if you are an adult involved in a mutually monogamous relationship). Not much, you're thinking. True, and yet those one hun-

Immunizations: What You Need

FLU

More than 35,000 deaths are attributed to the flu every year. I believe this number may be underreported by as much as two-thirds, as many of the deaths caused by influenza or pneumonia infections are attributed to other causes. Should you get a flu shot annually? Yes, according to the Centers for Disease Control and Prevention, everyone over the age of sixty-five should get an annual flu shot. The CDC also recommends that people who interact with the public, especially healthcare workers, who risk not only catching the influenza virus but also transmitting it, get annual flu shots. You should also get a flu shot if you have high blood pressure, arterial or coronary disease, lung disease, immune system dysfunction, or any metabolic disease such as diabetes or kidney disease, or if you are in close contact with people who have one of these conditions. Finally, if you spend time with individuals who are older than sixty-five, you should probably get a flu shot, too. In other words, pretty much everyone should get an annual flu shot. Why risk needless aging or infecting others?

Another benefit has been found in immunizing people against flu. In getting your flu shot, you reduce your risk of heart disease, because you reduce inflammation in your arteries. So, you are actually helping your arteries, which means less impotence, strokes, and wrinkling of the skin, as well. Perhaps if more people saw it in that light, more would obtain their flu shots. Getting the flu vaccine for the flu makes you about one-third day younger; getting it for health of your arteries makes you about four months younger.

Each year a new strain of influenza strikes, and each fall a new vaccine is developed to prevent that type of flu. Call your doctor or local public health agency to find out when the shots will be available; it's usually between September and November. Often local governments sponsor clinics for the public, and you can get a flu shot for free or at a reduced price.

Flu shots are about 70 percent effective at preventing the flu in populations under sixty-five years of age, and somewhat less effective in people over sixty-five. The shots reduce the severity of the symptoms in people who actually do get the flu. One study found that sleeping 8 hours the night before and after, taking vitamin E, and exercising, which boost the immune system, also seemed to improve the overall effectiveness of the vaccine.

PNEUMONIA

Pneumococcal infections cause as many as 70,000 deaths a year in the United States, primarily from pneumonia and blood infections. These diseases are extremely risky: 15 to 25 percent of those who have pneumococcal infections in their bloodstreams die, and 5 to 20 percent of those who have the most common type of pneumonia, a lung pneumococcal disease, may die. Mortality risks aside, pneumonia is extremely unpleasant.

The pneumococcus bacteria is an especially tricky germ, because it regularly changes its outer surface. Vaccines are designed to target specific surface configurations, and when the bacteria changes, the vaccine no longer works. Indeed, more than eighty pneumococcal strains are known to exist. The most common pneumonia vaccine protects against the twenty-three strains that account for 80 to 90 percent of all pneumococcal infections. The pneumonia vaccine is 70 to 80 percent effective in preventing infection in people under age sixty-five and somewhat less effective in preventing the disease among older people.

Who should be vaccinated against pneumonia? Everyone over sixty-five, plus people in high-risk groups, including those who have compromised immune systems, chronic coronary or lung disease, diabetes, or damage to their spleens. If you have human immunodeficiency virus (HIV) or leukemia, talk to your doctor about the pros and cons of getting the vaccine. Also, it is recommended that Native Americans and Alaskan Natives get this vaccine, as they are especially vulnerable to pneumonia. The pneumonia booster should be given every six years, because that is more or less the time the antibodies it produces will remain effective in the body. Once again, taking vitamin E and exercising help improve the body's receptivity to the vaccine.

HEPATITIS B

Two hundred thousand to 300,000 Americans become infected by the hepatitis B virus annually, and well over a million are chronic carriers. Acute hepatitis infection can be extremely painful, often requires hospitalization, and can be fatal. Chronic hepatitis B infection can lead to cirrhosis of the liver and liver cancers. In fact, hepatitis B infection is quickly becoming a silent epidemic.

The virus is transmitted primarily through blood and other body fluids, the major form of transmission being sexual contact. In general, hepatitis B is transmitted in the same ways as the HIV virus, except that hepatitis B is two hundred fifty times more contagious and can be transmitted in saliva. So, condoms do not provide the same level of protection for hepatitis B as they do for HIV. Even minimal contact with a hepatitis B carrier can cause infection. Because the vaccine is relatively new, the only population-wide immunization that has occurred has been for children under eight. Chances are, not you.

Groups at particular risk include those who are sexually active and not mutually monogamous; international travelers, especially those going to countries where hepatitis is common; men who have sex with men; intravenous drug users; healthcare workers or others who come in contact with blood or blood products; recipients of blood products, such as hemophiliacs; and those on kidney dialysis. Also at risk are the sex partners of any one at risk. Teenage and college-age individuals should be immunized, too.

If you have never received a hepatitis B vaccination, you will need to get an initial series of three shots (the same now goes for the recently introduced hepatitis A immunization). Ask your doctor or public health agency where you can get one for free or at reduced cost. Because the vaccine has only been available in the past fifteen years, it is unknown how often you will have to get booster vaccinations, although probably every five to ten years. Talk to your doctor, as new information will be coming out about this in the near future.

TETANUS AND DIPHTHERIA

Tetanus and diphtheria are usually given together with polio and MMR as part of immunization programs for children. Unlike many of the vaccines we are given during childhood, our immunity to tetanus and diphtheria wanes as we grow older, and many adults lack the appropriate levels of antitoxin against these two diseases. Several large screenings have shown that more than 50 percent of Americans over the age of thirty-nine, and 70 percent of those over age 70, need this combination vaccine. Admittedly, there's not much concern about tetanus or diphtheria these days. In 2001, only thirty-seven cases of tetanus and one case of diphtheria were reported in the United States. Nevertheless, these are serious bacterial diseases. Nearly a quarter of all patients who get tetanus die from the disease, and that number is probably an underestimation.

Just to be safe, you should get a tetanus-diphtheria (Td) booster shot every ten years or so. Usually we get these booster shots only if we go to the emergency room with a cut that needs stitches, so unless you've done that, you should probably get the Td booster. For those of us who patrol our own health, it is a quick, easy way to take out a little insurance policy against getting older fast.

MEASLES-MUMPS-RUBELLA (MMR)

If you were born after 1956 and do not know for sure if you were vaccinated for mumps, measles, and rubella, you should probably get an MMR immunization. Check with your doctor. Even if you know you've had one, if you work in settings where large groups of individuals (particularly young adults) congregate, such as schools and universities, you might want to consider getting a second one. If you were born before 1956 and never received an MMR vaccination, do not worry, as virtually everyone born before 1956 would have been exposed to these diseases and would have built up a natural immunity. The MMR vaccine is one of the safest and most effective vaccines we have, with an effectiveness of well over 90 percent.

dred twenty-six days can be pretty important. That's because this figure is misleading. Many of the diseases for which we have vaccines available, such as diphtheria or measles, rarely afflict adults. However, when they do, the effects can be devastating. Other diseases that are more common, such as the flu and pneumonia, are rarely fatal, so the mortality risk is low. Because RealAge calculations take into consideration both the number of people affected and the mortality risk, the RealAge differential for immunizations is somewhat skewed to a smaller effect, because if everyone gets the vaccinations, the chance of anyone getting this disease is extremely small. We call this "herd immunity." The entire herd doesn't, in general, get the disease. So even if one person is unvaccinated, it's unlikely that he or she will get the disease, because no one else in the herd has the disease with which to infect that person.

Ironically, in the United States and other developed countries, our vaccination programs have been so effective in preventing diseases such as mumps and measles among children that almost the only cases we see involve adults who have lapsed in keeping their immunizations current. However, other infectious diseases are still relatively common. In the United States, 55,000 to 70,000 deaths occur each year from pneumonia, influenza, and hepatitis B. Think about how many times you've caught the flu. Also think about how terrible it makes you feel. Five out of seven years, you can usually avoid the flu by getting your vaccinations (the other two years, the vaccination does not protect against that year's strain of influenza virus).

Vaccines and Side Effects

You may avoid getting immunizations because you fear side effects. However, the side effects are usually minimal. While there have been famous instances in which vaccines caused serious side effects such as paralysis, these occurred more than twenty years ago. The technology behind vaccine production has improved tremendously since then. Almost none of the vaccines prepared with current technology are associated with risks greater than placebo injection administration. In studies in which patients were given a vaccination in one arm and a placebo saline injection (no vaccine) in the other, the patients had equal side effects from both. In other studies, patients were given either one or the other, and again had equal complaints. Even side effects such as nausea or upset stomach did not correlate with the immunization, which indicates that people can feel sick on vaccination day just as they can on any other day.

Allergic reactions to vaccinations can occur, but are very rare. By far the most common type are allergic reactions to egg, as an egg protein makes up part of the measles, mumps, and yellow fever vaccines. If you are not allergic to eggs, these vaccines shouldn't cause problems for you. If you are allergic to eggs, tell your doctor. Occasionally, too, the antibiotic neomycin or streptomycin is included in various vaccines. If you are allergic to either of these antibiotics, alert your doctor just to make sure you receive an antibiotic-free vaccine. No vaccines currently contain penicillin, so if you are allergic to penicillin, you have no reason to avoid getting vaccinated.

However, when it comes to vaccinations and serious possible side effects, there is one marked exception: the smallpox vaccination. The current smallpox vaccination, part of the "War on Terrorism," is a throwback vaccine. That is, almost all the smallpox vaccines recently administered for "first responders" (for example, firefighters and police officers) were made by the old-fashioned vaccine development from more than twenty years ago. This vaccine apparently causes inflammation in the heart. The vessels or muscles in the heart cross-react with some substance that was used in production of the vaccine. You don't have to worry about this effect unless you're getting the smallpox vaccination. In fact, other current vaccines actually decrease the risk of inflammation in your arteries.

You may avoid getting vaccines because you feel you don't have the time. But getting vaccinated takes only about ten minutes. Finally, you may avoid keeping your vaccinations current because of the perceived cost. However, immunizations are not expensive and are usually covered by insurance. Medicare and about 35 percent of all health plans and HMOs pay for immunizations. In addition, many public health agencies routinely offer flu shots and other vaccinations free or at a relatively low cost.

So go ahead and make immunizations part of your RealAge plan. Call your doctor or nurse practitioner to set up an appointment each year between September and November to get your annual flu shot, and ask about any other vaccinations you might need. If your health plan doesn't pay for flu shots, remember that the small cost of a flu shot is probably less than a visit to the doctor once you get the flu or pneumonia. It is certainly worth avoiding the agony of the illness, not to mention the aging it can cause. Also, we now know that the flu shot protects against arterial aging.

Unfortunately, immunizations do not guarantee beyond a doubt that you won't get an illness. Although many immunizations ensure up to 90 percent resistance to a disease, flu shots, for example, are less reliable, offering only 45 to 70 percent benefit to predicted strains. Also, a person's resistance to disease often decreases as his or her RealAge increases, or if some other medical condition exists, meaning that an immunization may not be as effective. Nevertheless, when it comes to Age Reduction, nothing is as quick and easy as keeping your immunizations current.

Pill Popping and Mixing Medicines
Can Make You Old

When Sue C., one of my wife's good friends, phoned, she was in a near panic about her mother. "Mike," she said, "Mom's blood pressure is completely out of control. Sometimes it's at 150/80, but at other times it's as high as 220/150. She's on all this medication to control it, and she's good about taking them, but it seems like the medicine is just making things worse. She's been getting terrible headaches, too."

"Sue," I said, "if her blood pressure is as high as you say it is, it could be life-threatening. Bring her in immediately." It was hard to believe the blood pressure could be so high with medication. But when they arrived at my office, I saw that Sue was right. June's blood pressure was 220/150 mm Hg, a medical emergency.

After examining her, I asked June what medications she was taking, and she listed all five. I was puzzled. There were two drugs on the list that could have caused a negative drug reaction if taken together. But her symptoms—extremely high blood pressure and severe headaches—were not those that this particular interaction should have caused. I asked her about any vitamins or herbal supplements.

"Oh, I didn't even think of that. I'm taking several. But they're natural. They can't hurt me, can they?" Then she told me what they were.

"Bingo," I said. "We've found the culprit." An herbal remedy she was taking to alleviate sinus symptoms interacted with one of her medications, causing both terrible headaches and erratic blood pressure. They resulted in an explosive mixture that could cause a heart attack or a stroke.

I gave June some medication to bring her blood pressure down. I told her to immediately stop taking the herbal pills. Then I cut her blood pressure medications to just three, to eliminate the possible interactions. Within a week, her blood pressure was close to normal, ranging from 110/70 to 130/90. Her body adjusted to the medicine, and she started to feel great.

Then the second phone call came. It was Sue again. "Mike, Mom's been feeling super on her new blood pressure routine. In fact, she feels so good that she told me this morning she thought she would stop taking her medicine. I just wanted to double-check with you to make sure it's okay."

"You're kidding me!" I cried, not believing that I hadn't gotten my point across. "Going off that medicine so suddenly could put tremendous stress on her heart or the blood vessels in her brain. She could have a stroke or heart attack."

I called June and did something I almost never do: I yelled at a patient. I scolded her for putting herself in a possibly life-threatening situation, and I told her, in no uncertain terms, that she had to take her pills right away. June heard my message loud and clear. She didn't go off her medication, and she continues to do well.

Unfortunately, misuse of and misinformation about prescription drugs is not uncommon. In fact, it happens all the time: one doctor prescribes a medicine for a patient without knowing that another doctor has prescribed a second medicine for that same person. Somehow the information isn't communicated: The patient either forgets to tell the doctor what he or she is taking, or tells the doctor the wrong name for the medication (this is easy to do). The result can be a potentially life-threatening drug combination. Mixing drugs, taking medicines beyond their prescribed time, or taking them erratically can be hard on your body and can make you older rather than younger. This is a common American habit. Only 32 percent of statin drugs that are prescribed are taken as the doctor instructed; only 38 percent of antihypertensives (drugs that lower blood pressure) are taken as instructed. Is it the cost? No. Even when the medications are free, only 23 percent of people will take these drugs to reduce their blood pressure below 140/90 mm Hg, the American Heart Association's "danger zone." It is, I believe, the medical profession's failure. We do not communicate clearly enough how important it is to use medications properly, so that the patient is motivated to take the right medications and take them correctly.

Be an informed patient. Ask your doctors what your problem is, and why you should be taking the drug he or she prescribes. Then be sure to tell your doctors what you are already taking, even if they're just simple things like aspirin, over-the-counter drugs, vitamins, or supplements. Many patients forget to mention these, believing that because these substances are available to everyone, they must be harmless. This is not true. Also, don't forget to mention recent vaccinations you've had and antibiotics you've taken.

Taking pills can make you older if you don't know how to take them correctly. Table 12.3 shows the effect of taking a large number of pills. Statistics show that people who take too many pills without proper supervision have a RealAge as much as 4.5 years older. However, the fact that taking more pills makes your RealAge older doesn't mean you shouldn't take any medications. It's important to take the medicines you need, and to take them as instructed. Not taking necessary drugs, or taking them incorrectly, can make you many years older.

The surprising statistic is that on average, more than 15 percent of all hospital admissions are caused by the improper use of prescribed medications and the adverse interactions between drugs, or between drugs and supplements. In fact, one study calculated that in 2000, Americans spent one hundred forty billion

| Table 12.3 | The RealAge Effect of Pill Popping* | | | |

FOR MEN:

Number of Pills Taken Daily†

	0 to 4	5 to 7	8 to 14	More than 14
CALENDAR AGE		REALAGE		
35	34.9	35.1	35.3	35.7
55	54.9	55.1	55.4	55.9
70	69.8	70.1	70.4	70.9

FOR WOMEN:

Number of Pills Taken Daily†

	0 to 4	5 to 7	8 to 14	More than 14
CALENDAR AGE		REALAGE		
35	34.9	35.1	35.3	35.7
55	54.9	55.1	55.3	55.8
70	69.9	70.1	70.3	70.8

*These RealAge figures take into consideration only the effect of taking a large number of pills. They do not include the effects of nonadherence (not taking the medicines in the way prescribed) or the specific effects and interactions that occur from taking some medicines (such as sedative hypnotics) that increase aging when taken with other medications.
†Does not include vitamins.

dollars on prescription drugs, but that the costs due to adverse effects exceeded two hundred billion dollars. Hard to believe, isn't it? Does this mean we should quit prescribing or taking drugs? No. Drugs have saved a lot of dollars and years of life by controlling illness and preventing aging. It just means we all need to be more attentive to the problem of mixing drugs with other drugs, and with supplements.

The problem of drug interaction has gotten worse. The Food and Drug Administration (FDA), in an attempt to lower drug costs to consumers and to make medications more readily available, has increased the number of medications available without prescription. Drugs that just a few years ago required a prescription are now available to everyone, including such popular medicines as Pepcid (famotidine), Tagamet (cimetidine), nonsteroidal anti-inflammatory drugs (for example, ibuprofen [Advil, Motrin]), Rogaine (minoxidil), Imodium (loperamide), Prilosec (omeprazole), Allegra (fexofenadine), Claritin (loratadine), and nicotine chewing gum. Be sure to ask your doctor about these drugs, as they can have substantial adverse effects when mixed with various prescription drugs, herbs, or supplements.

Doctors themselves are at least partly responsible for many of the problems with drug interaction. The classic stereotype of the overworked and sleep-deprived doctor with incomprehensible handwriting is not far off: prescriptions can be difficult to read. There is a considerable industry push toward computerizing all order entries and prescription "writing," and these practices should minimize the problem. More important, however, is the fact that doctors and patients do not always communicate optimally or effectively. Doctors frequently think they are explaining things clearly but use technical terms and jargon that patients don't understand. Unfortunately, patients are often afraid to ask if they don't understand something, or they forget to ask, mainly because they are not feeling well or because being in a doctor's office can be a nerve-wracking experience. Several years ago, a patient checked off on her basic information form that she had had a hysterectomy. When I asked her about it, she told me she had had her tonsils out when she was six! I knew then that we were miscommunicating.

An informed patient is a better patient; ask your doctor about medication he or she has prescribed. In my opinion, there are seven basic questions to ask a physician any time a drug is prescribed for you:

1. What condition is this drug being prescribed to treat?
2. Do I have any condition other than the one this drug is being prescribed for?
3. Why should I take this particular drug?
4. What do I have to do so I do not need this drug after a period of time?
5. Does this drug interact with any of the other drugs, vitamins, minerals, supplements I am taking?
6. What interactions does this drug have with over-the-counter drugs or herbal remedies that I take regularly?
7. What side effects does this drug have that I should look for and call you about, and how do I minimize those side effects?

Don't feel self-conscious about taking up the doctor's time. You and your doctor should be partners in preserving your youth and your health. If there is something you forgot to ask while you were at the doctor's office, call back. You can also ask your pharmacist when you get your prescription filled. Pharmacists know about each drug and can help advise you on your overall medication regimen. Use your doctor and your pharmacist as cross-checks for each other: one might catch something the other one doesn't. Because the channels of information are different, one may have recently learned something the other doesn't yet know. In addition, the pharmacist who fills your prescriptions may be aware of medications you are taking that are prescribed by another physician.

Some people try to save money by keeping medication for possible future use, but this is a sure-fire way to get older. Once you have used a drug for its intended purpose, and in the manner prescribed, throw the rest away. Pills can change their composition over time. Also, by getting rid of extra bottles, you reduce the risk that you or others will take the wrong pill accidentally.

Prescription medications should not be used for anything other than their prescribed purposes. Never assume a medication that was good for one condition would be good for another. Don't take two pills when the instructions advise one; just because one is good doesn't mean that two will be better. And never take pills meant for animals—and the converse, never give animals medicine for humans, unless specifically prescribed by a veterinarian. I mention this because I had a patient whose sister-in-law was a jockey (horses, not music), and she took pills meant for horses all the time. Until she developed a complication. I guess it never occurred to her that horse meds might not be the same as people medications.

Remember, never discontinue taking a drug just because you are feeling better. The story of Ulysses D. will illustrate what can happen if you do.

Ulysses D. had a strong family history of heart disease. Although I was routinely taking care of his brother, Ulysses did not feel he needed a physician, even though his father, uncle, and brother had all died of coronary artery disease or strokes at ages younger than his. He himself did nothing to prevent arterial aging.

So, unlike his brother, Ulysses developed severe chest pain. Cardiac catheterization revealed a 95 percent narrowing in three coronary arteries, at sites not amenable to treatment with balloons or stents. He had two choices: bypass surgery or rigorous efforts to reverse arterial aging. He said he could do it, and he did. I was amazed at his discipline! He quit smoking immediately. He went to stress-reduction classes. He changed his diet radically. He started with one minute on a treadmill at two miles an hour and two degrees of elevation and built from there. He lost three pounds a week as he went on a diet and increased activity for the first four weeks. Then he lost about one pound a week until he had lost sixty-five pounds. Amazing! In addition, he took a drug called a beta-blocker to decrease his heart rate, stress, and blood pressure. He also took a diuretic for blood pressure, a statin drug for cholesterol, and an aspirin.

Then, one day, he decided he was feeling better. He had increased to thirty minutes on the treadmill at 3.6 miles per hour and twelve degrees, and after eighteen months, visualization of his coronary arteries showed real improvement at the narrowing. The narrowing of his arteries had not just stopped but had actually regressed: the three arterial areas that had been 95 percent blocked were now less than 60 percent blocked. He felt well enough to stop taking his beta-blocker without telling anyone.

You guessed it. A beta-blocker slows your heart rate. When he discontinued it abruptly, his heart rate and blood pressure shot up. Within a day, he was having severe chest pain, even though his coronary arteries were now in better shape than before. His heart rate was 120 beats per minute at rest. When he called me with chest pain, I went over his medications quickly. I couldn't believe it when he said, "Oh, by the way, I stopped the beta-blocker."

I said, "Take a pill immediately, call 911, and get an ambulance to the nearest hospital. I will meet you there." It was fifteen minutes in an ambulance for him. His blood pressure had gone from 120/80 with a heart rate of 60 just two weeks before, to a blood pressure of 210/110 with a heart rate of 140. That's what can happen when you suddenly stop taking a medicine you should not stop taking.

Ulysses was lucky: he didn't inadvertently kill himself. But what he did do was extremely dangerous. In fact, he came so close to a fatal heart attack that his doctor felt like he was going to have one, too. The moral of the story bears repeating: never go off medication abruptly, and never go off any medication without your physician's express permission. If you are prescribed antibiotics, for example, it is very important to take the entire amount prescribed. Do not stop after just a couple of days because you feel better. This is an exceedingly common and potentially very dangerous mistake, because the illness sometimes returns quickly and in a more virulent form. Because the bacteria causing the disease have already been exposed to the antibiotic, they often become resistant to it, and the drug no longer works effectively.

Another similar, highly dangerous practice is that people taking blood pressure medicine often quit taking it the minute their blood pressure dips into the normal range. What they don't realize is that doing so can be life-threatening. Stopping suddenly can cause a condition ("rebound tachycardia and rebound hypertension") in which your heart rate and blood pressure suddenly rise to levels that are higher than before the start of medication. Patients can put themselves in grave and mortal danger if they stop some medications suddenly. The subsequent changes can put enormous strain on the arteries and can trigger a heart attack or stroke. Even if they don't, they cause significant aging of the arteries.

To best serve you and to be your partner in your RealAge Makeover, a doctor needs your feedback. Your doctor can't know that a drug is causing a side effect unless you tell him or her. Therapy to normalize blood pressure provides a perfect example. Approximately 50 percent of patients who stop taking blood pressure medication do so without telling their physicians. The treatment is tricky. Because individuals react differently to different doses and combinations of medications, very often the dose and drug combinations need to be adjusted to find just the right drugs that work and don't produce bothersome side effects. By working with their doctor, most patients can find the right dosage and right combination that work for them.

Some patients hesitate to bring up side effects because they're embarrassing. For example, various drugs commonly cause two side effects that can be difficult to discuss with a doctor—impotence and loss of sexual desire. Several blood pressure medicines and depression medications such as Prozac have these side effects, as do other medications. Even though impotence and lack of sexual desire aren't mentioned to me much by patients, I try to search tactfully for these conditions. Male patients say impotence makes them feel and act older. Female patients also report changes in libido with various medications. Impotence and lack of sexual desire may be widespread, but they are very treatable conditions. If you notice that a medication is affecting you in this way, talk to your doctor. Don't be embarrassed. Usually, a different medicine can be prescribed. Virtually every week new information emerges about new ways to treat decreased libido. Testosterone creams and therapies appear to be a current mode that may actually make your RealAge younger by also decreasing aging of the arteries. Clearly as Dr. Lana Holstein (an expert on sexuality and women's health) says, you deserve magnificent sex, and it is possible and achievable for almost all of us, and should not be inhibited by drug therapy.

In summary, how can you keep your medications from aging you? The best way is to keep your drug regimen simple. Ask your doctor if you can reduce the number of medications you take.

Her are some simple steps for getting the RealAge benefit associated with taking medications.

- Develop a good relationship with your primary care doctor.
- Make sure you keep him or her updated on everything you're taking.
- Keep a list of medicines and dosages that you take either regularly or

occasionally, and bring it with you when you visit any doctor, drop-in-clinic, or emergency room.

- Choose a pharmacist you can trust and develop a long-term relationship with him or her. Your pharmacist will also have a record of all the drugs you are taking, or have taken, and can warn you about possible drug interactions. (Although many HMOs now provide drugs by mail, I prefer the old-fashioned drugstore with a new-fashioned computer, one where the pharmacist not only knows the patient but also has an up-to-the-minute record of his or her medication history.)

Now, of course, we must turn to the larger question: What if you have one of those conditions—heart disease, diabetes, arthritis, kidney malfunction—that require a lot of medicines and a lot of medical care? How can you prevent the aging effects of chronic illnesses?

Chronic Disease: Learning to Live with It

My friend D.K. Sui, a resident in neurosurgery, has a remarkable story to tell about his father. In February 2001, his father called him from Little Rock, Arkansas. He had gone to the hospital because he felt ill. For several months, when he talked with his son by phone, he had denied being ill. Now he had become very yellow and finally went to see a physician. The doctors did a series of tests, including a biopsy of the liver.

D.K. was annoyed. "Dad, why didn't you tell me? I would have come down there and gone with you."

"Son, I would have told you but I thought you were too busy. I didn't want to bother you."

"What did the biopsy show?" asked D.K.

"Liver cancer," said his father.

D.K. immediately flew to Little Rock to see his father and the cancer doctor. Over 50 percent of the liver, including the area where the liver receives all of its blood supply, was being invaded by cancer. The CT (computed tomography) scan of his father's lungs also showed nine spots in his lungs where the tumor had spread from his liver. The oncologist said that the average person with this cancer doesn't live for two months. In fact, in the experience of the Southwestern Oncology Group, a national clinical research group that studies cancer patients in the southwestern United States, the six-month survival rate was zero.

Then D.K. did something quite remarkable. He decided to give his father some nutritional therapies, as his father had lost about thirty pounds since D.K. had last seen him and was now down to 110 pounds. D.K. researched the alternative medicine, Chinese, and Vietnamese literature, and all the other literature on herbal, vitamin, and other therapies that have been shown to work for liver cancer. He started giving his father a specific mixture of ground-up fruits, vegetables, and vitamins. His father couldn't tolerate much else in his stomach.

Over the next two months, remarkable things started to happen. The cancer started to melt away and be replaced by normal tissue. Even eight of the nine metastases to his lungs (spots of cancer that are distant from the original site) seemed to go away. At nine months, the oncologist couldn't believe what she was seeing. She showed the films, the multiple CT scans, and the MRIs to other oncologists. No one had ever seen anything like it.

Every now and then miraculous cures occur. In the time course of the recovery—over eighteen months—the liver became totally normal and the lung spots vanished. This cancer became "immunology-sensitive": that is, the father's own body fought off the cancer.

Could that have happened without the vitamin and vegetable mixture that was given to him three times a day? Possibly. This miracle was so extraordinary that the oncologist started to treat all her end-stage cancer patients with the same specific mixture. The first five patients who were treated were all expected to die within two to three months. Yet three of the five experienced miraculous recoveries.

Coincidence? Possibly, but D.K. is now studying that specific mixture in a large randomized trial at one of the major cancer centers and has worked to obtain funding to examine this topic. He may have found a mixture of vitamins and vegetables that changes the proteins that this particular cancer produces. Those proteins may block the immunologic responsiveness of the cancer. Specifically, the vitamin mixture may change that protein into a different one solely through its physical and chemical means. That change may allow the cancer to be attacked by the normal immunologic responsiveness of the body.

What do I mean by that? Well, cancer is an unusual cell. It's not the normal thing, and so your immune system should fight it. If a proofreader gene doesn't spot the cancer cell and kill it at an early stage, the body should summon a system-wide immunologic response to the cell. However, we don't produce this response to some cancers, and those are the ones that kill us. Why don't we produce an immunologic response? It may be that the cancer secrets a protein that prevents the sites of immunologic action on the protein from being shown to our own immune system. It might be that the cancer protects itself by secreting protein. D.K.'s mixture may have knocked that protein protection away.

We will eventually find out whether the mixture that apparently helped

D.K.'s father so much will also help others. In the meantime, D.K.'s father had a wonderful outcome. He, like many other cancer patients, is living with cancer. Will the cancer come back? No one knows. Do most of the patients treated with cancer drugs get complete cures? No, many of them live with their cancer. You can live with cancer for many, many years. Learning to enjoy life, and living healthy even with cancer, can be a great joy to both you and your significant others.

Not surprisingly, I do not like the term "chronic disease." With the exception of a few contagious illnesses (HIV infection, for example), most of the chronic conditions that affect us as we age are not diseases in the way we generally think of the term—that is, infectious diseases. Nor are they usually purely inheritable genetic diseases, where the problem is something structurally wrong with us from the time we were born, and is therefore something we cannot influence. Rather, chronic conditions are examples of the body itself beginning to come undone as a result of aging. The image of a machine wearing down its parts is apt. These chronic conditions—heart disease, kidney disease, endocrine malfunction—are what we mean by age-related disease, or aging until calendar age ninety or so. Yet—and this is important—these conditions also serve to accelerate the rate at which other parts of us age, too. By managing such conditions, we can control, in large part, the degree to which whatever we mean by "aging"—for most of us, that's age-related disease—will age us.

Even though the ultimate goal of a RealAge Makeover is to prevent the kind of chronic conditions that cause us to age—heart disease, cancer, arthritis, Alzheimer's disease—the fact is that almost 80 percent of us will have a chronic condition at some point in our lives. You will know by the symptoms you experience that you have one. Since more than 95 percent of us will have osteoarthritis at least by x-ray at age 85, more than 80 percent will have symptoms of chronic condition. So the question remains: what happens if you get a chronic illness? How are you going to treat it? How can you prevent a chronic condition from aging you?

Perhaps the first issues one must address are psychological. It is vital not to succumb to depression or despondence, because a diagnosis of chronic disease is not a death sentence. Even with most forms of cancer, a person can still face a rich and vital future. Attitude, the so-called mind-body medicine of Chapter 7, matters—you can see that in the recovery from breast cancer of Patty Gelman—she wrote a book, *Humor After the Tumor* that is the series of e-mails she sent to her family and friends starting at time of diagnosis and during her period of living with the tumor and the treatment consequences. You can see that attitude helped her live with her tumor and its consequences. Every day we learn more about chronic diseases and more about staving off their effects. Such a diagnosis does not mean that you are now "old," but it does signal an important shift: you will have to learn how to live with the disease's "chronic-ness," and with the fact that it is a presence in your life, a presence that cannot be ignored without ill effect. Almost without exception, a diagnosis of chronic disease also signals that it's time to take your health much more seriously. If you are diagnosed as having a chronic and potentially debilitating illness, you will have to learn how to live healthily, and youthfully, in spite of it.

The fact that a person now has a chronic condition is certainly important, but how he or she chooses to manage that condition is perhaps even more important. For example, if diabetes is not managed properly, a diabetic can age at twice the expected rate: he or she will experience almost two years of biological aging for each passing calendar year. However, careful management of the disease can reduce the aging effect by over 50 percent, and as much as 80 percent. For type II diabetes (non-insulin-dependent diabetes), proper management can make manifestations of the disease virtually disappear, leaving no significant aging affect at all. Similarly, the aging effect of heart disease can be retarded by as much as 70 percent with proper vigilance, and, if the disease is diagnosed before significant structural damage occurs, the aging it causes can even be reversed. We see similar benefits of disease management for everything from kidney disease to neurologic disorders to thyroid problems. No matter what ails you, the aging damage that a chronic condition will have is always, always improved by proper management of the condition.

In fact, we should stop thinking about most of these conditions as diseases and start thinking about them as physical states of aging. States that accelerate the speed of aging. States that you can at least partly control. If cancer, heart disease, diabetes, or arthritis seem too remote to you, let's consider how you can live younger with a chronic condition most of us have or will have, diverticulosis.

Diverticula are small outpouchings (pockets) in the intestine that are filled with waste. By age sixty, 50 percent of us have them, and by age eighty, we all do. However, in the Nurse's Health Study, the subjects (most of them were women) who consumed the greatest amounts of insoluble fiber a day had 50 percent less diverticular disease than those who consumed the least amounts of fiber.

Diverticula do not necessarily cause disease. We can live with diverticula without the occurrence of diverticular disease. However, two hundred thousand Americans are hospitalized each year with obstruction of diverticula, a condition characterized by crampy abdominal pain, nausea, and fever. In the very worst cases, severe life-threatening infection can result from a rupture. So, how can you live with fewer symptoms and disease from your diverticula? Eat at least 5 grams of insoluble fiber a day. Insoluble fiber is found in many foods: grapefruit, oranges, grapes, raisins, dried fruit, sweet potatoes, peas, and zucchini, but espe-cially in whole wheat bread. Even nuts have fiber, and despite the old wives tale that you should not have nuts if you have diverticula, not even one case of a chewed nut causing diverticulitis exists. So, eating fiber (and any of the fifteen food choices shown to decrease aging that we discussed in Chapter 8) is another way you can live with a chronic condition that most of us have, and minimize the aging that that chronic condition causes.

Although diverticulosis may seem to be a simple and minor condition, in the twenty years between age sixty and age eighty, you could reduce your chance of hospitalization from diverticulitis from 18 percent to 9 percent. That's a pretty big result for just remembering to eat some great-tasting insoluble fiber every day, and a pretty easy way to keep your RealAge younger.

If you are suddenly diagnosed with heart disease, diabetes, arthritis, or some other age-accelerating condition—even cancer—what should you do? Your first challenge is to get into the right frame of mind. Instead of despairing or throwing in the towel, now is the time to take confidence in the fact that, with some plan-ning and care, you have the power to manage this condition. A positive attitude matters, and can make your RealAge substantially younger. Confront the situa-tion head on, do some research, and develop a plan. You will need to understand the disease in and out, and how it might affect and age you. Find a doctor who can work with you to develop a plan for disease management. (It matters less whether your doctor is a generalist or a specialist but, rather, that he or she is spe-cially knowledgeable about the condition and is caring toward you.) Read up on the condition yourself. Ask lots of questions. You can use the Internet or Internet support groups to find out a lot about the disease. The more you know and un-derstand, the better prepared you will be to fight the effects of the condition. Talk to your doctor about a well-rounded strategy for disease management, in-cluding diet, medications, exercise, stress reduction, and daily planning.

Great self-care is a vital part of the RealAge Makeover process, and never is self-care more important than when you are managing a chronic condition. That means not just focusing on the condition itself, but also treating your whole body with extra care. Those who suffer from almost every kind of chronic disease will want to pay extra special attention to retard or reverse more general aging processes throughout the body. Getting plenty of sleep, eating RealAge food choices, doing all three forms of physical activity, taking the right vitamins and avoiding the wrong ones, managing your weight, and avoiding cig-arettes and excess alcohol become key components of aging management for al-most all chronic diseases: these choices—each of them—change the proteins your genes make. Also, in a very real and a very large sense, they allow you to choose how much or how little that disease will age you. All of the things that can induce aging when you are healthy become amplified by a chronic condition. Whereas your body may have once been able to handle long working days, no breakfasts, insufficient exercise, or excessive drinking, the condition you now have will make the margin of error much lower, because your body won't tolerate as much abuse.

A Plan for Cardiovascular Disease

What should you do for cardiovascular disease? The plan below is what Sean (the patient I discussed at the start of this chapter) and his wife Susan have done, and you can, too. You can also slow down and reverse your arterial aging as Sean did, even if you haven't yet had symptoms. I suggest the following steps after you adopt a positive attitude:

1. See your physician and commit to working with him or her.
2. Control your blood pressure and learn techniques for relaxation and stress control.
3. If you smoke, quit (see the technique described in Chapter 6).
4. Start walking thirty minutes a day. Increase progressively but not more than 10 percent in any one week. After thirty days, add resistance exercise by working with a trainer for a period of time. Do twenty minutes of resistance exercises three times a week.
5. After sixty days of walking and thirty days of strength training, add stamina-building activities, under the guidance of your physician if you have coronary artery disease.
6. Talk to your physician about taking an aspirin a day, taking the correct vitamins and minerals, and avoiding the wrong ones.
7. Talk to your physician about adding coenzyme Q10 and a statin drug.
8. After thirty days of walking, buy yourself nine-inch dinner plates and work on portion control. Increase your intake of nuts, vegetables, fruits, olive oil, and whole grains, as well as flavonoids and tomato sauce. Decrease your intake of saturated and trans fats.
9. If you're not subject to alcohol or drug abuse, add a glass of red wine or your favorite alcoholic beverage every evening.
10. Work to find a job you love.
11. Find a partner who will work with you to keep you younger or educate your partner on how important it is to work with you on this project of reversing your arterial aging.

12. Make sure not to overdo it by trying to adopt too many habits all at once. Start small and then gradually work up.

You can take the RealAge test and think about other things to do. The most important aspects of managing cardiac disease are blood pressure control, stress control, diet, physical activity, taking the right vitamins and avoiding the wrong ones, reducing inflammation with regular dental checkups, and taking whatever medications your doctor prescribes (and never discontinuing them without that physician's permission).

A Plan for Diabetes

A RealAge Makeover Success Story: Elizabeth N.

Now let's consider diabetes, which is the sixth leading cause of death in this country, not to mention one of the most significant causes of premature aging. But it needn't be. The story of Elizabeth N. illustrates that point well.

Elizabeth found out she had type II diabetes. She was only thirty-four, and even though her mother and father both had type II diabetes, they didn't get it until they were sixty. She wondered why she got it so early. She didn't do much regular physical activity and was about twenty pounds over the weight she considered good for herself (her weight at age eighteen). She decided to be positive and to take action. Her first move was to see her physician. She was surprised to find she also had elevated blood pressure. She was even more surprised to find that controlling her blood pressure was the most effective way she could control how much aging her diabetes would cause her. Yes, she was very surprised when her doctor said that controlling blood pressure was three or four times more important than controlling her blood sugar levels.

Let's consider how all of us should manage diabetes, because Elizabeth N. did all of these things we will discuss, and she is now younger than she was when she first discovered she had diabetes, five years ago. In fact, she doesn't even know if she has it anymore, because her blood sugar is now normal, even two hours after a meal.

There are two types of diabetes, type I and type II. Although they have different causes, they have largely the same effect: high levels of sugar in the blood. Diabetes, if not treated properly, can cause arterial aging, blindness, kidney failure, liver damage, and, in advanced stages, limb loss and heart failure. Type I diabetes, sometimes called "juvenile diabetes" because the disease often begins in childhood, occurs when the body quits making insulin, the hormone necessary

Table 12.4	The RealAge Effect of Having Type II Diabetes*	

FOR MEN:

	Control of Diabetes	
	Poor Control	Tight Control and Exercise[†]
CALENDAR AGE	REALAGE	
35	37.5	35.3
55	67.5	57.0
70	90.0	73.2

FOR WOMEN:

	Control of Diabetes	
	Poor Control	Tight Control and Exercise[†]
CALENDAR AGE	REALAGE	
35	37.5	35.3
55	67.0	57.0
70	89.0	73.0

*Onset at age 30.
[†]Tight control of blood sugar levels and blood pressure, plus 30 minutes of physical activity a day.

to metabolize sugar in your food and to regulate glucose levels in your blood. In contrast, type II diabetes, or "adult-onset diabetes," usually develops after age thirty. Type II diabetes occurs when the cells in the body become insensitive to insulin. That is, the insulin receptors on the outside of each cell no longer react to the insulin molecule that signals the cell to break down glucose. Hence, blood glucose levels remain high because the sugar is not being taken in and broken down properly by the cell but is instead, staying in the blood. Type II diabetes can age your body approximately 1.46 years, or less than one year, for every year you have diabetes, depending on your lifestyle choices such as staying active and controlling blood pressure (see Table 12.4).

Type II diabetes occurs most often in people who are overweight. Although the reasons are unclear, excess weight seems to impede the body's ability to metabolize sugar properly. That fact would make one think that it was environmental causes—that is, overeating—that was to blame. But no, it's a genetically transmitted disease with what is called *variable penetrance*. Variable penetrance means is that if you're a twin and your twin gets type II diabetes, you have the genes for it, but how often one sees the clinical manifestations of diabetes and how much it ages you are governed to a large degree by your lifestyle choices. For example, when Elizabeth N. controlled her blood pressure, started eating less overall (and not any simple sugars), and did all three components of physical activity regularly, she managed to successfully normalize her blood sugar, even though she clearly has the genetic trait for type II diabetes. She probably won't see any aging from her diabetes as long as she keeps this regimen up. Pretty remarkable!

Type II diabetes affects 15 to 25 percent of adults over age fifty-five but is more prevalent among some groups of people than others, confirming that a genetic component is in operation. For example, African-Americans, particularly women, are much more susceptible to type II diabetes than other people their age. Indeed, 25 percent of African-Americans over the age of fifty-five have type II diabetes. Among certain Native American populations, the prevalence can be as high as 80 percent. In many cases the disease is triggered by the combination of genetic predisposition and lifestyle choices. If you "live young," you will have less chance of getting type II diabetes, no matter what genes you have.

Diabetic patients who take charge of their condition—vigilantly keeping their blood pressure low; doing all three forms of physical activity; flossing their teeth; and keeping their blood sugar levels within normal ranges by working with their physicians to find a regimen of pills and diet—experience very little premature aging. Even patients who do only some of these things—for example, lose excess weight, walk just thirty minutes a day, and lift weights ten minutes every other day—also benefit. Eating a balanced diet is important, too. That means decreasing simple sugars and increasing fish, fruit, vegetables, nuts, and whole grain intake. In addition, make sure you have some nuts or healthy fat about eight minutes before eating. Seventy calories of healthy fat (six walnuts, twelve almonds, twenty peanuts, or half a tablespoon of olive oil) is all you need to slow the emptying of your stomach so your blood sugar doesn't go sky high after fruit. Making these lifestyle changes can allow diabetics to reverse the aging effects of the disease altogether, suffering no more aging than their disease-free peers. Think of it this way: the diabetic's body can no longer create the conditions it needs for healthy existence all on its own. However, it is possible for the diabetic to make choices that create an environment inside the body that keeps him or her in an equally healthy state.

Diabetics should take the following steps:

1. Find a doctor who is a specialist in diabetes and will work with you to have tight control of your diabetes and no aging from your diabetes.
2. Prioritize yourself in your daily schedule. That means that you should not postpone your walk because of a deadline, but make sure the deadlines you accept take into account that you will walk every day.
3. Reduce your blood pressure to 115/75 mm Hg by whatever means possible (see Chapter 4).
4. Start doing all three forms of physical activity, first by walking thirty minutes a day, every day, no excuses.
5. After you have been walking for thirty days, go on the RealAge diet and reward yourself by buying a new set of nine-inch dinner plates for portion control.
6. After thirty days of walking every day, add strength training for ten to twenty minutes every other day.
7. After sixty days of walking and thirty days of strength training, start doing stamina activity for thirty minutes three times a week.
8. Add fruits, vegetables, fish, and whole grains to your diet and be sure to have nuts, olive oil, or some other healthy fat eight minutes before you eat. Avoid all simple sugars in your diet.
9. Add monounsaturated fat, and eliminate saturated and trans fats from your diet.
10. Learn how to measure your blood sugar levels and blood pressure and keep them normal.
11. Find a job that doesn't stress you or raise your blood pressure, or learn to manage the stress your job does cause.
12. Work with your mate or find a partner who will work with you on keeping yourself young, so your diabetes doesn't age you.

Although not all chronic diseases can be managed in the same way, many other types of diseases are similar to diabetes in the way they should be treated. Thyroid disease, kidney disease, endocrine disease, and many gastrointestinal diseases are analogous. The most important two elements in controlling the effects of these conditions are consistency and vigilance. Diabetics, and most others who have a chronic disease, have to monitor their condition each and every day.

One way to do this is to consider monitoring your condition as a job. Heather D. taught me that there are times when I don't want to manage my condition as there are times when I don't want to do my job, but I go to work every day because I know that's what I have to do. When it comes to exercise,

Table 12.5 The RealAge Effect of Sleep Apnea

FOR MEN:

Number of Apneic* Events Per Night

CALENDAR AGE	REALAGE			
	0	1 to 9	10 to 26	More than 26
35	35.0	36.6	38.2	39.6
55	54.7	57.1	59.0	60.4
70	69.4	72.6	74.7	75.9

FOR WOMEN:

Number of Apneic* Events Per Night

CALENDAR AGE	REALAGE			
	0	1 to 9	10 to 26	More than 26
35	35.0	35.9	37.9	39.3
55	54.7	56.3	58.1	60.1
70	69.4	71.6	73.6	74.9

*An apneic event is measured in a formal sleep study, and consists of the absence of air exchange (breathing) for ten seconds or more. Treatment of apneic events (for example, with a CPAP mask) reduces the aging, as the apneic events decrease or disappear.

it's even better if you can find a physically demanding game or activity that you really love, whether it's tennis, badminton, basketball, or swimming. Almost all of us have one activity that we love to do, and it's so much easier to be active when it's fun. But you have to do it.

A Plan for Sleep Apnea

Sleep apnea is another chronic condition that can be caused by excess weight, or that can occur for no reason. Five percent of men over the age of fifty have sleep apnea, which means they repeatedly wake up suddenly during sleep because their airway has been shut off and they are not getting enough oxygen. Most men don't realize they're actually waking up, although they may feel tired the next day. Sleep apnea ages you because it decreases your ability to have restorative sleep (see Chapter 11), raises your blood pressure, and adds to daytime somnolence, increasing accident risk. So it increases aging of your arteries, your immune system, and increases your risk of death or disability from accidents.

In most tests, snoring predisposes a person to sleep apnea. As you get older, the tissue at the back of your throat become less rigid and more loose. Surgery is one way to correct the problem. Another is to use a "CPAP mask," which stands for continuous positive airway pressure mask. The mask is tight fitting and pushes air into your airway. This air blows the soft tissue around your throat away from your airway. A third solution is to lose weight and reduce the "double-chin" inside your airway.

You can evaluate sleep apnea by undergoing a sleep study in which you sleep in a controlled environment with monitoring of respiration and brain waves. Analysis of twelve hours of periods of sleep shows how serious your sleep apnea is. People who have sleep apnea age faster (see Table 12.5).

If you have sleep apnea, it needs to be treated. Often you can know only if you get tested, because your partner says you sometimes don't breathe while sleeping, if you have daytime sleepiness, if you snore, or are overweight. Getting treatment will lessen the aging effect of sleep apnea.

Doing the Best You Can

Not all chronic conditions can be managed as well as Ulysses D.'s chest pain and heart problems, Elizabeth N.'s diabetes, and the liver cancer of D.K.'s father. However, all chronic conditions can be treated in some way that lessens the damage and aging that the condition would have caused if not treated. For arthritis, treatment means getting pain relief so you can continue to exercise and strengthen the muscles around the joint. It also means taking the right amount of vitamin C, calcium, and vitamin D, so that bone reconstruction is more normal. (In these ways, osteoarthritis can be less of a hazard.) And here a herbal remedy should become mainstream. The push that Dr. Jason Theodosakis started for glucosamine and chondroitin sulfate has been now demonstrated in four randomized studies. Since 95 percent of us will have osteoarthritis by the time calendar age 85 occurs, The RealAge scientific team has almost made this a RealAge benefit for all people. But the data are only for those with the diagnosis of osteoarthritis. This combination of "herbs" not only decreases pain substantially in over 50 percent of osteoarthritis patients by 3 months, but it slows and even reverses some of the clinical and radiologic symptoms and evidence of joint disease. Since so few preparations of glucosamine and chondroitin sulfate have the active ingredients on the label, see *drtheo.com* for the four or so preparations he has tested which actually contain what is listed on the label.

Even Alzheimer's disease, a condition with few effective treatments, can be managed in ways that slow the aging it can cause. For example, studies have found that Alzheimer's patients who participate in clinical trials, and hence are provided with quality medical care and better support systems, are half as likely to go to nursing homes within the same period of time as Alzheimer's patients who do not participate in such trials. Better disease management does not stop the disease, but does help stave off its most ruinous effects.

It's important, if you have a chronic condition, to consider in what ways the condition could make you more prone to other kinds of chronic conditions. For example, people who have arthritis may be less likely to exercise, for an obvious reason: it hurts. However, modest exercise relieves the symptoms of many types of arthritis. Furthermore, *not* exercising may cause the sudden appearance of arterial disease, arterial disease that has been put off because of exercise. That is, the response to one chronic illness (lack of exercise due to arthritis) may bring about another chronic illness (arterial disease).

Ask your doctor if there are any hidden symptoms that you should be looking for. Heart attack victims, for example, often have bouts of serious depression in their recovery period. It is unclear what the exact cause-and-effect relationship is. Does the heart attack cause a biological depression? Do depressed people have more heart attacks? Or is having a heart attack simply depressing? In any case, it is clear that those recuperating from heart attacks need to be aware of possible depression. Depression can undermine a recovery program, making it hard for a heart attack sufferer to muster the energy to change eating habits or begin a physical activity program—behaviors that speed recovery and help offset aging. Luckily, in most instances depression can be successfully treated.

It can be scary to be diagnosed with a chronic condition, and it's natural to react with anxiety and depression, which only makes the situation more difficult. After a lifetime of thinking of yourself as a healthy person, all of a sudden you have to reevaluate your self-image. However, because so many conditions can be managed well with close medical supervision and good self-care, much of this fear and bad feeling is unwarranted. Don't let a scary diagnosis derail you emotionally, or make you think that you have to go it alone. Instead, now is the time to lean on your support system of friends and family—or a support group of people who are going through the same thing (as we discussed in Chapter 7). Sadly, it is not at all uncommon for someone who is diagnosed as having a chronic condition to hide the news from loved ones, not wanting them to worry. This leaves the ill person feeling isolated, which creates needless suffering. Besides, those around the sick person always seem to know that something is wrong anyway, because such a diagnosis changes a person's behavior.

If you are diagnosed as having a chronic condition, use your social networks. There is a highly important choice for you to make here: buy a cell phone and use it for age reduction. Call friends and talk to them about your fears and worries. You will find that the people who care about you will want to help. They will help keep you on track, urging you to stay on that special diet, or joining you on your new physical activity routine. My wife enjoys giving people the book *Share the Care* that I mentioned in Chapter 7, because it's good not just for the caretakers, but also for the person who has the condition. It teaches you how to use a social network to live better and healthier when you have a chronic disease that requires the help of other people for care, such as some stages of cancer (often even the early treatment of cancer). In addition, don't hesitate to seek professional help from a therapist or counselor if you feel overwhelmed by a scary diagnosis. To ward off the aging effects of a chronic illness, you need to be prepared in both body and mind.

Be Eighty, Feel Fifty-Two

Eight Not-So-Secret Steps to Stay Young and Have the Energy You Want

The book is over, but the rest of your life is about to begin. How will you choose to live it? You now know what your RealAge is, and how to make it even younger through a RealAge Makeover. You have essential information to make informed choices about your health and aging. You know what factors accelerate aging and what factors slow it down. Evaluate your health behaviors and lifestyle. What will you do to age-proof yourself? You can reduce the rate of aging. In the end, the choice is up to you.

A RealAge Makeover Success Story: My Dad and His Friends

When I was writing the first edition of this book, my ninety-one-year-old father traveled from his home in upstate New York to spend the winter in Arizona, living in a community of other retirees, the youngest of them in their mid-seventies. I sent him drafts of the chapters, and he began sharing what he had learned with his friends. More and more of them developed an interest.

They formed the equivalent of a "RealAge Club": they'd get together and read selections, finding out what each of them could do to stay young longer. They started taking the right vitamins in the right amounts, avoiding vitamin A, eating more fruits and vegetables, and incorporating new "get-young" strategies as new sections of the book arrived. After reading about the three forms of physical activity, they jumped to action. The whole group—not one of them younger than seventy-five—raided the local WalMart. They bought out the entire supply of two- to fifteen-pound free weights, much to the amazement of the open-mouthed twenty-two-year-old salesclerk who looked on as twenty-five retirees in jogging shoes departed, barbells in hand. As a group, they hired a personal trainer to show them how to lift the weights correctly and to guide them through a fitness routine. They started lifting weights three days a week, went mall-walking another three days a week, and met for "happy hour" every evening to have a drink and spend time with their new "young" friends. They egged one another on to get younger and celebrated one another's successes.

They had a blast. They got younger, lived more vigorously, and almost certainly lived with more fun and less dependence than they would have had. Each day they were getting younger and having fun doing it. They read more, took more trips, and danced more. My dad changed from someone who was focusing on the end to someone who saw the future, was willing to explore and be adventurous. One day my father called to tell me all the different things he was doing to make his RealAge younger. Then he said, "I'm a negative ten years old, and waiting to be born."

All I could do was laugh; he had me on the floor. Then I said "No, Dad. Each number is the age benefit you would get if you did that choice optimally, and by itself. If you did two choices, you get less benefit from each individually, but more overall. The most benefit you can have, since you're a man, is about twenty-seven years. A woman can get about twenty-nine years."

He then said, with relief, "You mean I don't have to go back to acne?"

I said, "No, you won't have to go back to acne."

My father was so busy, sometimes I had problems tracking him down: he was often out on the town. He frequently went to New York City and traveled by himself. He knew more about the Internet than I did. He had friends, social engagements, and freedom, and there was no stopping him. When Mom, his wife of sixty-two years, died at age ninety-one, he didn't date for a year or two but then remarried. People always said to me, "He's amazing. To think, at his age."

Sure, he was amazing, but not because of his age. When my dad was ninety-one, his RealAge was seventy-six. Dad died at age ninety-six. I was happy that I could help him live happy and healthier. He had only a short period of age-related disability before his death. It seemed like a long time—two years—but that's much less than it probably would have been. The hospice movement in central New York is predicated on the idea "All of Life's Stages Are Important." Nothing could be more true: living as young as you can and making the end of life meaningful is what Dad did.

Following in my dad's footsteps (and hoping to go just a little bit further), I want to be the youngest ninety-eight-year-old I can be. Remember back to your youth: we once considered sixty-five old. Now it's seventy-five or eighty-five that we consider older. Many people live to ninety or ninety-five years of age, and doing so with vigor and energy should be the rule, not the exception.

Ninety-eight is really a remarkable increase in focus in just thirty or forty years. That's about the rate we're now increasing the healthy life span: about two-tenths to four-tenths of a year for every year we live. That means that at the present rate of change, twenty years from now you will probably be able to achieve a quality life span that is four to eight years longer than it is today. Also, that increase would occur without the radical breakthrough I spoke of in Chapter 1, the ability to keep the nonnuclear DNA much younger and thus influence the basic rate of aging (the mitochondrial aging theory). The data increasingly show that as long as you make changes before the point of irreversibility—such as the entry of calcium into the plaques in your arteries, or the propagation of too many cancer cells—the changes you make today will make a huge difference in your RealAge within ninety days. It is almost never too late to start to get younger. You can actually pull the lipid out of calcified plaque; it is just that while the calcium in the plaque will not prohibit you from making the artery younger, it will not be as young an artery as it once was. It really is almost never too late to start to get younger.

The RealAge program allows you to buy time and to understand what your biological potential is. The younger your RealAge, the more possibilities, choices, and freedom you will have, to do what you want with your life. The younger you make your RealAge, the more time you will have to spend with your friends and family, to develop new interests, and to do whatever it is that makes you enjoy life. For me, a younger RealAge gives me more energy to let you and others know that you can control your genes and be younger if you want to be—to make sure you know the choice is yours, and that it's not that tough to do. Don't let ill health keep you from being who you want to be.

As life expectancy has increased dramatically in the past century, especially in the past thirty years, medical researchers have been faced with a major ethical dilemma: are we extending the quantity of life at the expense of quality of life? With expensive life support machines and new technologies that can keep people alive longer and longer, doctors have worried that perhaps all this effort has only extended suffering, making patients endure painful diseases longer, living out their final years in misery. But this is not true.

New studies show that most Americans can expect to live long lives (that is, to the national averages) without major illness or disability. However, there is enormous variation within the population. When studies have examined those who live the longest with the greatest mobility and independence, they have found that individuals at the top of the curve tended to make the same behavioral choices. Even at the end of their lives, these people had less illness, and briefer illnesses, than those who didn't make those choices. The period of decline tended to be compressed and lessened, as in my dad's case. In these same studies, those who had the most illness and incapacitation didn't adopt those healthy behaviors, and they got older faster. They had shorter life expectancies and spent more time in hospitals and doctors' offices.

Clearly, there are no sound statistical measures of "quality of life." It is a subjective indicator. Some people are always happy no matter what; others are never happy. However, by looking at the data, we can draw certain conclusions. A person who is healthy has a better quality of life than the person who needs to be under strict medical supervision. Also, a person who is mobile, lives independently, and is disease-free has a better quality of life than the person who is hospitalized. Those aren't giant leaps of logic.

Before you even picked up this book, you were probably aware of all kinds of behavioral choices that were "good" for you. Did you adopt those behaviors? I hope this book has helped you to view your health in a new light. Rather than seeing these decisions as prevention of disease, I hope you now see them as preventing aging. Thinking about "disease prevention"—the classic way preventive medicine has modeled itself—is disheartening. Perhaps it's too daunting a project, or its benefits seem too far off. Moreover, we think of disease in black or white terms: you're either sick or you're not. However, this description doesn't fit the reality of human health. Most of the "old-age" diseases are not actually diseases so much as manifestations of the aging process itself. And you can largely control how almost any disease affects you.

RealAge is a way of understanding that everything you do—from walking the dog to brushing your teeth—affects your rate of aging. Adopting healthy habits means not just that you prevent disease, but that you live longer—and younger. By giving yourself a RealAge Makeover, you increase the length of that part of your life that's vigorous and productive.

When I think about why I became a doctor in the first place, I realize that my decision can be summed up in one word: prevention. I never wanted to cure people after they were already ill; I wanted to help them avoid illness in the first place. Life is too much fun to spend time being sick. Yet, until now, prevention has been thought of in terms of far-off, negative goals. "I won't eat unhealthy foods today so that I don't have a heart attack thirty years from now." However, prevention isn't a negative goal but a positive one. Preventing aging is gaining health. The payoff is not thirty years in the future but right now. I'll eat RealAge-smart foods today so I'll have more energy today and tomorrow. I'll fix that dripping faucet today so that I'll have less stress now and more energy now and tomorrow. I'll fill out that expense report on the airplane while traveling home rather than let it linger and naggingly stress me for three more days.

If you've made it this far through this book, you know in tangible and practical terms how you can prevent and even reverse aging. So where should you start?

- First, write down your RealAge. Look at that number. Are you happy with it, or would you like to make it younger? What will you do to change it?
- Second, review your Age-Reduction Plan (see Chapter 3). What choices can you make to make your RealAge younger? Are they practical choices for you? In light of what you've read, are you willing to make choices that two hundred pages ago you wouldn't have made?
- Third, establish priorities. Consider how and when you want to add new Age-Reduction strategies to your life. Set realistic goals and decide what steps you can take to meet them. What are the quick-and-easy strategies you can adopt for getting younger with hardly any effort at all? What are those antiaging strategies that require more work? How will you integrate them into your life?
- Fourth, start small. Don't overwhelm yourself by trying to do too much at once. Begin with the "quick fixes," integrating new Age-Reduction practices slowly, especially if they are in the "most difficult" category. After all, you're in this for the long run. It's more important that you stick with your Age-Reduction Plan than that you do every possible Age-Reduction step right now, only to give them all up after a few weeks or months. Where do I start, for example, when advising my own patients? I recommend that they start with thirty minutes of walking a day, adding an aspirin a day, and taking the right vitamins and avoiding the wrong ones. Thirty days later I ask my patients to reward themselves by buying small dinner plates and hiring a personal trainer to teach them how to do resistance exercises, or by taking a class at a local health club.
- Fifth, reevaluate. Often. Review your Age-Reduction Plan every few months. Is it time to add a new strategy? I have patients who add one new antiaging practice to their life every year—a kind of New Year's resolution.
- Sixth, don't give up, even if you slip up. Eddie E. (see Chapter 6) called me about seven weeks into his smoking cessation program and said, "Doc, I had a cigar last night. What do I do?" I said, "Eddie, it's not the end of the world. You fell off the wagon with one cigar. Go

back and keep walking and put the patch on and keep taking the pill. You'll make it." Eddie hasn't had a cigar or cigarette in more than a year since. Don't give up. Keep pushing younger. Getting younger is not that hard. A few simple choices can help make you five to seven years younger in just a few months. Other choices can help reduce your RealAge by as much as twenty-nine years. Most of the benefits can be achieved by making simple choices that do not take much time or effort, just some practice.

- Seventh, you are never too old to start getting young. It doesn't matter if you're a lifelong smoker, if you've had a heart attack, or if you've suffered any number of other conditions. You can undo much of the aging that you have already incurred by making changes now. Our bodies are remarkably resilient, and it is within your power to undo years of unnecessary aging. When Drs. John Wallis Rowe and Robert L. Kahn interpreted the results of the long-term, multidisciplinary MacArthur Foundation Study of Successful Aging, they said, "There is increasing evidence of the remarkable capacity to recover lost function." Yes, you can get young again.

- Eighth, and most important, celebrate successes. Reward yourself for becoming younger. Whether you decide to throw yourself a "year-younger" party or to treat yourself to a massage after a month of daily workouts, you need to congratulate yourself for getting younger. People will say you look younger, too; and you will. Making your arteries younger makes your skin look younger from the inside out. And if you choose all three forms of exercise your muscles will be firmer, helping you look younger still. (Don't forget to celebrate the year-younger successes of those around you, too. By encouraging someone close to you to get younger, you are giving yourself a gift. You are helping those you care about to stay young with you.)

Think of RealAge planning as retirement planning. Most of us spend time in our forties and fifties making investments and setting up a pension fund or an individual retirement account, planning for that day when we no longer have to go to the office. RealAge is retirement planning for your body, an age-insurance plan. Your RealAge is a calculation of your net present value. It is a way of calculating how old your body really is. The choices you make affect that value. You build value by building youth.

Several years ago, my friend Simon called me. (Remember him from Chapter 1? He was the first person I convinced to stop smoking using the RealAge concept.) "Mike," he shouted exuberantly into the phone, "I'm a grandfather!"

At age sixty-two (and a RealAge of fifty-seven), he had lived to see the birth of his first grandson. It was nothing short of a miracle.

Thirteen years earlier, when Simon was barely able to walk and in need of a dangerous operation, none of us—not his family, not me, and not Simon—would have believed that he'd live to see the day when he'd become a grandfather. Much less, live to see that day as an energetic, physically fit, and young grandfather. "Simon," I laughed, "you're not old enough to be a grandfather."

Simon made choices that did not merely save his life but actually gave him back his life. Eighteen years ago (his first grandchild is now five years old) he couldn't walk across a room without pain. Now he's playing tennis and challenging me to squash matches. He's tackled some of the toughest challenges in Age Reduction: cessation of smoking, exercising, and eating a more healthful diet. He's done it slowly, adding bit by bit. Each year, he reevaluates his antiaging plan, integrating new choices and behaviors. He's living younger now than he did eighteen years ago. The payoff has been huge. He's seen his kids get married, he's traveled, and he's enjoying his life. He even retired early, so he could have more fun. (Now he's feeling so young, he's been threatening to come out of retirement!)

There is a debate in the medical scientific community on aging: whether you can only slow it, or actually reverse it. I believe that the data indicating you can reverse aging are so strong that I'd bet on it. Not all of my colleagues have always agreed. University of Illinois biodemographer Jay Olshansky, one of the proponents of the nonreversal theory, stated in 1993 that we would never extend the average life span in the United States by more than a trivial amount, because it's already as long as it will get. Of course, by 2002, he had already been proved wrong. In that nine years, we have extended the life span by 2.9 years on average in America. And that's about the rate we're doing it. We're gaining two to four years every ten years. The data are clear: the studies of Dean Ornish, the Cleveland Clinic, the Cooper Clinic, and many other groups show that you can actually diminish plaque size and reverse arterial aging. You can pull the LDL cholesterol out. I've seen reversal with Ulysses D., Kevin D., Maureen K., Eddie E., Sean, and many, many, patients. It isn't just slowing your rate of aging; you can actually reverse aging. I hope this book will inspire you to do just that.

In my own practice, and even in my own life, I see that RealAge motivates people to change their behaviors and to choose youth. I see how my own patients have stopped smoking, lost weight, and made choices that helped them stay young. I see how it has helped me learn to eat a healthier diet and be more balanced in my exercise regimen. RealAge has encouraged my friends to start lifting weights and has helped my wife to start taking her calcium regularly. RealAge helps us place a value on our daily choices, choices that are easy to overlook but that help us stay young. (Every time I take the stairs instead of the elevator, I remember that it is helping me stay younger. Every time I choose an apple over a cookie, I think that, too.) I hope that RealAge helps motivate you. By giving yourself a RealAge Makeover, you are buying time to do more and be more, to enjoy life like you've always wanted. What could be more promising than that? Stay young from the inside out—for the rest of your life.

Key References

CHAPTER 1

Baird J, Osmond C, Bowes C. Mortality from birth to adult life: a longitudinal study of twins. *Early Human Development* 1998;53:73–79.

Fraser GE, Shavlik DJ. Risk Factors for All-Cause and Coronary Heart Disease Mortality in the Oldest-Old. *Archives of Internal Medicine* 1997;157:2249–2258.

Greenland P, Knoll MD, Stamler J, et al. Major Risk Factors as Antecedents of Fatal and Nonfatal Coronary Heart Disease Events. *JAMA* 2003;290:891–897.

Harrap SB, Stebbing M, Hopper JL, et al. Familial Patterns of Covariation for Cardiovascular Risk Factors in Adults. The Victorian Family Heart Study. *American Journal of Epidemiology* 2000;152:704–715.

Khot UN, Khot MB, Bajzer CT, et al. Prevalence of Conventional Risk Factors in Patients with Coronary Heart Disease. *JAMA* 2003;290:898–904.

Reed T, Carmelli D, Swan GE, et al. Ten-Year Follow-Up for Male Twins Divided into High or Low Risk Groups for Ischemic Heart Disease Based on Risk Factors Measured 25 Years Previously. *Annals of Epidemiology* 2000;10:278–284.

Vaupel JW, Carey JR, Christensen K, et al. Biodemographic trajectories of longevity. *Science* 1998;280:855–860.

Vita AJ, Terry RB, Hubert HB, et al. Aging, health risks, and cumulative disability. *New England Journal of Medicine* 1998;338:1035–1041.

Wright JC, Weinstein MC. Gains in life expectancy from medical interventions standardizing data on outcomes. *New England Journal of Medicine* 1998;339:380–386.

Zdravkovic S, Wienke A, Pedersen NL, et al. Heritability of death from coronary heart disease: a 36-year follow-up of 20,966 Swedish twins. *Journal of Internal Medicine* 2002;252:247–254.

CHAPTER 2

Fraser GE, Lindsted KD, Beeson WL. Effect of risk factor values on lifetime risk of and age at first coronary event. The Adventist health study. *American Journal of Epidemiology* 1995;142:746–758.

Goldberg RJ, Larson M, Levy D. Factors associated with survival to 75 years of age in middle-aged men and women. The Framingham study. *Archives of Internal Medicine* 1996;156:505–509.

Gulati M, Pandey DK, Arnsdorf MF, et al. Exercise Capacity and the Risk of Death in Women. *Circulation* 2003;108:1554–1559.

Hu FB. The Mediterranean Diet and Mortality. Olive Oil and Beyond. *New England Journal of Medicine* 2003;348:2595–2596.

Lindqvist P, Bengtsson C, Lissner L, et al. Cholesterol and triglyceride concentration as risk factors for myocardial infarction and death in women, with special reference to influence of age. *Journal of Internal Medicine* 2002;251:484–489.

Sharrett AR, Ballantyne CM, Coady SA, et al. Coronary Heart Disease Prediction from Lipoprotein Cholesterol Levels, Triglycerides, Lipoprotein (a), Apolipoproteins A-I and B, and HDL Density Subfractions. The Atherosoclerosis Risk in Communities (ARIC) study. *Circulation* 2001;104:1108–1113.

CHAPTER 3

Canto JG, Iskandrian AE. Major Risk Factors for Cardiovascular Disease. *JAMA* 2003;290:947–949.

Trichopoulou A, Costacou T, Bamia C, Trichopoulos D. Adherence to a Mediterranean diet and survival in a Greek population. *New England Journal of Medicine* 2003;348:2599–2608.

Tunstall-Pedoe H, Woodward M, Tavendale R, et al. Comparison of the prediction by 27 different factors of coronary heart disease and death in men and women of the Scottish heart health study: cohort study. *BMJ* 1997;315:722–729.

CHAPTER 4

Blood Pressure

Anonymous. Prevention of stroke by antihypertensive drug treatment in older persons with isolated systolic hypertension. Final results of systolic hypertension in the elderly program (SHEP). *JAMA* 1991;265:3255.

Antihypertensive and Lipid-Lowering Treatment to Prevent Heart Attack Trial Collaborative Research Group. Diurtetic Versus alpha-blocker as First-Step Antihypertensive Therapy: Final Results From the Antihypertensive and Lipid-Lowering Treatment to Prevent Heart Attack Trial (ALLHAT). *Hypertension* 2003;42:239–246.

Curb JD, Pressel SL, Cutler JA, et al. Effect of diuretic-based antihypertensive treatment on cardiovascular disease risk in older diabetic patients with isolated systolic hypertension. *JAMA* 1996;276:1886–1892.

Fowkes FGR, Price JF, Leng GC. Targeting subclinical atherosclerosis has the potential to reduce coronary events dramatically. *BMJ* 1998;316:1764.

Hardy R, Kuh D, Langenberg C, et al. Birthweight, childhood social class, and change in adult blood pressure in the 1946 British birth cohort. *Lancet* 2003;362:1178–1183.

Kornitzer M, Dramaix M, Sobolski J, et al. Ankle/arm pressure index in asymptomatic middle-aged males: an independent predictor of ten-year coronary heart disease mortality. *Angiology* 1995;46:211–219.

Stamler J, Dyer AR, Shekelle RB, et al. Relationship of baseline major risk factors to coronary and all-cause mortality, and to longevity: Findings from long-term follow-up of Chicago cohorts. *Cardiology* 1993;82:191–222.

Stamler J, Stamler R, Neaton JD; Blood pressure, systolic and diastolic, and cardiovascular risks. US population data. *Archives of Internal Medicine* 1993;153:598–615.

Wilson PW, Hoeg JM, D'Agostino RB. Cumulative effects of high cholesterol levels, high blood pressure, and cigarette smoking on carotid stenosis. *New England Journal of Medicine* 1997;337:516–522.

Inflammation

Bronstrup A, Hages M, Prinz-Langenohl R, et al. Effects of folic acid and combinations of folic acid and vitamin B-12 on plasma homocysteine concentrations in healthy, young women. *The American Journal of Clinical Nutrition* 1998;68:1104–1110.

Burke AP, Fonseca V, Kolodgie F, et al. Increased Serum Homocysteine and Sudden Death Resulting from Coronary Atherosclerosis with Fibrous Plaques. *Arteriosclerosis Thrombosis & Vascular Biology* 2002;22:1936–1941.

Chan AW, Bhatt DL, Chew DP, et al. Relation of inflammation and benefit of statins after percutaneous coronary interventions. *Circulation* 2003;107:1750–1756.

Eichholzer M, Luthy F, Moser U, et al. Folate and the risk of colorectal, breast and cervix cancer: the epidemiological evidence. *Swiss Medical Weekly* 2001;131:539–549.

Feigelson HS, Jonas CR, Robertson AS, et al. Alcohol, Folate, Methionine, and Risk of Incident Breast Cancer in the American Cancer Society Cancer Prevention Study II Nutrition Cohort. *Cancer Epidemiology, Biomarkers & Prevention* 2003;12:161–164.

Giles WH, Kittner SJ, Croft JB, et al. Serum Folate and Risk for Coronary Heart Disease: Results from a Cohort of US Adults. *Annals of Epidemiology* 1998;8:490–496.

Mennen LI, de Courcy GP, Guilland JC, et al. Homocysteine, cardiovascular disease risk factors, and habitual diet in the French Supplementation with Antioxidant Vitamins and Minerals Study. *The American Journal of Clinical Nutrition* 2002;76:1279–1289.

Pancharuniti N, Lewis CA, Sauberlich HE, et al. Plasma homocysteine, folate and vitamin B_{12} concentration and risk for early onset coronary artery disease. *The American Journal of Clinical Nutrition* 1994;59:940–948.

Rice JB, Stoll LL, Li WG, et al. Low Level Endotoxin Induces Potent Inflammatory Activation of Human Blood Vessels. *Arteriosclerosis Thrombosis & Vascular Biology* 2003;23:1576–1582.

Ridker PM, Hennekens CH, Buring JE, Rifai N. C-Reactive Protein and other Markers of Inflammation in the Prediction of Cardiovascular Disease in Women. *New England Journal of Medicine* 2000;342:836–843.

Selhub J, Jacques PJ, Bostom AG, et al. Association between plasma homocysteine concentrations and extracranial carotid-artery stenosis. *New England Journal of Medicine* 1995;332:286–291.

Selhub J, Jacques PF, Wilson PWF, Rush D, Rosenberg IH. Vitamin Status and Intake as Primary Determinants of Homocysteinemia in an Elderly Population. *JAMA* 1993;270; 2693–2698.

Shrubsole MJ, Jin F, Dai Q, et al. Dietary Folate Intake and Breast Cancer Risk: Results from the Shaghai Breast Cancer Study. *Cancer Research* 2001;61:7136–7141.

Tanne D, Haim M, Goldbourt U, et al. Prospective Study of Serum Homocysteine and Risk of Ischemic Stroke Among Patients with Preexisting Coronary Heart Disease. *Stroke* 2003;34:632–636.

Terry P, Jain M, Miller AB, et al. Dietary Intake of Folic Acid and Colorectal Cancer Risk in a Cohort of Women. *International Journal of Cancer* 2002;97:864–867.

Van Oort FV, Melse-Boonstra A, Brouwer IA, et al. Folic acid and reduction of plasma homocysteine concentrations in older adults: a dose-response study. *The American Journal of Clinical Nutrition* 2003;77:1318–1323.

Voutilainen S, Rissanen TH, Virtanen J, et al. Low Dietary Folate Intake Is Associated with an Excess Incidence of Acute Coronary Events. *Circulation.* 2001;103: 2674–2680.

Wald DS, Law M, Morris JK. Homocysteine and cardiovascular disease: evidence on causality from a meta-analysis. *BMJ* 2002;325:1202–1206.

Aspirin

Giovannucci E, Egan KM, Hunter DJ, et al. Aspirin and the risk of colorectal cancer in women. *New England Journal of Medicine* 1995;333:609–614.

Eidelman RS, Hebert PR, Weisman SM, Hennekens CH. An Update on Aspirin in the Primary Prevention of Cardiovascular Disease. *Archives of Internal Medicine* 2003;163: 2006–2010.

Pennisi E. Building a Better Aspirin. *Science* 1998;280:1191–1192.

Steering Committee of the Physicians' Health Study Research Group. Final report on the aspirin component of the on-going Physicians' Health Study. *New England Journal of Medicine* 1989;321:129–135.

Hormone Replacement Therapy

Barrett-Connor E, Goodman-Gruen D, Patay B. Endogenous Sex Hormones and Cognitive Function on Older Men. *Journal of Clinical Endocrinology & Metabolism* 1999; 84:3681–3685.

Cherrier MM, Asthana S, Plymate S, et al. Testosterone supplementation improves spatial and verbal memory in healthy older men. *Neurology* 2001;57:80–88.

Ettinger B, Friedman GD, Bush T. Reduced mortality associated with long-term postmenopausal estrogen therapy. *Obstetrics & Gynecology* 1996;87:6–12.

Grady D, Yaffe K, Kristof M, et al. Effect of postmenopausal hormone therapy on cognitive function: the Heart and Estrogen/Progestin Replacement Study. *American Journal of Medicine* 2002;113:543–548.

Greendale G, Reboussin B, Hogan P, et al. Symptom relief and side effects of postmenopausal hormones: results from the Post-menopausal Estrogen/Progestin Interventions Trial. *Obstetrics & Gynecology* 1998;92:982–988.

Hlatky MA, Boothroyd D, Vittinghoff E, et al. Quality of life and depressive symptoms in postmenopausal women after receiving hormone therapy: results from the Heart and Estrogen/Progestin Replacement Study (HERS) trial. *JAMA* 2002;287:591–597.

MacLennan A, Lester S, Moore V. Oral estrogen replacement therapy versus placebo for hot flushes: a systematic review. *Climacteric* 2001;4:58–74.

Sih R, Morley JE, Kaiser FE, et al. Testosterone Replacement in Older Hypogonadal Men: A 12-Month Randomized Controlled Trial. *Journal of Clinical Endocrinology & Metabolism* 1997;82:1661–1667.

Van den Beld AW, Bots ML, Janssen JA, et al. Endogenous Hormones and Carotid Atherosclerosis in Elderly Men. *American Journal of Epidemiology* 2003;157:25–31.

Wiklund I, Karlberg J, Mattsson LA. Quality of life of postmenopausal women on a regimen of transdermal estradiol therapy: a double-blind placebo-controlled study. *American Journal of Obstetrics and Gynecology* 1993;168:824–830.

CHAPTER 5

Brusselmans K, De Schrijver E, Heyns W, et al. Epigallocatechin 3-Gallate is a potent natural inhibitor of fatty acid synthase in intact cells and selectively induces apoptosis in prostate cancer cells. *International Journal of Cancer* 2003;106:856–862.

Chung FL, Schwartz J, Herzog CR, Yang YM. Tea and Cancer Prevention: Studies in Animals and Humans. *Journal of Nutrition* 2003;133:3268S–3274S.

Davies MJ, Judd JT, Baer DJ, Clevidence BA, Paul DR, Edwards AJ, Wisemen SA, Muesing RA, Chen SC. Black Tea Consumption Reduces Total and LDL Cholesterol in Mildly Hypercholesterolemic Adults. *American Society for Nutritional Sciences* 2003;133: 3298S–3302S.

Harris R, Lohr, K. Screening for Prostate Cancer: An Update of the Evidence for the U.S. Preventive Services Task Force. *Annals of Internal Medicine* 2002;137:917–929.

Tomato or Spaghetti Sauce

Gann PH, Ma J, Giovannucci E, et al. Lower Prostate Cancer Risk in Men with Elevated Plasma Lycopene Levels: Results of a Prospective Analysis. *Cancer Research* 1999;59: 1225–1230.

Giovannucci E, Ascherio A, Rimm EB, et al. Intake of carotenoids and retinol in relation to risk of prostate cancer. *Journal of the National Cancer Institute* 1995;87:1767–1776.

Giovannucci E, Rimm EB, Liu Y, Stampfer MJ, Willett WC. A Prospective Study of Tomato Products, Lycopene, and Prostate Cancer Risk. *Journal of the National Cancer Institute* 2002;94:391–398.

Rissanen T, Voutilainen SA, Nyyssönen K, Salonen JT. Lycopene, Atherosclerosis, and Coronary Heart Disease. *Experimental Biology and Medicine* 2002;227:901–907.

Rissanen TH, Voutilainen S, Nyyssönen K, Lakka TA, Sivenius J, Salonen R, Kaplan GA, Salonen JT. Low serum lycopene concentration is associated with an excess incidence of acute coronary events and stroke: the Kuopio Ischaemic Heart Disease Risk Factor Study. *British Journal of Nutrition* 2001;85:749–754.

Sato R, Helzlsouer KJ, Alberg AJ, Hoffman SC, Norkus EP, Comstock GW. Prospective

Study of Carotenoids, Tocopherols, and Retinoid Concentrations and the Risk of Breast Cancer. *Cancer Epidemiology, Biomarkers & Prevention* 2002;11:451–457.

Tzonou A, Signorello B, Lagiou P, Wuu J, d. Trichopoulos D, Trichopoulou A. Diet and Cancer of the Prostate: a case-control study in Greece. *International Journal of Cancer* 1999;80:704–708.

Sun Exposure and Vitamin D

Groth FM, Gundberg CM, Hollis BW, Haddad JG, Tobin JD. Vitamin D Deficiency in Homebound Elderly Persons. *JAMA* 1995;274:1683–1686.

McCullough ML, Robertson AS, Rodriguez C, et al. Calcium, vitamin D, dairy products, and risk of colorectal cancer in the Cancer Prevention Study II Nutrition Cohort (United States). *Cancer Causes and Control* 2003;14:1–12.

Shin, MH, Holmes MD, Hankinson SE, et al. Intake of Dairy Products, Calcium, and Vitamin D and Risk of Breast Cancer. *Journal of the National Cancer Institute* 2002; 94:1301–1311.

Stern RS, Weinstein MC, Baker SG. Risk reduction for nonmelanoma skin cancer with childhood sunscreen use. *Archives of Dermatology* 1986;122:537–545.

Studzinski GP, Moore DG. Sunlight—Can it prevent as well as cause cancer? *Cancer Research* 1995;55:4014–4022.

Watson KE, Abrolat ML, Malone LL, et al. Active serum vitamin D levels are inversely correlated with coronary calcification. *Circulation* 1997;96:1755–1760.

Webb AR, Kline L, Holick MF. Influence of season and latitude on the cutaneous synthesis of vitamin D_3: Exposure to winter sunlight in Boston and Edmonton will not promote vitamin D_3 synthesis in human skin. *Journal of Clinical Endocrinology & Metabolism* 1998;67:373–378.

Zittermann A, Schleithoff SS, Tenderich G, et al. Low Vitamin D Status: A Contributing Factor in the Pathogenesis of Congestive Heart Failure? *Journal of American College of Cardiology* 2003;41:105–112.

Dental Disease

Cao JJ, Thach C, Manolio TA, et al. C-Reactive protein, carotid intima-media thickness, and incidence of ischemic stroke in the elderly. The Cardiovascular Health Study. *Circulation* 2003;108:166–170.

DeStefano F, Anda RF, Kahn HS, et al. Dental disease, and risk of coronary heart disease and mortality. 1993;306:688–691.

Huittinen T, Leinonen M, Tenkanen L, et al. Synergistic effect of persistent chlamydia pneumoniae infection, autoimmunity, and inflammation on coronary risk. *Circulation* 2003;107:2566–2570.

Joshipura KJ, Hung HC, Rimm EB, et al. Periodontal disease, tooth loss, and incidence of ischemic stroke. *Stroke* 2003;34:47–52.

Kalayoglu MV, Galvan C, Mahdi OS, Byrne GI, Mansour S. Serological Association Between Chlamydia pneumoniae Infection and Age-Related Macular Degeneration. *Archives of Opthalmology* 2003;121:478–482.

Smith GC, Pell JP, Walsh D. Spontaneous loss of early pregnancy and risk of ischaemic heart disease in later life: retrospective cohort study. *BMJ* 2003;326:423–424.

CHAPTER 6

Smoking

Skolnick ET, Vomvolakis MA, Buck KA, et al. Exposure to environmental tobacco smoke and the risk of adverse respiratory events in children receiving general anesthesia. *Anesthesiology* 1998;88:1141–1142.

West RR. Smoking: Its influence on survival and cause of death. *Journal of the Royal College of Physicians of London* 1992;26:357–366.

Driving

Hemmelgarn B, Suissa S, Huang A, et al. Benzodiazepine use and the risk of motor vehicle crash in the elderly. *JAMA* 1997;278:27–31.

Rowe JW, Kahn RI. Chapter 2, section on avoiding disease and disability. In Rowe JW, Kahn RL, (ed.): *Successful Aging*. New York, Random House, 1998, p. 69.

Seat Belt and Vehicle Safety

Graham JD, Thompson KM, Goldie SJ, Seigu-Gomez M, Weinstein MC. The cost-effectiveness of air-bags by seating position. *JAMA* 1997;278:1418–1425.

Jacobsen PI. Safety in numbers: more walkers and bicyclists, safer walking and bicycling. *Injury Prevention* 2003;9:205–209.

Servadei F, Begliomini C, Gardini E, et al. Effect of Italy's motorcycle helmet law on traumatic brain injuries. *Injury Prevention* 2003;9:257–260.

Air Pollution

Dockery DW, Pope CA III, Xu X, et al. An association between air pollution and mortality in six U.S. cities. *New England Journal of Medicine* 1993;329:1753–1759.

EPA website for 594 metropolitan regions:
www.epa.gov/ttn/airs/airsaqs/archived%20data/downloadaqsdata.ht.

National Resources Defense Council. *Breathtaking: Premature Mortality Due to Particulate Air Pollution in 239 American Cities*. May, 1996.

Pope CA III, Thun MJ, Namboodiri MM, et al. Particulate air pollution as a predictor of mortality in a prospective study of US adults. *American Journal of Respiratory Critical Care Medicine* 1995;151:669–674.

Rothkamm K, Lobrich M. Evidence for a lack of DNA double-strand break repair in human cells exposed to very low x-ray doses. *Proceedings of the National Academy of Sciences of the United States of America* 2003;100:5057–5062.

Tsai SS, Goggins WB, Chiu HF, et al. Evidence for an Association Between Air Pollution and Daily Stroke Admissions in Kaohsiung, Taiwan. *Stroke* 2003;34:2612–2616.

Sex-ercise, Casual Sex, Sexually Transmitted Diseases

Davey Smith Gd, Frankel S, Yarnell J. Sex and death: are they related? Findings from the Caerphilly cohort study. *BMJ* 1997;315:1641–1644.

Downs AM, De Vincenzi I. Probability of heterosexual transmission of HIV: Relationship to the number of unprotected sexual contacts. *Journal of Acquired Immune Deficiency Syndromes and Human Retrovirology* 1996;11:388–395.

Sparrow MJ, Lavill K. Breakage and slippage of condoms in family planning clients. *Contraception* 1994;50:117–129.

Wiley JA, Herschkorn SJ, Padian NS. Heterogeneity in the probability of HIV transmission per sexual contact: The case of male to female transmission in penile-vaginal intercourse. *Statistics in Medicine* 1989;8:93–102.

CHAPTER 7

Stress

Cartwright M, Wardle J, Steggles N, et al. Stress and Dietary Practices in Adolescents. *Health Psychology* 2003;22:362–369.

Hayashi K, Hayashi T, Iwanaga S, et al. Laughter lowered the increase in postprandial blood glucose. *Diabetes Care* 2003;26:1651–1652.

Karlin WA, Brondolo E, Schwartz J. Workplace social support and ambulatory cardiovascular activity in New York City traffic agents. *Psychosomatic Medicine* 2003; 65:167–176.

Kivimaki M, Vahtera J, Elovainio, et al. Death or illness of a family member, violence, interpersonal conflict, and financial difficulties as predictors of sickness absence: Longitudinal cohort study on psychological and behavioral links. *Psychosomatic Medicine* 2002;64: 817–825.

Lee S, Colditz GA, Berkman LF, et al. Caregiving and risk of coronary heart disease in U.S. women. A prospective study. *American Journal of Preventive Medicine* 2003;24:113–119.

Lillberg K, Verkasalo PK, Kaprio J, et al. Stressful life events and risk of breast cancer in 10,808 women: A cohort study. *American Journal of Epidemiology* 2003;157:415–423.

Rosengren A, Orth-gomer K, Wedel HL: Stressful life events, social support and mortality in men born in 1933. *BMJ* 1993;307:1102–1105.

Truelsen T, Nielsen N, Boysen G, et al. Self reported stress and risk of stroke. The Copenhagen city heart study. *Stroke* 2003;34:1–7.

Social Contacts

Berkman LF, Syme SI. Social networks, host resistance and mortality: A nine-year follow-up study of Alameda County residents. *American Journal of Epidemiology* 1979;109:186–204.

Fineberg HV, Wilson ME. Social vulnerability and death by infection. *New England Journal of Medicine* 1996;334:828–833.

Marital Status

Coker AL, Davis KE, Arias I, et al. Physical and mental health effects of intimate partner violence for men and women. *American Journal of Preventive Medicine* 2002;23:260–268.

Ebrahim S, Wannamethee G, McCallum A, Walker M, Shaper AG. Marital status, change in marital status and mortality in middle-aged British men. *American Journal of Epidemiology* 1985;142:834–842.

Gordon HS, Rosenthal GE. Impact of marital status on outcomes in hospitalized patients: Evidence from an academic medical center. *Archives of Internal Medicine* 1995;155(22): 2465–2471.

Sorlie PD, Backlund MS, Keller JB. US mortality by economic, demographic, and social characteristics: The National Longitudinal Mortality Study. *American Journal of Public Health* 1995;85:949–956.

Your Parents' Divorce
Cherlin AJ, Frustenberg FF Jr., Chase-Lansdale L. Longitudinal studies of effects of divorce on children in Great Britain and the United States. *Science* 1991:252;1386–1399.

Educational Level
Fox AJ, Goldblatt PO, Jones DP. Social class mortality differentials: Artifact, selection or life circumstances. In Wilkenson RG (ed): *Class & Health*. New York, NY. Tavistock Publications, 1986.

Heaney DC, MacDonald BK, Everitt A, et al. Socioeconomic variation in incidence of epilepsy: prospective community based study in south east England. *BMJ* 2002;325: 1013–1016.

Sorlie PD, Backlund MS, Keller JB. US mortality by economic, demographic, and social characteristics: The National Longitudinal Mortality Study. *American Journal of Public Health* 1995;85:949–966.

CHAPTER 8

Bazzano LA, He J, Ogden LG, Loria CM, Whelton PK. Dietary Fiber Intake and Reduced Risk of Coronary Heart Disease in US Men and Women. *Archives of Internal Medicine* 2003;163:1897–1904.

Freedman JE. High Fat Diets and Cardiovascular Disease. *Journal of the American College of Cardiology* 2003;41:1750–1751.

Fung TT, Hu FB. Plant-based diets: what should be on the plate. *The American Journal of Clinical Nutrition* 2003;78:357–358.

Giammattei J, Blix G, Marshak HH, Wollitzer AO, Pettitt DJ. Television Watching and Soft Drink Consumption associations with obesity in eleven- to twelve-year-old school-children. *Archives of Pediatric Adolescent Medicine* 2003;157:882–886.

Michels KB, Giovannucci E, Joshipura KJ, et al. Prospective Study of Fruit and Vegetable Consumption and Incidence of Colon and Rectal Cancers. *Journal of the National Cancer Institute* 2000;92:1740–1752.

Nutrition Examination Survey (NHANES III). *Journal of the American College of Nutrition* 2003;22:296–302.

Smith-Warner SA, Elmer PJ, Fosdick L, et al. Fruits, Vegetables, and Adenomatous Polyps. *American Journal of Epidemiology* 2002;155:1104–1113.

Tangvoranuntakul P, Gagneux P, Diaz S, Bardor M, Varki N, Varki A, Muchmore E. Human uptake and incorporation of an immunogenic nonhuman dietary sialic acid. *Proceedings of the National Academy of Sciences of the United States of America* 2003;100: 12045–12050.

Dietary Diversity

Gillman MW, Cupples LA, Millen BE, et al. Inverse Association of Dietary Fat With Development of Ischemic Stroke in Men. *JAMA* 1997;278:2145–2150.

Harris HH, Pickering IJ, George GN. The Chemical Form of Mercury in Fish. *Science* 2003;301:1203.

Kant AK, Schatzkin A, Ziegler RG. Dietary diversity and subsequent cause-specific mortality in the NHANES I epidemiologic follow-up study. *Journal of the American College of Nutrition* 1995;14:233–238.

Leon W, DeWaal CS. Is Our Food Safe? Environmental Working Group; Monterey Bay Aquarium; Environmental Defense; Natural Resources Defense Council. (see *www. nrdc.org*).

Steffen LM, Jacobs DR, Stevens J, et al. Associations of whole-grain, refined-grain, and fruit and vegetable consumption with risks of all-cause mortality and incident coronary artery disease and ischemic stroke: The Atherosclerosis Risk in Communities (ARIC) Study. *The American Journal of Clinical Nutrition* 2003;78:383–390.

Total Cholesterol

Hamilton VH, Racicot FE, Zowall H, et al. The cost-effectiveness of HMG-CoA reductase inhibitors to prevent coronary artery disease. *JAMA* 1995;273:1032–1038.

Hu FB, Stampfer MJ, Manson JE, et al. Dietary fat intake and the risk of coronary heart disease in women. *New England Journal of Medicine* 1997;337:1491–1499.

Muldoon MF, Manuck SB, Matthews KA. Lowering cholesterol concentrations and mortality: Does cholesterol lowering increase non-illness related mortality. *Archives of Internal Medicine* 1991;151:1453–1454.

Randomized trial of cholesterol lowering in 4444 patients with coronary artery disease: The Scandinavian Simvastatin Survival Study. *Lancet* 1994;344;1383–1389.

von Muhlen D, Langer RD, Barrett-Connor E. Sex and Time Differences in the Associations of Non-High Density Lipoprotein Cholesterol Versus Other Lipid and Lipoprotein Factors in the Prediction of Cardiovascular Death (The Rancho Bernardo Study) *American Journal of Cardiology* 2003;91:1311–1315.

Yang CC, Jick SS, Jick H. Lipid-Lowering Drugs and the Risk of Depression and Suicidal Behavior. *Archives of Internal Medicine* 2003;163:1926–1932.

HDL Cholesterol

Downs JR, Clearfield M, Weis S, et al. Primary prevention of acute coronary events with lovastatin in men and women with average cholesterol levels. Results of AFCAPS/TexCAPS. *JAMA* 1998;279:1615–1622.

Rosenson RS, Tangney CC. Antiatherothrombotic properties of statins. Implications for cardiovascular event reduction. *JAMA* 1998;279:1643–1650.

Saturated Fat

Cho E, Spiegelman D, Hunter DJ, Chen WY, Stampfer MJ, Colditz GA, Willett WC. Premenopausal Fat Intake and Risk of Breast Cancer. *Journal of the National Cancer Institute* 2003;95:1079–1085.

Hu FB, Stampfer MJ, Manson JE, et al: Dietary fat intake and the risk of coronary heart disease in women. *New England Journal of Medicine* 1997;337:1491–1499.

Kromhout D, Bloemberg B, Feskens E, et al. Saturated fat, vitamin C and smoking predict long-term population all-cause mortality rates in the Seven Countries Study. *International Journal of Epidemiology* 2000;29:260–265.

Triglycerides

Eberly LE, Stamler J, Neaton JD, et al. Relation of Triglyceride Levels, Fasting and Non-fasting, to Fatal and Nonfatal Coronary Heart Disease. *Archives of Internal Medicine* 2003;163:1077–1083.

Gaziano JM, Hennekens CH, O'Donnell CJ, Breslow JL, Baring JE. Fasting triglycerides, high-density lipoprotein, and the risk of myocardial infarction. *Circulation* 1997;96: 2520–2525.

Talmud PJ, Hawe E, Miller GJ, et al. Nonfasting Apolipoprotein B and Triglyceride Levels as a Useful Predictor of Coronary Heart Disease Risk in Middle-Aged UK Men. *Arteriosclerosis Thrombosis & Vascular Biology* 2002;22:1918–1923.

Trans Fats

Gaziano JM, Hennekens CH, O'Donnell CJ, et al. Fasting triglycerides, high-density lipoprotein, and the risk of myocardial infarction. *Circulation* 1997;96:2520–2525.

Hu FB, Stampfer MJ, Manson JE, et al. Dietary fat intake and the risk of coronary heart disease in women. *New England Journal of Medicine* 1997;337:1491–1499.

Mensink RP, Katan MB. Effect of dietary trans fatty acids on high-density and low-density lipoprotein cholesterol levels in healthy subjects. *New England Journal of Medicine* 1990; 323:439–445.

Body Mass Index

Linsted K, Tonstad S, Kusma JW. Body mass index and patterns of mortality among Seventh Day Adventist men. *International Journal of Obesity* 1991;15:397–406.

CHAPTER 9

Physical Activity

Blair SN, Kohl HW, Paffenbarger RS, et al. Physical fitness and all-cause mortality. A prospective study of healthy men and women. *JAMA* 1989;262:2395–2401.

Hakim AA, Petrovich H, Burchfield CM, et al. Effects of walking on mortality among nonsmoking retired men. *New England Journal of Medicine* 1988;338:94–99.

Kujala UM, Kaprio J, Sarna S, Koskenvuo M. Relationship of leisure-time physical activity and mortality. The Finnish twin cohort. *JAMA* 1998;279:440–444.

Paffenbarger RS, Hyde RT, Wing AL, et al: The association of changes in physical-activity level and other lifestyle characteristics with mortality among men. *New England Journal of Medicine* 1993;328:538–545.

Paffenbarger RS, Kampert JB, Lee IM, Hyde RT, Leung RW, Wing AL. Changes in physical activity and other lifeway patterns influence longevity. *Medicine and Science in Sports and Exercise* 1994;26:852–865.

Patel AV, Press MF, Meeske K, et al. Lifetime recreational exercise activity and risk of breast carcinoma in situ. *Cancer* 2003;98:2161–2169.

Verghese J, Lipton RB, Katz MJ, Hall CB, Derby CA, Kuslansky G, Ambrose AF, Sliwinski M, Buschke H. Leisure Activities and the Risk of Dementia in the Elderly. *New England Journal of Medicine* 2003;348:2508–2516.

Strength-Building Exercise

Province MA, Hadley EC, Hornbrook MC, Lipsitz LA. The effect of exercise on falls in elderly patients. A preplanned metaanalysis of the FICSIT trials. *JAMA* 1995;273:1341–1347.

Seguin R, Nelson ME. The Benefits of Strength Training for Older Adults. *American Journal of Preventive Medicine* 2003;25:141–149.

Tinetti ME, Williams CS. Falls, injuries due to falls, and the risk of admission to a nursing home. *New England Journal of Medicine* 1997;337:1279–1284.

Stamina-Building Exercise

Blair SN, Kohl HW III, Barlow CE, Paffenbarger RS, et al. Changes in physical fitness and all-cause mortality. A prospective study of healthy men and unhealthy men. *JAMA* 1995;273:1093–1098.

Gulati M, Pandey DK, Arnsdorf MF, Lauderdale DS, Thisted RA, Wicklund RH, Al-Hani AJ, Black HB. Exercise Capacity and the Risk of Death in Women. *Circulation* 2003;108:1554–1559.

Lee CD, Folsom AR, Blair SN. Physical Activity and Stroke Risk A Meta-Analysis. *Stroke* 2003;34:2475–2482.

CHAPTER 10

Abbott RD, Ando F, Masaki KH, et al. Dietary Magnesium Intake and the Future Risk of Coronary Heart Disease (The Honolulu Heart Program). *American Journal of Cardiology* 2003;92:665–669.

Baron JA, Cole BF, Mott L, et al. Neoplastic and Antineoplastic Effects of beta-carotene on Colorectal Adenoma Recurrence: Results of a Randomized Trial. *Journal of the National Cancer Institute* 2003;95:717–722.

Bleske BE, Willis RA, Anthony M, et al. The effect of pravastatin and atorvastatin on coenzyme Q10. *American Heart Journal* 2001;142:E2.

Fairfield KM, Fletcher RH. Vitamins for Chronic Disease Prevention in Adults. *JAMA* 2002;287:3116–3127.

Heart Protection Study Collaborative Group. MRC/BHF Heart Protection Study of antioxidant vitamin supplementation in 20536 high-risk individuals: a randomized placebo-controlled trial. *Lancet* 2002;360:23–33.

Todd S, Woodward M, Tunstall-Pedoe H, et al. Dietary Antioxidant Vitamins and Fiber in the Etiology of Cardiovascular Disease and All-Causes Mortality: Results from the Scottish Heart Health Study. *American Journal of Epidemiology* 1999;150:1073–1080.

Van Hoydonck PG, Temme EH, Schouten EG, et al. A Dietary Oxidative Balance Score of Vitamin C, beta-carotene, and Iron Intakes and Mortality Risk in Male Smoking Belgians. *Journal of Nutrition* 2002;132:756–761.

Vivekananthan DP, Penn MS, Sapp SK, et al. Use of antioxidant vitamins for the prevention of cardiovascular disease: meta-analysis of randomized trials. *Lancet* 2003;361:2017–2023.

Wong WY, Merkus HM, Thomas CM, et al. Effects of folic acid and zinc sulfate on male factor subfertility: a double blind, randomized, placebo-controlled trial. *Fertility and Sterility* 2002;77:491–498.

Yong LC, Brown CC, Schatzkin A, et al. Intake of Vitamins E, C, and A and Risk of Lung Cancer. *American Journal of Epidemiology* 1997;146:231–243.

Vitamin C

Enstrom JE, Kanin LE, Klein MA. Vitamin C intake and mortality among a sample of United States population. *Epidemiology* 1992;3:194–202.

Khaw KT, Bingham S, Welch A, et al. Relation between plasma ascorbic acid and mortality in men and women in EPIC-Norfolk prospective study: a prospective population study. *Lancet* 2001;357:657–663.

Kromhout D, Bloemberg B, Feskens E, et al. Saturated fat, vitamin C and smoking predict long-term population all-cause mortality rates in the Seven Countries Study. *International Journal of Epidemiology* 2000;29:260–265.

Loria CM, Klag MJ, Caulfield LE, et al. Vitamin C status and mortality in US adults. *The American Journal of Clinical Nutrition* 2000;72:139–145.

Osganian SK, Stampfer MJ, Rimm E, et al. Vitamin C and Risk of Coronary Heart Disease in Women. *Journal of the American College of Cardiology* 2003;42:246–252.

Plotnick GD, Corretti MC, Vogel RA, et al. Effect of Supplemental Phytonutrients on Impairment of the Flow-Mediated Brachial Artery Vasoactivity After a Single High-Fat Meal. *Journal of the American College of Cardiology* 2003;41:1744–1749.

Sahyoun NR, Jacques PF, Russell RM. Carotenoids, Vitamins C and E, and Mortality in an Elderly Population. *American Journal of Epidemiology* 1996;144:501–511.

Simon JA, Hudes ES, Tice JA, et al. Relation of Serum Ascorbic Acid to Mortality Among US Adults. *Journal of the American College of Nutrition* 2001;20:255–263.

Vitamin E

Chan JM, Stampfer MJ, Ma J, et al. Supplemental Vitamin E Intake and Prostate Cancer Risk in a Large Cohort of Men in the United States. *Cancer Epidemiology, Biomarkers & Prevention* 1999;8:892–899.

Hodis HN, Mack WJ, LaBree L, et al. Alpha-Tocopherol Supplementation in Healthy Individuals Reduces Low-Density Lipoprotein Oxidation but Not Atherosclerosis. *Circulation* 2002;106:1453–1459.

Hodis HN, Mack WJ, LaBree L, et al. Serial coronary angioplastic evidence that antioxidant vitamin intake reduces profession of coronary artery atherosclerosis. *JAMA* 1995;273:1845–1854.

Stampfer MJ, Hennekens CH, Manson JR, et al. Vitamin E consumption and the risk of coronary disease in women. *New England Journal of Medicine* 1993;328:1444–1449.

Calcium and Vitamin D

Feskanich D, Willett WC, Colditz GA. Calcium, vitamin D, milk consumption, and hip fractures: a prospective study among postmenopausal women. *The American Journal of Clinical Nutrition* 2003;77:504–511.

Harel Z, Riggs S, Vaz R, et al. Adolescents and calcium: What they do and do not know and how much they consume. *Journal of Adolescent Health* 1998;22:225–228.

Ishitani K, Itakura E, Goto S, et al. Calcium Absorption from the Ingestion of Coral-Derived Calcium by Humans. *Journal of Nutritional Science and Vitaminology* 1999;45:509–517.

National Institutes of Health Consensus Statement. Optional calcium intake. *JAMA* 1994;272:1942–1948.

Watson KE, Abrolat ML, Malone LL, et al. Active serum vitamin D levels are inversely correlated with coronary calcification. *Circulation* 1997;96:1755–1760.

Shevde NK, Plum LA, Clagett-Dame M, et al. A potent analog of 1,alpha, 25-dihydroxy-vitamin D3 selectively induces bone formation. *Proceedings of the National Academy of Sciences of the United States of America* 2002;99:13487–13491.

Trivedi DP, Doll R, Khaw KT. Effect of four monthly oral vitamin D_3 (cholecalciferol) supplementation on fractures and mortality in men and women living in the community: randomised double blind controlled trial. *BMJ* 2003;326:469.

Folate

Choi SW, Mason JB. Folate and Carcinogenesis: An Integreted Scheme. *Nutrition* 2000;130:129–132.

French AE, Grant R, Weitzman S, Ray JG, Vermeulen MJ, Sung L, Greenberg M, Koren G. Folic acid food fortification is associated with a decline in neuroblastoma. *Clinical Pharmacology & Therapeutics* 2003;74:288–294.

George L, Mills JL, Johansson ALV, et al. Plasma Folate Levels and Risk of Spontaneous Abortion. *JAMA* 2002;288:1867–1873.

Hernandez-Diaz S, Werler MM, Louik C, et al. Risk of Gestational Hypertension in Relation to Folic Acid Supplementation during Pregnancy. *American Journal of Epidemiology* 2002;156:806–812.

Heude B, Ducimetiere P, Berr C. Cognitive decline and fatty acid composition of erythrocyte membranes—The EVA Study. *The American Journal of Clinical Nutrition* 2003; 77:703–708.

La Vecchia C, Negri E, Pelucchi C, et al. Dietary Folate and Colorectal Cancer. *International Journal of Cancer* 2002;102:545–547.

Liem A, Reynierse-Buitenwerf G, Zwinderman H, et al. Secondary Prevention With Folic Acid: Effects on Clinical Outcomes. *Journal of the American College of Cardiology* 2003;41:2105–2113.

Lim U, Cassano PA. Homocysteine and Blood Pressure in the Third National Health and Nutrition Examination Survey, 1988–1994. *American Journal of Epidemiology* 2002;156:1105–1113.

Loria CM, Ingram DD, Feldman JJ, et al. Serum Folate and Cardiovascular Disease Mortality Among US Men and Women. *Archives of Internal Medicine* 2000;160: 3258–3262.

Markus RA, Mack WJ, Azen SP, et al. Influence of lifestyle modification on atherosclerotic progression determined by ultrasonographic change in the common carotid intima-media thickness. *The American Journal of Clinical Nutrition* 1997;65; 1000–1004.

McIlroy SP, Dynan KB, Lawson, JT, et al. Moderately Elevated Plasma Homocysteine, Methylenetetrahydrofolate Reductase Genotype, and Risk for Stroke, Vascular Dementia, and Alzheimer Disease in Northern Ireland. *Stroke* 2002;33:2351–2356.

Quinlivan EP, Gregory JE. Effect of food fortification on folic acid intake in the United States. *The American Journal of Clinical Nutrition* 2003;77:221–225.

Pancharumiti N, Lewis CA, Sauberlich HE, et al. Plasma homocysteine, folate and vitamin B_{12} concentration and risk for early onset coronary artery disease. *The American Journal of Clinical Nutrition* 1994;59:940–948.

Ray JG, Meier C, Vermeulen MJ, et al. Association of neural tube defects and folic acid food fortification in Canada. *Lancet* 2002;360:2047–2048.

Selhub J, Jacques PJ, Bostom AG, et al. Association between plasma homocysteine concentrations and carotid-artery stenosis. *New England Journal of Medicine* 1995;332:286–291.

Su LJ, Arab L. Nutritional Status of Folate and Colon Cancer Risk: Evidence from NHANES I Epidemiologic Follow-up Study. *Annals of Epidemiology* 2001;11:65–72.

Vitamin B_6

Giovannucci E, Rimm EB, Ascherio A, et al. Alcohol, Low-Methionine-Low-Folate Diets, and Risk of Colon Cancer in Men. *Journal of the National Cancer Institute* 1995; 87:265–273.

Giovannucci E, Stampfer MJ, Colditz GA, et al. Multivitamin Use, Folate, and Colon Cancer in Women in the Nurses' Health Study. *Annals of Internal Medicine* 1998;129: 517–524.

Jacobs EJ, Connell CJ, Chao A, et al. Multivitamin Use and Colorectal Cancer Incidence in a US Cohort: Does Timing Matter? *American Journal of Epidemiology* 2003;158: 621–628.

Medrano MJ, Sierra MJ, Almazan J, et al. The Association of Dietary Folate, B_6, and B_{12}, With Cardiovascular Mortality in Spain: An Ecological Analysis. *American Journal Of Public Health* 2000;90:1636–1638.

Rimm EB, Willett WC, Hu FB, Simpson L, Colditz GA, Manson JE, Hennekens C, Stampfer MJ. Folate and vitamin B_6 from diet and supplements in relation to risk of coronary heart disease among women. *JAMA* 1998;279:359–64.

Zhang SM, Willett WC, Selhub J, et al. Plasma Folate, Vitamin B_6, Vitamin B_{12}, Homocysteine, and Risk of Breast Cancer. *Journal of the National Cancer Institute* 2003;95:373–380.

CHAPTER 11

Sleep

Ayas NT, White DP, Manson JE, et al. A Prospective Study of Sleep Duration and Coronary Heart Disease in Women. *Archives of Internal Medicine* 2003;163:205–209.

Belloc N. Relationship of health practices and mortality. *Preventive Medicine* 1973;2:67–81.

Gottlieb DJ, Whitney CW, Bonekat WH, et al. Relation of Sleepiness to Respiratory Disturbance Index. The Sleep Heart Health Study. *American Journal of Respiratory & Critical Care Medicine* 1999;159:502–507.

Kaplan GA, Seeman TE, Cohen RD, Knudson G, et al. Mortality among the elderly in the Alameda County Study: Behavioral and demographic risk factors. *Journal of Public Health* 1987;77:307–312.

Kripke DF, Garfinkel L, Wingard DL, et al. Mortality Associated with Sleep Duration and Insomnia. *Archives of General Psychiatry* 2002;59:131–136.

Liu Y, Tanaka H, The Fukuoka Heart Study Group. Overtime work, insufficient sleep, and risk of non-fatal acute myocardial infarction in Japanese men. *Occupation and Environmental Medicine* 2002;59:447–451.

Mallon L, Broman JE, Hetta J. Sleep complaints predict coronary artery disease mortality in males: a 12-year follow-up study of a middle-aged Swedish population. *Journal of Internal Medicine* 2002;251:207–216.

Mooe T, Franklin KA, Holmstrom K, et al. Sleep-disordered Breathing and Coronary Artery Disease. Long-term Prognosis. *American Journal of Respiratory & Critical Care Medicine* 2001;164:1910–1913.

Nieto FJ, Young TB, Lind BK, et al. Association of Sleep-Disordered Breathing, Sleep Apnea, and Hypertension in a Large Community Based Study. *JAMA* 2000; 283:1829–1836.

Scher AI, Lipton RB, Stewart WF. Habitual snoring as a risk factor for chronic daily headache. *Neurology* 2003;60:1366–1368.

Snacking

Belloc N. Relationship of health practices and mortality. *Preventive Medicine* 1973;2:67–81.

Eating Breakfast

Belloc N. Relationship of health practices and mortality. *Preventive Medicine* 1973;2:67–81.

Cho S, Dietrich M, Brown CJP, et al. The Effect of Breakfast Type on Total Daily Energy Intake and Body Mass Index: Results from the Third National Health and Nutrition Examination Survey (NHANES III). *Journal of the American College of Nutrition* 2003;22:296–302.

Kaplan GA, Seeman TE, Cohen RD, Knudson G, et al. Mortality among the elderly in the Alameda County Study: Behavioral and demographic risk factors. *Journal of Public Health* 1987;77:307–312.

Alcohol Consumption

Carluccio MA, Siculella L, Ancora MA, Massaro M, Scoditti E, Storelli C, Visiolo F, Distante A, De Caterina R. Olive Oil and Red Wine Antioxidant Polyphenols Inhibit Endothelial Activation-Antiatherogenic Properties of Mediterranean Diet Phytochemicals. *Arteriosclerosis Thrombosis & Vascular Biology* 2003;23:622–629.

Fuchs CS, Stampfer MJ, Colditz GA, et al. Alcohol consumption and mortality among women. *New England Journal of Medicine* 1995;332:1245–1250.

Klatsky AL, Armstrong MA. Alcohol and Mortality. *Annals of Internal Medicine* 1992;117:646–654.

US Government Dietary Guidelines for Americans, January 8, 1996.

Dog Ownership

Beck AM, Meyers NM. Health enhancement and companion animal ownership. *Annual Review of Public Health* 1996;17:247–257.

Friedmann E, Thomas SA. Pet ownership, social support, and one-year survival after acute myocardial infarction in the Cardiac Arrhythmia Suppression Trial (CAST). *American Journal of Cardiology* 1995;76:1213–1217.

CHAPTER 12

Patrolling Your Own Health

Brunelli A, Refai MA, Monteverde M, Borri A, Salati M, Fiachini A. Stair Climbing Test Predicts Cardiopulmonary Complications After Lung Resection. *Chest* 2002;121: 1106–1110.

Conaway DG, House J, Bandt K, et al. The Elderly: Health Status Benefits and Recovery of Function One Year After Coronary Artery Bypass Surgery. *Journal of American College of Cardiology* 2003;42:1421–1426.

Fearon KC, Von Meyenfeldt MF, Moses AG et al. Effect of a protein and energy dense N-3 fatty acid enriched oral supplement on loss of weight and lean tissue in cancer cachexia: a randomised double blind trial. *Gut* 2003;52:1479–1486.

Hash RB, Munna RK, Vogel RL, et al. Does Physician Weight Affect Perception of Health Advice? *Preventive Medicine* 2002;36:41–44.

Poldermans D, Bax JJ, Kerai MD, et al. Statins are associated with a reduced incidence of perioperative mortality in patients undergoing major noncardiac vascular surgery. *Circulation* 2003;107:1848–1851.

Reilly DF, McNeely MJ, Doerner D, Greenberg DL, Staiger TO, Geist MJ, Vedovatti PA, Coffey JE, Mora MW, Johnson TR, Guray ED, Van Norman GA, Fihn SD. Self-reported Exercise Tolerance and the Risk of Serious Periopertive Complications. *Archives of Internal Medicine* 1999;159:2185–2192.

Rumsfeld JS. Valve Surgery in the Elderly. *Journal of the American College of Cardiology* 2003;42:1208–1217.

Schoenfeld DE, Malmorse LC, Brazer DG, Gold DT, Seeman TE. Self-rated health and mortality in the high-functioning elderly—a closer look at healthy individuals: McArthur Field Study of Successful Aging. *Journal of Gerontology* 1994;49:M109–115.

Tabar L, Yen MF, Vitak B, Chen HHT, Smith RA, Duffy SW. Mammography service screening and mortality in breast cancer patients: 20-year follow-up before and after introduction of screening. *Lancet.* 2003;361:1405–1410.

Age of Parents at Their Time of Death

Brand FN, Kiely DK, Kannel WB, Myers RH. Family patterns of coronary heart disease mortality: The Framingham longevity study. *Journal of Clinical Epidemiology* 1992;45: 169–174.

Chen W, Srinivasan SR, Bao W, et al. The Magnitude of Familial Associations of Cardiovascular Risk Factor Variables between Parents and Offspring Are Influenced by Age: The Bogalusa Heart Study. *Annals of Epidemiology* 2001;11:522–528.

Frederiksen H, McGue M, Jeune B, et al. Do Children of Long-Lived Parents Age More Successfully? *Epidemiology* 2002;13:334–339.

Vandenbrouke JP, Matroos AW, van der Heide-Wessel C, van der Heide RM. Parental survival, an independent predictor of longevity in middle-aged persons. *American Journal of Epidemiology* 1984;119:742–750.

Yarnell J, Yu S, Patterson C, et al. Family history, longevity, and risk of coronary heart disease: the PRIME Study. *International Journal of Epidemiology* 2003;32:71–77.

Pill Popping

Johnson JA, Bootman JL. Drug related morbidity and mortality. A cost-of-illness model. *Archives of Internal Medicine* 1995;155:1949–1956.

Lazarou J, Pomeranz BH, Corey PN. Incidence of adverse drug reactions in hospitalized patients. A meta-analysis of prospective studies. *JAMA* 1998;279:1200–1205.

Murphy GM, Kremer C, Rodriques HE, Schatzberg AF. Pharmacogenetics of Antidepressant Medication Intolerance. *American Journal of Psychiatry* 2003;160:1830–1835.

Yuan Y, Jay JW, McCombs JS. Effects of ambulatory-care pharmacist consultation on morality and hospitalization. *American Journal of Managed Care* 2003;9:45–56.

Immunizations

Gardner P, Schaffner W. Immunization of adults. *New England Journal of Medicine* 1993;328:1252.

McQuillan GM, Kruszon-Moran D, Deforest A, et al. Serologic Immunity to Diphtheria and Tetanus in the United States. *Annals of Internal Medicine* 2002;136:660–666.

Chronic Disease Management

Mangano DT, Layug EL, Wallace A, et al. Effect of Atenolol on mortality and cardiovascular morbidity after noncardiac surgery. *New England Journal of Medicine* 1996;335:1713–1720.

Arthritis

Chiang EI, Bagley PJ, Selhub J, Nadeau M, Roubenoff R. Abnormal Vitamin B_6 Status Is Associated with Severity of Symptoms in Patients with Rheumatoid Arthritis. *The American Journal of Medicine* 2003;114:283–287.

Pagnano MW, McLamb LA, Trousdale RT. Primary and Revision Total Hip Arthroplasty for Patients 90 Years of Age and Older. *Mayo Clinic Proceedings* 2003;78:285–288.

Diabetes

The Diabetes Control and Complications Trial Research Group. The effect of intensive treatment of diabetes on the development and progression of long-term complications in insulin-treated diabetes mellitus. *New England Journal of Medicine* 1993;329:977–986.

Schauer PR, Burguera B, Ikramuddin S, et al. Effect of Laparoscopic Roux-En Y Gastric Bypass on Type 2 Diabetes Mellitus. *Annals of Surgery* 2003;238:467–485.

CHAPTER 13

Freedman VA, Martin LG, Schoeni RF. Recent Trends in Disability and Functioning Among Older Adults in the United States. *JAMA* 2002;288:3137–3146.

Greenland P, Knoll MD, Stamler J, et al. Major Risk Factors as Antecedents of Fatal and Nonfatal Coronary Heart Disease Events. *JAMA* 2003;290:891–897.

Luft FC. Bad Genes, Good People, Association, Linkage, Longevity and the Prevention of Cardiovascular Disease. *Clinical and Experimental Pharmacology and Physiology* 1999;26: 576–579.

Perls T, Terry D. Understanding the Determinants of Exceptional Longevity. *Annals of Internal Medicine* 2003;139:445–449.

Index

Page numbers in *italics* refer to charts, figures, and tables.